Topics in Equine Anesthesia

Editor

STUART C. CLARK-PRICE

VETERINARY CLINICS OF NORTH AMERICA: EQUINE PRACTICE

www.vetequine.theclinics.com

Consulting Editor
A. SIMON TURNER

April 2013 • Volume 29 • Number 1

ELSEVIER

1600 John F. Kennedy Boulevard ● Suite 1800 ● Philadelphia, Pennsylvania, 19103-2899

http://www.vetequine.theclinics.com

VETERINARY CLINICS OF NORTH AMERICA: EQUINE PRACTICE Volume 29, Number 1
April 2013 ISSN 0749-0739, ISBN-13: 978-1-4557-7346-6

Editor: John Vassallo; j.vassallo@elsevier.com
Developmental Editor: Teia Stone

Veterinary Clinics of North America: Equine Practice (ISSN 0749-0739) is published in April, August, and December by Elsevier Inc., 360 Park Avenue South, New York, NY 10010-1710. Business and Editorial Offices: 1600 John F. Kennedy Blvd., Suite 1800, Philadelphia, PA 19103-2899. Subscription prices are $267.00 per year (domestic individuals), $397.00 per year (domestic institutions), $126.00 per year (domestic students/residents), $299.00 per year (Canadian individuals), $496.00 per year (Canadian institutions), $346.00 per year (international individuals), $496.00 per year (international institutions), and $172.00 per year (international and Canadian students/residents). To receive student/resident rate, orders must be accompanied by name of affiliated institution, date of term, and the signature of program/residency coordinator on institution letterhead. Orders will be billed at individual rate until proof of status is received. Foreign air speed delivery is included in all *Clinics* subscription prices. All prices are subject to change without notice. **POSTMASTER:** Send address changes to *Veterinary Clinics of North America: Equine Practice*, 3251 Riverport Lane, Maryland Heights, MO 63043. Customer Service (orders, claims, online, change of address): Elsevier Health Sciences Division, Subscription Customer Service, 3251 Riverport Lane, Maryland Heights, MO 63043. Tel: 1-800-654-2452 (U.S. and Canada); 314-447-8871 (outside U.S. and Canada). Fax: 314-447-8029. E-mail: journalscustomer service-usa@elsevier.com (for print support); E-mail: journalsonlinesupport-usa@elsevier (for online support).

Reprints. For copies of 100 or more of articles in this publication, please contact the Commercial Reprints Department, Elsevier Inc., 360 Park Avenue South, New York, NY 10010-1710. Tel.: 212-633-3812; Fax: 212-462-1935; E-mail: reprints@elsevier.com.

Veterinary Clinics of North America: Equine Practice is covered in *MEDLINE/PubMed (Index Medicus)*, *Excerpta Medica*, *Current Contents/Agriculture, Biology and Environmental Sciences*, and *ISI*.

Printed and bound by CPI Group (UK) Ltd, Croydon, CR0 4YY

Transferred to digital print 2012

Contributors

CONSULTING EDITOR

A. SIMON TURNER, BVSc, MS, DVSc
Diplomate, American College of Veterinary Surgeons; Professor Emeritus, Department of Clinical Sciences, College of Veterinary Medicine and Biomedical Sciences, Colorado State University, Fort Collins, Colorado

EDITOR

STUART C. CLARK-PRICE, DVM, MS
Diplomate, American College of Veterinary Internal Medicine – Large Animal; Diplomate, American College of Veterinary Anesthesiologists; Assistant Professor, Anesthesia and Analgesia; Head, Clinical Service, Department of Veterinary Clinical Medicine, College of Veterinary Medicine, University of Illinois, Urbana, Illinois

AUTHORS

LORI A. BIDWELL, DVM
Diplomate, American College of Veterinary Anesthesiologists; Assistant Professor, Veterinary Medical Center, College of Veterinary Medicine, Michigan State University, East Lansing, Michigan

JORDYN M. BOESCH, DVM
Diplomate, American College of Veterinary Anesthesiologists; Lecturer, Department of Clinical Sciences, College of Veterinary Medicine, Cornell University, Ithaca, New York

ROBERT J. BROSNAN, DVM, PhD
Diplomate, American College of Veterinary Anesthesiologists; Department of Surgical and Radiological Sciences, School of Veterinary Medicine, University of California-Davis, Davis, California

STUART C. CLARK-PRICE, DVM, MS
Diplomate, American College of Veterinary Internal Medicine - Large Animal Internal Medicine; Diplomate, American College of Veterinary Anesthesiologists; Assistant Professor of Anesthesia and Pain Management, Clinical Service Head of Anesthesia and Pain Management, Department of Veterinary Clinical Medicine, College of Veterinary Medicine, University of Illinois Urbana-Champaign, Urbana, Illinois

FRANK GASTHUYS, DVM, PhD
Diplomate, European College of Veterinary Anaesthesia and Analgesia; Dean and Professor of Veterinary Anaesthesiology, Faculty of Veterinary Medicine, University of Ghent, Belgium

AMBER L. LABELLE, DVM, MS
Diplomate, American College of Veterinary Ophthalmologists; Assistant Professor, Department of Veterinary Clinical Medicine, College of Veterinary Medicine, University of Illinois Urbana-Champaign, Urbana, Illinois

PHILLIP LERCHE, BVSc, PhD
Diplomate, American College of Veterinary Anesthesiologists; Assistant Professor, Veterinary Clinical Sciences, College of Veterinary Medicine, The Ohio State University, Columbus, Ohio

MANUEL MARTIN-FLORES, DVM
Diplomate, American College of Veterinary Anesthesiologists; Assistant Professor of Anesthesiology, College of Veterinary Medicine, Cornell University, Ithaca, New York

YVES MOENS, DVM, PhD, Priv Doz
Diplomate, European College of Veterinary Anaesthesia and Analgesia; Anaesthesiology and Perioperative Intensive Care, University of Veterinary Medicine, Vienna, Austria

STIJN SCHAUVLIEGE, DVM, PhD
Diplomate, European College of Veterinary Anaesthesia and Analgesia; Head of Anaesthesia Service, Faculty of Veterinary Medicine, University of Ghent, Belgium

JONATHAN MARK SENIOR, BVSc, PhD, CertVA, MRCVS
Diplomate, European College of Veterinary Anaesthesia and Analgesia; Senior Lecturer in Veterinary Anaesthesia, Philip Leverhulme Equine Hospital, School of Veterinary Science, University of Liverpool, Neston, South Wirral, United Kingdom

ANDRE SHIH, DVM
Diplomate, American College of Veterinary Anesthesiologists; Assistant Professor, Department of Large Animal Clinical Sciences, College of Veterinary Medicine, University of Florida, Gainesville, Florida

LINDSEY B.C. SNYDER, DVM, MS
Diplomate, American College of Veterinary Anesthesiologists; Clinical Assistant Professor, Anesthesia and Pain Management, Department of Surgical Sciences, School of Veterinary Medicine, University of Wisconsin-Madison, Madison, Wisconsin

ALEXANDER VALVERDE, DVM, DVSc
Diplomate, American College of Veterinary Anesthesiologists; Associate Professor, Department of Clinical Studies, Ontario Veterinary College, University of Guelph, Guelph, Ontario, Canada

ERIN WENDT-HORNICKLE, DVM
Diplomate, American College of Veterinary Anesthesiologists; Clinical Instructor, Anesthesia and Pain Management, Department of Surgical Sciences, School of Veterinary Medicine, University of Wisconsin-Madison, Madison, Wisconsin

Contents

General anesthesia in horses carries an increased risk of morbidity and mortality compared with other species. In recent years the number and complexity of epidemiologic studies in equine anesthesia has increased. The ability to interpret such studies and understand epidemiologic terminology is vital for veterinarians for them to make potential improvements to their anesthetic practice and to allow them to communicate effectively the findings of such studies to colleagues and owners. This article provides the equine clinician with a basic understanding of the methodologies that can be used in observational epidemiologic studies, and reviews the literature on equine anesthetic morbidity, mortality, and risk.

Despite the use of balanced anesthesia and fluids, drugs for cardiovascular support are often needed in anesthetized horses. Antimuscarinics can be used to treat bradycardia unrelated to hypertension. Vasopressors can be useful when hypotension is caused by vasodilation and/or when the effect of fluids and inotropes is insufficient. In most cases, however, inotropes, including sympathomimetics, calcium salts, and phosphodiesterase inhibitors, are preferred. Of the β-sympathomimetics, dobutamine remains the agent of choice. Calcium salts are mainly useful in hypocalcemic patients. Phosphodiesterase inhibitors may offer an alternative solution, but more research is needed.

The mechanical ventilation of horses during anesthesia remains a crucial option for optimal anesthetic management, if the possible negative cardiovascular side effects are managed, because this species is prone to hypercapnia and hypoxemia. The combined use of capnography and pitot-based spirometry provide complementary information on ventilation and respiratory mechanics, respectively. This facilitates management of mechanical ventilation in conditions of changing respiratory system compliance (ie, laparoscopy) and when investigating new ventilatory strategies including alveolar recruitment maneuvers and optimization of positive expiratory pressure.

Inhaled agents represent an important and useful class of drugs for equine anesthesia. This article reviews the ether-type anesthetics in contemporary use, their uptake and elimination, their mechanisms of action, and their desirable and undesirable effects in horses.

Balanced anesthetic techniques are commonly used in equine patients, and include the combination of a volatile anesthetic with at least one injectable anesthetic throughout the maintenance period. Injectable anesthetics used in balanced anesthesia include the α_2-agonists, lidocaine, ketamine, and opioids, and those with muscle-relaxant properties such as benzodiazepines and guaifenesin. Administration of these injectable anesthetics is best using constant-rate infusions based on the pharmacokinetics of the drug, which allows steady-state concentrations and predictable pharmacodynamic actions. This review summarizes the different drug combinations used in horses, and provides calculated recommended doses based on the pharmacokinetics of individual drugs.

Total intravenous anesthesia (TIVA) is the mainstay of short-term (up to 60 minutes) and field anesthesia in horses. This article discusses the pros and cons of TIVA, commonly used TIVA protocols, and their use, monitoring during, and recovery from, TIVA.

This article briefly reviews the physiology of the neuromuscular junction and the pharmacologic mechanisms of neuromuscular blocking agents. The clinical use of modern agents is discussed. Monitoring techniques used to assess the level of neuromuscular block and to exclude residual paralysis at the end of an anesthetic procedure are reviewed.

Cardiac output (CO) is the volume of blood pumped out by the heart in 1 minute. Monitoring of CO can guide therapy and improve clinical outcome in critically ill patients and during anesthesia. Although there is increasing research into clinically useful methods of monitoring CO in equine patients, there are limitations to the available methods. There are 4 basic methods of measuring CO: (1) indicator methods, (2) a derivation of the Fick principle, (3) arterial pulse wave analysis, and (4) imaging diagnostic techniques. This article discusses the importance of CO, available technology, and challenges of monitoring CO in equine medicine.

The purpose of this article is to update the community of veterinarians performing general anesthesia in horses on fluid therapy. The rationale behind intraoperative fluid therapy, fluid dynamics, and various fluid options (crystalloids, hypertonic saline, colloids) is discussed. Additionally, electrolytes (calcium, potassium, and sodium) are included in the discussion in relation to general anesthesia and intraoperative fluid management.

VETERINARY CLINICS OF NORTH AMERICA: EQUINE PRACTICE

Preface

Topics in Equine Anesthesia

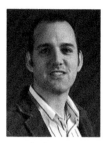

Stuart C. Clark-Price, DVM, MS
Editor

Care, and not fine stables, makes a good horse.
— *Danish proverb*

It has been an honor and privilege to help develop this edition of *Veterinary Clinics of North America: Equine Practice* devoted to Topics in Equine Anesthesia. This endeavor could not have been achieved without the tireless effort of the pioneers of equine anesthesia, who, out of desire to provide better care for horses, put us on the road of developing clinically useful anesthetics and anesthetic techniques. As far as the veterinary community has come with equine anesthesia, I cannot help but believe that we are still in our infancy and that bigger and better ideas, approaches, and techniques are yet to come.

Anesthetic management of the equine patient continues to evolve and improve. This can be seen in the decrease in the rates of morbidity and mortality of today as compared to the past and is directly related to the dedication of the clinician-scientists who contribute to the body of knowledge that is equine anesthesia. It has been 11 years since the last edition of *Veterinary Clinics of North America: Equine Practice* was dedicated to the topic of anesthesia. That seminal edition compiled and delivered a large amount of information to the practicing equine anesthetist and many of the authors of this issue were either trained or heavily influenced by the authors of that previous issue. It is our sincere hope that the information in this issue will continue in the tradition of providing useful and relevant materials to veterinarians in the field and in equine hospitals, to specialists around the world, and to residents training in anesthesia.

I would personally like to extend my deepest thanks to the authors who have helped bring this edition together and to the great people at Elsevier, and to John Vassallo in particular, for his help and guidance. The goal was to gather an international author list that had a balance of established equine veterinary scientists at the top of their respective fields and newer scientists that are establishing their careers.

Vet Clin Equine 29 (2013) ix–x
http://dx.doi.org/10.1016/j.cveq.2013.01.001
0749-0739/13/$ – see front matter © 2013 Published by Elsevier Inc.

vetequine.theclinics.com

Readers may note that this issue is not a complete overview of equine anesthesia; rather, the emphasis was to bring discussion to topics that have recently emerged in the research literature or continue to be a significant clinical problem. The result may allow for improvements in standard of care and research methodology. Readers looking for more general information on the practice of equine anesthesia are referred to the many excellent textbooks on equine anesthesia that are available as that was beyond the scope of this issue.

Finally, I would like to dedicate this issue to our students, who we endeavor to enrich, our clients, who we endeavor to serve faithfully, and to that which is our inspiration, our equine patients. Winston Churchill once said, "There is something about the outside of a horse that is good for the inside of a man."

Stuart C. Clark-Price, DVM, MS
Assistant Professor, Anesthesia and Analgesia
Head, Clinical Service
Department of Veterinary Clinical Medicine
College of Veterinary Medicine
University of Illinois
1008 West Hazelwood Drive, MC-004
Urbana, IL 61802, USA

E-mail address:
sccp@illinois.edu

Morbidity, Mortality, and Risk of General Anesthesia in Horses

Jonathan Mark Senior, BVSc, PhD, CertVA, MRCVS

KEYWORDS

- Equine • Anesthesia • Morbidity • Mortality • Risk • Epidemiology • Review

KEY POINTS

- Equine anesthesia is more likely to result in morbidity and mortality compared with other commonly anesthetized animal species.
- Epidemiology is well suited to the study of the frequency and causes of equine anesthetic-related morbidities and mortalities.
- It is therefore important that the equine anesthetist is familiar with epidemiologic study design and how to interpret the results of such studies.
- Equine anesthesia can boast several well-designed and powerful studies into risk factors for anesthetic-related mortality but the data from the last multicenter study are now more than 13 years old prompting calls for a new multicenter study.
- Further epidemiologic studies into common anesthetic-related morbidities are also needed.
- The value of clinical audit within one's own hospitals, with one's own unique population of horses, and unique clinical practice should not be overlooked.

INTRODUCTION

In the author's experience, when discussing anesthesia in horses, many owners seem to readily understand that horses are more likely to suffer morbidities and mortality compared with people, dogs, and cats, and that anesthesia in the horse is inherently risky. Owners may ask what the level of risk is and what will be done to ameliorate that risk in their horses. The answers to those questions are more complex than at first they may seem.

It is important that clinicians continue to strive to determine the frequency, and understand the causes of, anesthetic-related morbidities and mortalities (ARMMs). By determining the frequencies of ARMMs, the benefits of performing a procedure can be considered against the potential for complications, and baselines for assessing future developments in case management are established. Understanding the causes

Philip Leverhulme Equine Hospital, School of Veterinary Science, University of Liverpool, Leahurst Campus, Neston, South Wirral CH64 7TE, UK
E-mail address: J.M.Senior@liverpool.ac.uk

Vet Clin Equine 29 (2013) 1–18
http://dx.doi.org/10.1016/j.cveq.2012.11.007   **vetequine.theclinics.com**
0749-0739/13/$ – see front matter © 2013 Elsevier Inc. All rights reserved.

of ARMMs also informs case management where causes are avoidable or modifiable, and risk assessment where they are not. A discussion between the veterinarian and owner about ARMMs is also an important part of gaining informed consent to undertake anesthesia in the owner's horse.

In recent years, the number and complexity of epidemiologic studies in equine anesthesia has increased, potentially resulting in some veterinarians with little or no epidemiologic training struggling to critically interpret data from these studies. The ability to interpret such studies and understand epidemiologic terminology is vital for veterinarians in order for them to make potential improvements to their anesthetic practice and to allow them to communicate effectively the findings of such studies to colleagues and owners.

This article provides the equine clinician with a basic understanding of the methodologies that can be used in observational epidemiologic studies, and reviews the literature on equine anesthetic morbidity, mortality, and risk. The overview and description of epidemiologic methodologies and terminologies is aimed at readers with a limited understanding of the subject and is not intended to be a comprehensive review. For further details the interested reader is strongly encouraged to review any veterinary epidemiology textbook (eg,[1,2]).

EPIDEMIOLOGY

Epidemiology is the study of disease in (animal) populations and of factors that determine its occurrence.[1] It equips clinicians with the tools to analyze the frequency and causes of ARMMs. However, it is important to remember that because epidemiology involves the study of two complex and dynamic entities (populations and disease), sometimes epidemiology can only inform as to where studies should be focused and may not provide a definitive answer straight away.

MEASURES OF DISEASE FREQUENCY

One of the most important aims of any study into ARMMs is to know how often they occur. This allows one to estimate risk and also allows analysis of associations of hypothesized causal factors. There are different ways that the frequency of disease (eg, death or new morbidity) can be measured. Prevalence refers to the number of cases in a population at a single specific time point. Incidence refers to the number of new cases in a defined population within a set time period. Importantly, incidence can be used to estimate risk.[1,2]

RISK

Risk is the chance of something bad happening. In terms of an adverse event (eg, death), one could say that the risk of death in a population is the number of animals that die during a defined time period divided by the total number of animals in that population.[2] In epidemiologic studies risk is used to describe several subtly but importantly different things. It is important to use the correct terms and to understand what each term means. An example of mixed terminologies is when the term "mortality rate" is often used to imply the risk of mortality; however, strictly speaking, mortality rate relates to the incidence rate of death,[2] which would be the number of new deaths per unit of animal time. The difficulty is that the animal time function should be the period through which the animal is exposed to the risk of disease, and how this is defined is subjective (eg, per hour of anesthesia or number of hours per days in the perianesthetic period).

Individual Risk or Population Risk?

Risk may be an overall risk for the study population (eg, the proportion of horses that suffer anesthetic-related deaths within a study period) or an individual horse's risk (eg, the probability of a horse dying if it is anesthetized). An animal may be exposed to several types of risk at the same time, and the risks or risk factors that are presented in epidemiologic studies may not reflect the true or overall exposure to risk of an individual. For example, many equine anesthetists use the American Society of Anesthesiologists (ASA) physical status risk classification system (http://www.asahq.org/For-Members/Clinical-Information/ASA-Physical-Status-Classification-System.aspx) to estimate the risk of death during anesthesia, and there is epidemiologic evidence that prior physical status correlates to anesthetic-related death. However, the ASA system does not take into account risk associated with surgery (eg, a healthy horse may be undergoing a procedure where severe intraoperative hemorrhage is possible). There may also be risks that the horse is exposed to that most of the equine population may not be, and so the population risk does not reflect the risk for that horse (eg, hyperkalemic periodic paralysis in quarter horses).

Risk in Epidemiologic Studies

Risk can also be used to evaluate the association of causal factors with a disease. Studies attempting to estimate the influence or association of a hypothesized causal factor on the occurrence of a disease can do this by expressing risk as relative risks.[1,2]

Relative risks are calculated from the ratio of disease occurrence between the exposed and nonexposed groups. Ratios are relative measures and are only meaningful to interpret risk within groups. Two terms widely used are risk ratio (RR) and odds ratio (OR).[1,2]

RR is normally used in cohort studies and is the ratio of the incidence of disease in exposed animals to the incidence in nonexposed animals. An RR greater than 1 indicates a positive association between the exposed factor and the disease; an RR equal to 1 suggest no association between the factor and disease; and an RR less than 1 suggests a negative (protective) association between the factor and the disease.

OR is normally used in case-control studies and in this context is the ratio of the odds of exposure to a factor in the cases to the odds of exposure in the control subjects. An OR greater than 1 indicates a positive association between the exposed factor and the disease; an OR equal to 1 suggest no association between the factor and disease; and an OR less than 1 suggests a negative (protective) association between the factor and the disease.

The subtle difference in how RR and OR are calculated is important because if a causal factor is associated with a disease that is not rare, RR is preferred because OR will overestimate the magnitude of association.[1,2]

Because RR or OR are relative measures they are always expressed in relation to a reference variable and the value is only relative to that reference variable. The reference variable always has an RR or OR value of 1 and is often the subset with the largest number of cases or a biologically/clinically relevant subset. See the example in **Table 1** . From the data one can infer that:

- The RR of mortality within 7 days of anesthesia in horses is around half, either half as likely to die or twice as likely to be alive, for left lateral recumbency compared with dorsal recumbency (RR, 0.4; 95% confidence interval [CI], 0.3–0.8; $P = .002$). The RR of mortality within 7 days of anesthesia in horses is around a third for right lateral compared with dorsal recumbency (RR, 0.3; 95% CI, 0.2–0.6; $P = .0004$). One can say that right lateral has slightly less risk of death within 7 days of anesthesia than left lateral compared with dorsal recumbency.

Table 1
Example of output of univariable chi-square analysis for the relative risk of different body positions during anesthesia to mortality within 7 days of anesthesia

Body Position During Anesthesia	Total Number	Number that Died	Number Alive	Relative Risk (95% Confidence Interval[a])	P Value
Dorsal	2768	70	2698	1 (reference variable)	
Left lateral	1521	17	1504	0.4 (0.3–0.8)	0.002
Right lateral	1281	11	1270	0.3 (0.2–0.6)	0.0004
Others	352	4	348	0.5 (0.2–1.2)	0.2

[a] 95% confidence interval is the range within which one is confident that if the population is sampled 100 times, that 95 times the RR value one would calculate would fall within that range.[1,2]

Data from Johnston GM, Taylor PM, Holmes MA, et al. Confidential Enquiry of Perioperative Equine Fatalities (CEPEF-1): preliminary results. Equine Vet J 1995;27:193–200.

- It is inappropriate to interpret the data in **Table 1** as also indicating that right lateral is less likely to result in death within 7 days of anesthesia compared with left lateral because the RR ratio for right lateral recumbency is lower. This is because the RRs for either lateral recumbency are relative to the risk of death in horses that were in dorsal recumbency. To accurately estimate the relative risks of death within 7 days of anesthesia between right and left lateral, one would have to recalculate the RR with either lateral recumbency being the reference variable.
- One also cannot interpret the RR for the "others" subset. The P value is higher than that which is normally taken as being significant (P<.05) and also the RR 95% CI range is either side of 1, implying that this subset could be either positively or negatively associated with death.

STUDY DESIGN

In simple terms, differences in study design affect what results will be obtained from that study. Understanding different ways that studies can be designed is useful for the researcher and for those trying to interpret the research.

Intervention Studies

Intervention studies, especially when the intervention is randomized, are less prone to confounding, and when masked, less prone to bias than observational studies, and provide the best chance of producing evidence for causation.[3] In addition, by their nature they are also prospective and longitudinal (see later). However, intervention studies can be expensive to undertake and may be ethically difficult to justify, especially if the intervention (or lack of) exposes animals to an increased risk of disease. Confidential Enquiry of Perioperative Equine Fatalities (CEPEF)-3[4] is an example of a large-scale, multicenter, randomized intervention epidemiologic intervention study.

Observational Study Types

In contrast, observational studies avoid many of the ethical problems of intervention studies, can be conducted on clinical populations, and if well-designed can lead to identification of frequencies and risk factors for ARMMs. However, observational studies tend to identify potential causal factors and cannot conclusively prove them; often concurrent or subsequent interventional studies are required to establish conclusive causal factors.[3]

Case studies and case series

Case studies and case series are descriptive reports of ARMMs and tend to be limited to hypothesizing possible causal factors.[5,6] However, their value should not be underestimated, particularly when further case reports review previous reports and update current (lack of) understanding[7] or case series begin to elucidate likely causal factors.[8]

Case-control studies

These compare groups of diseased animals with groups of nondiseased animals that have shared exposure to the factors of interest. Case-control studies allow for evaluation of risk factors for developing the disease, in that if the diseased cases report greater exposure to certain factors, then it suggests that those factors influence the likelihood of developing the disease. Case-control studies are particularly suited to studying rare diseases, such as anesthetic mortality, that have multiple causal factor exposures[2]; they also produce substantial amounts of data relatively inexpensively.[3] Case-control studies are susceptible to many different types of study bias, and appropriate study design is important to minimize these (eg, selection of appropriate control subjects).[2]

Cohort studies

These studies compare a group exposed to the hypothesized causal factors of a disease with a group not exposed to those factors. The studies are sometimes called follow-up studies, in that a cohort of subjects of interest are observed or followed for a period of time to determine whether they develop any disease. These studies are most commonly prospective but can be retrospective if sufficient records are available (eg, until discharge from hospital). The risk of developing the disease can then be related to exposure to the hypothesized causal factors.[1,2] Cohort studies are not suited to studying rare diseases because the number of subjects needing to be followed would be huge to gather enough disease events. Cohort studies are suited to studying common diseases (or diseases with multiple outcomes) and rare exposures to causal factors and hence are suited to morbidity studies with multiple complications.[1,2] Cohort studies also have their own problems, such as sample selection.[1,2]

Nested case-control studies

Nested case-control studies are amalgamations of case-control and cohort studies. They predefine a cohort to follow over time and then, when cases appear, select control subjects from the cohort and provide many of the advantages of the cohort study, with the efficiency of the case-control study, allowing multiple exposures and risk factors to be studied.[2] The Confidential Enquiry into Perioperative Small Animal Fatalities[9] is an example of a nested case-control study in veterinary anesthesia.

Prospective and Retrospective Studies

Prospective studies collect data going forward in time from a defined start point in a study. Importantly, the data collection methods may be specifically designed for the purposes of the study.[4,10,11] Retrospective studies collect data that refer to (eg, questionnaires or recall) or were recorded during past events.[1] Often data collected in retrospective studies rely on data collection systems that may not have been designed to accurately obtain the data required by the study or the ability of study participants to recall events from the past. In general, data from retrospective studies are considered less reliable.[1]

Longitudinal and Cross-sectional Studies

Longitudinal studies investigate changes over time and can be interventional or observational.[1] They can look back over time. For example, in a retrospective case-control study into anesthetic mortality, animals were exposed to the risk of anesthesia; some (cases) died at some time point later, and many (control subjects) did not.[12] Or, they can look forward over time.[4,10,13] Cross-sectional studies select a sample population from a larger population at a given time point and then assess presence or absence of disease for each individual in the sample on a single occasion. Many cross-sectional studies are descriptive and are often called surveys.[1] Sample selection is again important.[1]

Single-center and Multicenter Studies

Single-center studies

Single-center studies are generally considered to provide weaker evidence compared with multicenter studies, for two main reasons. First, single-center studies tend to have a homogenous study population, and so comparing data and results between studies may be problematic (eg, a first opinion practice, performing mainly elective anesthesia in healthy horses compared with a large referral hospital dealing with a greater proportion of sick horses and undertaking more emergency anesthetics). Second, in single-center studies it can take several years to collect data from enough cases to be able to undertake meaningful analysis, and during this time changes may take place either in the study population or the standard anesthetic practice. A good example of this is the retrospective study of Young and Taylor,[14] where during the study period of 7 years, the standard management of hypotension in anesthetized horses changed in response to studies[15,16] highlighting the importance of hypotension in the development of myopathy.

Multicenter studies

Multicenter studies have the advantages of being likely to introduce more heterogeneity into the study population and being able to generate sufficient case numbers over a shorter period of time.[3] However, using multicenter study designs can also introduce problems. Although overall the study population may be more heterogeneous and more similar to the overall population, individual centers may still contribute homogenous subpopulations into the overall study population and depending on the size of the subpopulation may introduce varying degrees of bias. Another source of bias is different centers may contribute predictable (eg, level of experience of main anesthetist) and unpredictable (eg, an unknown or unmeasured difference in perianesthetic management) confounding variables. For these reasons multicenter studies often analyze their data using statistical methods that take into account that individual center data may be correlated to or confounded by that center.[4,11] In multicenter intervention studies where an intervention is randomized, both study populations should be checked to ensure their baseline characteristics are similar because simple randomization may result in differences (eg, in age distribution) between the study groups purely by chance. One approach to improve the balance of measured factors between the study populations in a multicenter intervention study is to use stratified randomization.[3]

Univariable and Multivariable Statistical Analysis

Many different statistical methods can be used to demonstrate an association between a causal factor and the occurrence of a disease (eg, Student *t* test, correlation, chi-square, Fisher exact test). The problem in studying ARMMs is that there is likely to be two or more causal factors contributing to the outcome of the disease. If one measures the association between just one of these causal factors (eg, age) and the disease (eg, anesthetic-related death) (univariable analysis), the result obtained also includes the effects of the other unmeasured or confounding factors and does not accurately reflect the association between the causal factor of interest and the disease. Often one may well have a good idea of what some of the other causal factors contributing to a disease may be (eg, physical status, anesthetic agent, length of anesthesia, surgery type, and so forth), either because of previous studies, case reports, clinical impression, or hypothesis. If the study is designed to measure multiple causal factors (called predictor variables) it is possible to tease out how the measured causal factors may confound each other using multivariable models (most commonly multiregression models), which can analyze multiple variables at the same time. The standard practice is to analyze the association of all the measured variables to the disease individually using univariable analysis, and then those showing a reasonable association, then go into the multivariable model. It is common that variables that had an apparently strong association with the disease drop out of the model because they are strongly confounded by another variable (eg, dorsal recumbency and exploratory laparotomy may both be strongly associated with anesthetic-related death after univariable analysis, but only one of the predictor variables would remain in the multivariable model because they confound so strongly).

Because many ARMMs are likely to have multiple causal factors, it is important to interpret epidemiologic studies that use univariable approaches alone cautiously because they will not account for confounding factors.

Even multivariable studies need to be interpreted carefully because multivariable models can only attempt to explain the data using the measured variables and do not account for confounding by unmeasured or unknown predictor variables. This is why multivariable models sometimes produce results that seem difficult to explain.

For example, in the second CEPEF study,[13] after colics were excluded time of surgery remained as a strong predictor variable (overall $P<.001$) in the final multivariable model for the probability of death within 7 days of anesthesia. Surgery undertaken between 6 AM and 1 PM was the reference variable, "out-of-hours" surgeries were associated with an increased risk of death compared with surgeries performed between 6 AM and 1 PM (6 PM to midnight: OR, 2.15; 95% CI, 1.35–3.46; $P<.002$; midnight to 6 AM: OR, 7.61; 95% CI, 2.16–26.74; $P<.002$), as were surgeries performed in the afternoon (1–6 PM: OR, 1.46; 95% CI, 1.15–1.85; $P = .002$). That out-of-hours surgeries were relatively more likely to result in an anesthetic-related death compared with surgeries in the morning may be explained as at least some of the cases anesthetized during these hours were likely to be (noncolic) emergencies, and although the model accounted for confounding factors, such as protocol, duration of operation, and type of procedure, the CEPEF-2 data collection form did not include data on other potential causal factors, such as whether horses were starved, whether the horses had traveled on a long journey, or if the personnel working out-of-hours were working earlier in the day. That surgery in the afternoon is also more likely to result in an anesthetic-related death compared with surgeries in the morning is less easy to explain, but suggests that once again there are likely unknown and unmeasured contributing and confounding factors; maybe horses that have surgery in the afternoon are more likely to have concurrent infections because the "clean" surgeries are likely to be put on the list first or perhaps diurnal rhythm has a role to play in ARMMs.

MORBIDITY AND MORTALITY STUDIES

Anesthetic-related complications can result in an illness or disease (morbidity) that was not present before anesthesia. Such morbidities can vary in severity but can always be considered to have a deleterious impact on the horse's welfare, prolong hospitalization, and increase costs of care. Anesthetic-related complications can also lead to the death of a horse either directly or indirectly if the horse is euthanized on humane, economic, or other grounds. When discussing individual deaths it is correct to discuss fatalities; when discussing deaths among a population the terms "mortality" or "mortalities" are often used.

There are relatively fewer studies into anesthetic-related morbidities compared with mortalities. The amount of subjectivity that surrounds the study of morbidities makes meaningful interpretation of studies and comparisons between them difficult.[17] The severity of morbidity that should be studied is subjective (eg, minor wounds in recovery or transient pyrexia or severe myopathies). The lack of universally agreed definitions for many morbidities means that definitions may be arbitrarily chosen that are open to question. In contrast, death is a well-defined and recognizable outcome that is also a dichotomous variable. For this reason, most ARMM studies are focused on mortality. However, even in mortality studies, meaningful comparisons between studies can be problematic.

MORTALITY STUDIES
Comparative Mortality

Apart from the differences in study design outlined previously the following consider-ations affect interpretation of and comparison between mortality studies. First, most studies that refer to mortality rates actually mean mortality risks. Second, although the definition of the outcome of death is likely to be rigorous and well-understood across all studies, many studies vary as to what is defined as an anesthetic-related death. Some studies only include those deaths where anesthesia was judged to be the sole cause of death, or no other cause for death could be found, whereas other studies include any death that may occur in relation to anesthesia even though other factors likely had a strong influence in the outcome (eg, physical status, surgery-related risk). Studies also differ in the length of time they follow cases for. Some studies only follow cases until the patient has regained consciousness; these studies are less likely to lose data but are likely to exclude some causes of anesthetic-related deaths. Other studies regard the perianesthetic period as lasting for many days; these studies tend to lose data because the outcomes of some patients may not be recorded, and may inadvertently include nonanesthetic-related deaths. Finally, it is important to appreciate the nature of the study population and the centers involved in the study.

Anesthetic-related mortality in people

Retrospective and prospective studies conducted during the last 30 years reveal a mortality risk of approximately 0.05% to 0.001% where death was considered primarily as a result of anesthesia, and of approximately 0.02% to 0.005% where anesthesia played a contributory role but was not the sole cause.[18–22] Most reviewers of human studies quote an overall figure of around 0.01% (1 in 10,000).[23,24] Although the study populations and types of procedures performed vary markedly between studies the mortality rates are similar. One consequences of such a low anesthetic-related mortality rate in people is that future studies will likely need to be very large, involving many centers, and many cases, and therefore very expensive to have enough power to detect risk factors.[24]

Anesthetic-related mortality in small animals

Retrospective questionnaire-based multicenter cohort studies have been under-taken[25,26] and report anesthetic-related mortality risks of around 0.1%. Three prospective multicenter studies into small animal anesthetic mortality have been undertaken. Two were cohort studies[27,28] and the most recent was a nested case-control study.[9] The first study[27] recruited 53 practices in the United Kingdom and recorded data from 41,881 anesthetics over 2 years. The overall mortality risk was 0.23% in dogs and 0.29% in cats. If pre-existing physical status was taken into account: the mortality risks were 0.11% (1 in 870) in dogs and 0.18% (1 in 552) in cats for healthy animals (ASA 1–2), and 3.13% in dogs and 3.33% in cats for sick animals (ASA 3–5). The second study[28] recruited 76 practices in Canada and recorded data from 16,789 anesthetics over a 6-month period. The overall mortality risk was 0.11% in dogs and 0.09% in cats. For healthy animals (ASA 1–2), the mortality risks were 0.07% (1 in 1428) in dogs and 0.05% (1 in 2000) in cats. The total number of deaths in this study was low (nine dogs and eight cats) and so the figures are likely to be approximate. The most recent study recruited 117 practices in the United Kingdom, and over the 2-year study period, 98,036 dog, 79,178 cat, and 8209 rabbit anesthetics and sedations took place. The overall anesthetic and sedation mortality risks were estimated to be 0.17% (1 in 601) in dogs, 0.24% (1 in 419) in cats, and 1.39% (1 in 72) in rabbits within 48 hours of the procedure. In healthy animals (ASA 1–2), the risks were estimated to be 0.05% (1 in 1849) for dogs; 0.11% (1 in 895) for cats; and 0.73% (1 in 137) for rabbits. In sick (ASA 3–5) dogs, cats, and rabbits, the risks were estimated to be 1.33% (1 in 75), 1.40% (1 in 71), and 7.37% (1 in 14), respectively.[9] A comparison of the data collection for both of the two large UK studies[9,27] shows that mortality risks have improved for dogs and cats over the 20-year period.

Anesthetic-related mortality in horses

Most studies performed in horses have been done in university teaching or referral hospitals. In contrast to small animal studies, equine study populations are often subdivided into elective or emergency anesthesia cases rather than health status, with most emergency cases comprised of anesthesia for surgical colic. **Table 2** summarizes several studies performed into equine anesthesia-related mortality risks since the 1960s. Overall, the studies outlined in **Table 2** suggest that the anesthesia-related mortality risk for horses is around 1%, increasing to between 2% and 10% in horses undergoing emergency laparotomies.[12,33]

It is clear that the comparative anesthesia-related mortality risk in horses (~1%) is much higher than that in people (~0.01%), and in most other commonly anesthetized veterinary species (dog ~0.05%, cat 0.11%), with only rabbits having a similar mortality risk (0.73%). The higher mortality risk in horses is likely caused by species differences. Some of the causes of and risk factors for anesthetic-related mortality are discussed next. It is also interesting to note that the mortality risk has not changed much over the 40 years of studies outlined in **Table 2**, suggesting that improvements in standards of anesthesia are likely offset by increasingly complex procedures being undertaken.

Causes of Anesthetic-related Mortality in Horses

Documenting the causes of anesthetic-related death in horses allows for a more thorough evaluation into risk factors for death and also allows potential underlying mechanisms to be identified and investigated. Often the death of a horse in the perianesthetic period may be caused by several contributing factors, such as pre-existing disease, surgical complications, anesthetic complications, and human error. Veterinary literature contrasts sharply with medical literature in that human error is rarely investigated, or even listed, as a potential cause of death. One large multicenter prospective study documented different examples of human error (eg, insufficient

Table 2
Summary of several studies published detailing anesthesia mortality risk for horses

	Number of Anesthetics	Study Duration	Study Population	Elective or Emergency	Prospective or Retrospective	Single Center or Multicenter	Anesthetic-related Mortality Risk (%)
Mitchell[29] 1969	473	7 y	Mainly clinical cases, 29 cases were research cases	Mainly elective	Retrospective	Single	1.47
Heath[30] 1973	275	3 y	Clinical cases	Mixed	Retrospective	Single	1.69
Tevik[31] 1983	1216	17 y	Clinical cases	Mixed	Retrospective	Single	2.2 (all cases) 1.5 (after sick horses were excluded)
Young and Taylor[14] 1993	1314	7 y	Clinical cases	Mixed but colics were excluded	Retrospective	Single	0.68
Mee et al[32] 1998a	1279	3 y 10 mo	Clinical cases	Elective	Retrospective	Single	0.63 0.08 (where anesthesia was sole cause of death)
Mee et al[33] 1998b	995	3 y 10 mo	Clinical cases	Emergency	Retrospective	Single	2 (noncolic) 4.3 (colic)
Johnston et al[10] 1995	6255	2 y 1 mo	Clinical cases	Mixed	Prospective	Multicenter: 62 UK clinics	1.6% (after colics and delivery of foals were excluded) 0.9% (after colics were excluded)
Johnston et al[13] 2002	41,824	6 y	Clinical cases	Mixed	Prospective	Multicenter: 62 UK clinics	0.9% (after colics were excluded)
Johnston et al[4] 2004	11,366	2 y 4 mo	Clinical cases	Mixed	Prospective randomized intervention	Multicenter: 35 clinics in seven countries	1.6% 0.9% (after colics were excluded)
Bidwell et al[12] 2007	17,961	5 y	Clinical cases	Mixed	Retrospective	Single	0.24%

knowledge, failure to apply knowledge, and inexperience) as playing a role in 75% of anesthetic-related deaths in people.[22] Interestingly, one of the few veterinary studies to take human error into account also found that errors in case management played a role in 75% of deaths in healthy (ASA 1–2) dogs and cats, with airway complications causing most deaths.[27]

In equine studies, where causes of death have been documented, they tend to relate to body systems. In veterinary studies a judgment on the likely cause of an anesthetic-related death is either made by the person making the records at the time[13] or by an individual[4] or group of individuals reviewing the case records at a later stage.[9]

Cardiovascular causes of death

Ultimately, the lack of delivery of oxygen to the heart and brain results in death, so failure of the cardiac pump or circulatory collapse is always involved in death at some stage. Normally, when death has been recorded as being caused by cardiovascular factors it is when failure of the cardiovascular system was considered to be the primary or initial cause of death. It is likely, however, that some anesthetic-related deaths are misclassified as being caused by cardiovascular factors in the absence of any other information that could explain death (eg, in cases where minimal anesthetic monitoring was being undertaken). Taking some level of overreporting into account, anesthetic-related death is attributed to cardiovascular causes in 20% to 50% of cases.[4,12–14,32,33] Although some cardiovascular causes of anesthetic-related death may be related to disease or surgical procedure in horses (eg, hypovolemia after hemorrhage),[33] such causes as fatal arrhythmias can occur in apparently healthy animals.[12]

Respiratory causes of death

In human[22] and small animal studies[27] respiratory causes of anesthetic-related death, such as airway problems, ventilation problems, or delivery of hypoxic gas mixtures, are as least as common as cardiovascular causes of death. In equine studies, where respiratory causes of anesthetic-related death are listed, they contribute to only 4% to 25% of cases.[4,13,14,32] The reasons for this are unclear but may be related in some part to the relative security of the horse's airway (eg, laryngeal spasm and regurgitation or aspiration is unlikely, in contrast to people and small animals).

Other causes of death

The equine literature is again divergent from human or small animal literature in that other noncardiorespiratory causes of death are commonly listed, and also account for most anesthetic-related deaths,[4,12–14,31–33] again reflecting the unique challenges of anesthetizing horses.

Fractures on recovery contributed to death in 12.5% to 38% of anesthetic-related deaths.[4,12–14,32] The figures for fractures on recovery seem to be reasonably stable over the 18 years that the quoted studies cover.

In contrast, postanesthetic myopathy (PAM) is reported as being a cause of death in 7% to 44% of anesthetic-related deaths,[4,12–14] with the highest incidence in the earlier study.[14] Later studies report lower incidences of myopathy contributing to anesthetic-related death of 7%[4,13] and 14.3%,[12] likely reflecting changes to anesthetic management to reduce the likelihood of myopathy. One study spanned a period where intraoperative hypotension (<9.3 kPa [<70 mm Hg]) began to be monitored for and treated using intravenous fluid therapy and dobutamine infusions, with the result that between the two periods of the study the incidence of myopathy did not change but the severity of myopathies occurring after more aggressive management of hypotension were less (five of seven horses developing myopathy died in the early period and none of the seven horses that developed myopathy in the late period died).[14]

Abdominal complications, such as colitis or peritonitis, are reported as causing 13% of anesthetic-related deaths in noncolic cases in CEPEF-2 and CEPEF-3.[4,13] The same studies also report that central nervous system disease or spinal cord myelomalacia contributed to 5% (18 deaths)[13] and 4% (five deaths)[4] of anesthetic-related death in noncolic cases. Details of the numbers contributing cases to either the central nervous system or spinal cord myelomalacia classification were not given and the overall number of cases was low, but the number of case reports into spinal cord myelomalacia–like pathology after anesthesia in horses suggest that these figures may be a reasonable estimate of the incidence of this perplexing catastrophic complication.[6,34–42]

Risk Factors for Anesthetic-related Mortality

The identification of risk factors for anesthetic-related mortality is important in informing case management where the risk factors are avoidable or modifiable, and risk assessment where they are not. In some respects, veterinary and equine anesthesia in particular is well placed to take advantage of case-control or cohort study methodologies because anesthetic-related mortalities are rare. As a result risk factors for mortality can be identified with a reasonable level of confidence and detail. Indeed the CEPEF series of studies,[4,10,13] especially CEPEF-2[13] and CEPEF-3[4] where multivariable analysis of data was undertaken to account for confounding variables, provide valuable information.

Surgery or procedure risk factors

Several single-center retrospective studies established that anesthesia for emergency abdominal surgery was associated with anesthetic-related deaths.[12,31,33] In the first large-scale multicenter cohort study (CEPEF-1), emergency abdominal surgery had a strong association with mortality under anesthesia compared with ear, nose, and throat (ENT) surgeries after univariable analysis.[10] In CEPEF-2[13] emergency abdominal procedures were excluded from further analysis, but in the multivariable analysis undertaken in CEPEF-3 they were associated with a greater risk of death compared with the ENT, urogenital, and miscellaneous procedures group (OR, 2.48; 95% CI, 1.4–4.5; $P = .002$).[4] Further analyses of why emergency abdominal procedures are an increased risk are confined to single-center studies, but various studies have indicated that physical status,[33,43] intraoperative hypotension, and long duration of anesthesia[44] may be associated with mortality risks.

Orthopedic surgery, especially such invasive surgery as fracture repair, is associated with an increased risk of anesthetic-related death. After multivariable analysis in CEPEF-2, fracture repair surgeries had a greater risk of death compared with the ENT group (OR, 5.50; 95% CI, 3.37–5.50; $P<.001$).[13] In CEPEF-3 fracture repair surgeries were relatively riskier than emergency abdominal surgeries compared with the urogenital and miscellaneous procedures group (OR, 4.80; 95% CI, 2.2–10.6; $P<.001$), and other types of orthopedic surgery were also associated with an increased risk of mortality relative to the reference group (OR, 1.77; 95% CI, 1.06–2.90; $P = .03$).[4]

After multivariable analysis, when surgery takes place is also associated with increased risk of anesthetic-related mortality. Relative to those taking place between 6 AM and 1 PM, surgeries taking place between 1 and 6 PM, 6 PM and midnight, and midnight and 6 AM showed an increasing risk of mortality[13] (see also **Table 1**). In addition, surgeries taking place at weekends were also associated with an increased risk of mortality relative to those occurring during the week (OR, 1.52; 95% CI, 1.02–2.28; $P = .04$).[13]

Horse-related risk factors
After multivariable analysis (CEPEF-2), horses aged between 12 months and 5 years are at a lower risk of anesthetic-related mortality relative to horses aged between 5 and 14 years (OR, 0.67; 95% CI, 0.51–0.87; P = .004).[13] In CEPEF-3, age remained in the final multivariable model but did not become significant as a variable until it was entered as a mixed effects function (of age × treatment) and even here none of the subdivisions of age showed a significant association relative to any other subdivision.[4] This suggests that age likely does play a role in anesthetic-related mortality but either the way that age groups were stratified was not able to show the relationship, or there are other confounding factors that are obscuring the associations between the subdivisions. The physical status of the horse also remained in the final multivariable model for all deaths in CEPEF-3, with horses evaluated as medium risk (OR, 2.28; 95% CI, 1.40–3.70; P = .001) or high risk (OR, 6.34; 95% CI, 3.4–11.9; $P<.001$) being at more risk of death relative to those assessed as being low risk.[4]

Anesthesia-related risk factors
After univariable analysis in CEPEF-1, the following risk factors were significantly associated with anesthetic-related death: premedication type (relative to the use of detomidine alone, acepromazine and detomidine in combination decreased the risk and the use of xylazine alone or the lack of premedication increased risk of death), induction agent (relative to the use of intravenous guaiphenesin and thiopentone, the use of intravenous guaiphenesin and ketamine or inhalation inductions using halothane increased the risk of death), and maintenance type (relative to the use of halothane, not using an maintenance agent decreased the risk of death), and increasing duration of anesthesia increased the risk of death.[10]

After multivariable analysis in CEPEF-2[4] only the following risk factors remained in the random effects model: induction and maintenance, and preoperative sedative. Induction and maintenance agent was strongly significant ($P<.001$) at the variable level and relative to an intravenous induction followed by halothane or other inhalational maintenance, total intravenous anesthesia decreased the risk of death (OR, 0.48; 95% CI, 0.18–0.93; P = .03) and total inhalational anesthesia increased the risk of death (OR, 4.84; 95% CI, 2.25–10.44; $P<.001$). The cases receiving total intravenous anesthesia had apparently shorter anesthetics than the reference group, but the numbers of cases in this group was too small to allow statistical comparison of anesthesia time between groups. The total inhalational anesthesia (including inhalation induction) group was comprised entirely of foals, which were a high-risk group after univariable analysis for anesthetic-related death in CEPEF-1.[10] Preoperative sedative was not significant at the variable level (P = .08) (although the authors report it was in the ordinary logistic regression model), nor were any of the subgroups significantly associated to the reference group.[4] However, the fact that the variable remained in the model (ie, that the variable preoperative sedative must have improved the fit of the model, helped the model explain the data) suggests that this variable has some association with anesthetic-related death but what that association is cannot be said for certain.

CEPEF-3[4] was designed to evaluate whether the use of halothane or isoflurane as maintenance agents affected risk of anesthetic-related mortality, and although it found no overall difference between the two agents, it did find that isoflurane significantly reduced risk of mortality in horses between of 2 and 5 years of age (OR, 0.18; 95% CI, 0.06–0.50; $P<.001$). When data for cardiac-related anesthetic deaths were analyzed as a subpopulation, isoflurane (in relation to halothane) (OR, 0.4; 95% CI, 0.2–0.8; P = .02) and blood pressure monitoring (in relation to no blood pressure monitoring) (OR, 0.1; 95% CI, 0.06–0.30; $P<.001$) were associated with a decreased risk of cardiac-related death in the final multivariable model.[4] These results support those from experimental studies that suggest that isoflurane causes less cardiovascular depression compared with halothane when used as a maintenance agent.[45–47] Because there was no significant difference in overall anesthetic-related mortality between isoflurane and halothane, yet isoflurane significantly reduced the risk of mortality in young horses and reduced the risk of cardiac-related deaths, one can infer that isoflurane may increase the risk of mortality in other age groups or be more likely to be associated with other causes of anesthetic-related death (eg, central nervous system); however, no significant associations between isoflurane and mortality were found in these other categories.[4]

MORBIDITY STUDIES

Epidemiologic morbidity studies are fewer in number and suffer from lack of universally agreed case definitions. Problems also occur in how to analyze data for morbidities that may also result in mortality. Morbidities may also be species specific, limiting interspecies comparisons.

Anesthetic-related morbidities in horses

Only a few studies have published overall morbidity risk for populations of horses undergoing anesthesia. In a single-center retrospective study of 1314 anaesthetics,[14] serious anesthetic-related problems were reported in 1.4% of cases of which 0.68% resulted in death. Fifteen of the nineteen serious complications (79%) were reported as having PAM–postanesthetic neuropathy involved in the complications.[14] CEPEF-3[4] was also designed to detect nonfatal perioperative complications and reported that nonfatal complications occurred in approximately 2.7% of cases but the morbidity classifications were not reported. In a much smaller multicenter prospective study of 861 anesthetics where morbidity definitions were predefined, morbidities were reported in 13.7% of cases.[48]

Postanesthetic myopathy

Early studies estimated myopathy risk at between 1% and 6.4%.[14,49,50] More recently, myopathy risk has been estimated to be between 0.8% and 1.6% by one retrospective[51] and two prospective studies.[4,48] Experimental studies have suggested that PAM is caused by decreased muscle perfusion secondary to sustained hypotension or raised intracompartmental muscle pressures.[15,16,50,52,53]

Epidemiologic studies that have been designed to identify risk factors for PAM are rare. In a single-center retrospective study comparing myopathy in horses anesthetized for surgery or magnetic resonance imaging, body weight was the only variable associated with developing myopathy after multivariable analysis, but the total number of cases was low so the power of the study was weak.[51] CEPEF-3 identified duration of anesthesia and body position during anesthesia as risk factors for PAM after final random effect multivariable analysis.[4] In relation to anesthetics of less than 45 minutes, anesthetics of more than 90 minutes led to an increased risk of developing PAM (OR, 9.7; 95% CI, 2.9–31.7; $P<.001$).[4] Increased duration of anesthesia has been demonstrated to cause progressive increases in detected levels of muscle enzymes.[52] In relation to dorsal recumbency for nonabdominal procedures, lateral recumbency was associated with an increased risk of developing PAM (OR, 2.3; 95% CI, 1.2–4.4; $P = .01$).[4] Lateral recumbency may lead to increased compression and isolation of dependent muscle groups (eg, triceps) and may also reduce perfusion of the upper nondependent limb.[47] Interestingly, in CEPEF-3, blood pressure monitoring did not decrease the risk of developing myopathy, and the use of intraoperative inotropic agents was not recorded.[4] Other retrospective studies have indicated that more aggressive treatment of hypotension with intravenous fluid therapy and the use of dobutamine to maintain mean arterial blood pressure higher than 9.3 kPa (70 mm Hg) did not affect the incidence of myopathy but did reduce the severity in those that occurred.[14,54]

Other risk factors that are unlikely to be detected at a population level, such as hyperkalemic periodic paralysis and equine polysaccharide storage disease, are also likely to increase risk of myopathy in certain susceptible animals.

Postanesthetic colic
The risk of developing postanesthetic colic (PAC) has been estimated to be between 2.8% and 12% in retrospective single-center studies,[11,55–58] and in a prospective multicenter study the risk of developing PAC was estimated to be 5.2% (95% CI, 2.8–8).[11] PAC was also reported as the most common type of recorded morbidity.[48]

The two retrospective studies that had just enough cases to identify risk factors for the development of PAC identified several potential risk factors as increasing the risk of developing PAC including the use of morphine (relative to butorphanol),[57] out-of-hours surgery,[57] maintenance with isoflurane (relative to other agents),[58] and the use of sodium penicillin or ceftiofur (relative to not using them)[58]; and some factors associated with a reduction in risk of developing PAC including increasing duration of anesthesia and the use of romifidine as a preanesthetic sedation (relative to the use of other sedatives).[58] Both these studies had limited power to evaluate risk factors. A prospective multicenter study with more power identified that the risk for PAC differed between the centers and when center identity was included in the final multivariable model as a random effect, nonseptic orthopedic surgeries (relative to nonorthopedic surgeries) had an increased risk of developing PAC. Some other factors (whether horses had been fasted before anesthesia, or the use of opioids) remained in the model because they improved the fit of the model but they did not reach significance in the final model ($P<.05$).[11]

Other morbidities
Other studies have attempted to indicate the types of and incidence of other types of morbidities[48] but the case numbers were too low to allow statistical analysis. Currently, the understanding of other morbidities relies on the evaluation of case reports,[59] case series,[60] or experimental studies.[61]

SUMMARY

General anesthesia in horses carries an increased risk of morbidity and mortality compared with other species. It is important for the equine anesthetist to be able to understand and interpret epidemiologic studies into ARMMs, allowing them to communicate effectively with owners and colleagues. Although equine anesthesia can boast several well designed and powerful studies into risk factors for anesthetic-related mortality, the data collected from the last of these are now more than 13 years old,[4] and recent changes to equine anesthesia, such as the increasing number of horses anesthetized in private veterinary clinics, the increasing use of partial intravenous anesthesia or balanced anesthesia, and more interventional approaches to recovery, have led to calls for another large-scale multicenter epidemiologic study.[62] Further epidemiologic studies into common morbidities are also needed to inform case management.

Clinicians should value clinical audit within their own hospitals, with their population of horses and clinical practice for identifying potential unique risks for morbidity and mortality. Such tools as morbidity and mortality rounds are often the only place where the role of human error in morbidity and mortality is considered.

REFERENCES

1. Thrusfield M. Veterinary epidemiology. 2nd edition. Oxford (United Kingdom): Blackwell Science; 1997. p. 15, 39–44, 220–2, 224–6.
2. Dohoo I, Martin W, Stryhn H. Veterinary epidemiologic research. 2nd edition. Prince Edward Island (Canada): VER Inc; 2009. p. 75–82, 137–43, 167–80, 182–98.
3. Altman DG. Practical statistics for medical research. 1st edition. London (United Kingdom): Chapman & Hall; p. 86–93, 152.
4. Johnston GM, Eastment JK, Taylor PM, et al. Is isoflurane safer than halothane in equine anaesthesia? Results from a prospective multicentre randomised controlled trial. Equine Vet J 2004;36:64–71.
5. Pearson H, Gibbs C. Review of sixty equine laparotomies. Equine Vet J 1970;2: 60–3.
6. Blakemore WF, Jefferies A, White RA, et al. Spinal cord malacia following general anaesthesia in the horse. Vet Rec 1984;114:569–70.
7. Joubert KE, Duncan N, Murray SE. Post-anaesthetic myelomalacia in a horse. J S Afr Vet Assoc 2005;76:36–9.
8. Trim CM, Mason J. Post-anaesthetic forelimb lameness in horses. Equine Vet J 1973;5:71–6.
9. Brodbelt DC, Blissitt KJ, Hammond RA, et al. The risk of death: the confidential enquiry into perioperative small animal fatalities. Vet Anaesth Analg 2008;35: 365–73.
10. Johnston GM, Taylor PM, Holmes MA, et al. Confidential enquiry of perioperative equine fatalities. (CEPEF-1): preliminary results. Equine Vet J 1995;27: 193–200.
11. Senior JM, Pinchbeck GL, Allister R, et al. Post anaesthetic colic in horses: a preventable complication? Equine Vet J 2006;33:479–84.
12. Bidwell LA, Bramlage LR, Rood WA. Equine perioperative fatalities associated with general anaesthesia at a private practice: a retrospective case series. Vet Anaesth Analg 2007;34:23–30.
13. Johnston GM, Eastment JK, Wood JL, et al. The confidential enquiry into perioperative equine fatalities (CEPEF): mortality results of Phases 1 and 2. Vet Anaesth Analg 2002;29:159–70.
14. Young SS, Taylor PM. Factors influencing the outcome of equine anaesthesia: a review of 1,314 cases. Equine Vet J 1993;25:147–51.
15. Grandy JL, Steffey EP, Hodgson DS, et al. Arterial hypotension and the development of postanesthetic myopathy in halothane-anesthetized horses. Am J Vet Res 1987;48:192–7.
16. Lindsay WA, Robinson GM, Brunson DB, et al. Induction of equine postanesthetic myositis after halothane-induced hypotension. Am J Vet Res 1989;50:404–10.
17. Johnston GM. Confidential enquiry into perioperative equine fatalities. Equine Vet Educ 1991;3:5–6.
18. Lunn JN, Mushin WW. Mortality associated with anaesthesia. Anaesthesia 1982; 37:856.
19. Tikkanen J, Hovi-Viander M. Death associated with anaesthesia and surgery in Finland in 1986 compared to 1975. Acta Anaesthesiol Scand 1995;39:262–7.

20. Eagle CC, Davis NJ. Report of the Anaesthetic Mortality Committee of Western Australia 1990-1995. Anaesth Intensive Care 1997;25:51-9.
21. Biboulet P, Aubus P, Doubourdieu J, et al. Fatal and non fatal cardiac arrest related to anesthesia. Can J Anaesth 2001;48:326-32.
22. Buck N, Devlin HB, Lunn JN. The report of a confidential enquiry into perioperative deaths 1987. London (United Kingdom): Nuffield Provincial Hospitals Trust, The King's Fund; 1988.
23. Jones RS. Comparative mortality in anaesthesia. Br J Anaesth 2001;87:813-5.
24. Johnston GM. Findings from the CEPEF epidemiological studies into equine perioperative complications. Equine Vet Educ 2005;7:64-8.
25. Dodman NH, Lamb LA. Survey of small animal anesthetic practice in Vermont. J Am Anim Hosp Assoc 1992;28:439-44.
26. Joubert KE. Routine veterinary anaesthetic management practice in South Africa. J S Afr Vet Assoc 2000;71:166-72.
27. Clarke KW, Hall LW. A survey of anaesthesia in small animal practice: AVA/BSAVA report. J Assoc Vet Anaesth 1990;17:4-10.
28. Dyson DH, Maxie MG, Schnurr D. Morbidity and mortality associated with anesthetic management in small animal veterinary practice in Ontario. J Am Anim Hosp Assoc 1998;34:325-35.
29. Mitchell B. Equine anaesthesia: an assessment of techniques used in clinical practice. Equine Vet J 1969;1:261-75.
30. Lumb WV, Jones EW. Veterinary anesthesia. In: Lumb WV, Jones EW, editors. Philadelphia: Lea & Febiger; 1973. p. 611-31.
31. Tevik A. The role of anesthesia in surgical mortality in horses. Nord Vet Med 1983; 35:175-9.
32. Mee AM, Cripps PJ, Jones RS. A retrospective study of mortality associated with general anaesthesia in horses: elective procedures. Vet Rec 1998;14:275-6.
33. Mee AM, Cripps PJ, Jones RS. A retrospective study of mortality associated with general anaesthesia in horses: emergency procedures. Vet Rec 1998;142:307-9.
34. Schatzmann U, Meister V, Fankhauser R. Akute hamatomyelie nach langerer Ruckenlage beim Pferd. Schweiz Arch Tierheilkd 1979;121:149-55.
35. Zink MC. Postanesthetic poliomyelomalacia in a horse. Can Vet J 1985;26:275-7.
36. Yovich JV, LeCouteur RA, Stashak TS, et al. Postanesthetic hemorrhagic myelopathy in a horse. J Am Vet Med Assoc 1986;188:300-1.
37. Brearley JC, Jones RS, Kelly DF. Spinal cord degeneration following general anaesthesia in a Shire horse. Equine Vet J 1986;18:222-4.
38. Lerche E, Laverty S, Blais D, et al. Hemorrhagic myelomalacia following general anesthesia in a horse. Cornell Vet 1993;83:267-73.
39. Wan PY, Latimer FG, Silva-Krott I, et al. Hematomyelia in a colt: a post anesthesia/surgery complication. J Equine Vet Sci 1994;14:495-7.
40. Lam KH, Smyth JB, Clarke K, et al. Acute spinal cord degeneration following general anaesthesia in a young pony. Vet Rec 1995;136:329-30.
41. Raidal SR, Raidal SL, Richards RB, et al. Acute paraplegia in a Thoroughbred race-horse after general anaesthesia. Aust Vet J 1997;75:178-9.
42. van Loon JP, Meertens NM, van Oldruitenborgh-Oosterbaan MM, et al. Post-anaesthetic myelopathy in a 3-year-old Friesian gelding. Tijdschr Diergeneeskd 2010;135:272-7.
43. Proudman CJ, Dugdale AH, Senior JM, et al. Pre-operative and anaesthesia-related risk factors for mortality in equine colic cases. Vet J 2006;171:89-97.
44. Trim CM, Adams JG, Cowgill LM, et al. A retrospective survey of anaesthesia in horses with colic. Equine Vet J Suppl 1989;7:84-90.

45. Steffey EP, Howland D Jr. Comparison of circulatory and respiratory effects of isoflurane and halothane anesthesia in horses. Am J Vet Res 1980;41:821–5.
46. Grosenbaugh DA, Muir WW. Cardiorespiratory effects of sevoflurane, isoflurane and halothane anesthesia in horses. Am J Vet Res 1998;59:101–6.
47. Raisis AL, Young LE, Blissitt KJ, et al. A comparison of the haemodynamic effects of isoflurane and halothane anaesthesia in horses. Equine Vet J 2000;32:318–26.
48. Senior JM, Pinchbeck GL, Allister R, et al. Reported morbidities following 861 anaesthetics given at four equine hospitals. Vet Rec 2007;160:407–8.
49. Johnson BD, Heath RB, Bowman B, et al. Serum chemistry changes in horses: a pilot study investigating the causes of post-anesthetic myositis in horses. J Equine Med Surg 1978;2:109–23.
50. Richey MT, Holland MS, McGrath CJ, et al. Equine post-anesthetic lameness: a retrospective study. Vet Surg 1990;19:392–7.
51. Franci P, Leece EA, Brearley JC. Post anaesthetic myopathy/neuropathy in horses undergoing magnetic resonance imaging compared to horses undergoing surgery. Equine Vet J 2006;38:497–501.
52. Lindsay WA, McDonell W, Bignell W. Equine postanesthetic forelimb lameness: intracompartmental muscle pressure changes and biochemical patterns. Am J Vet Res 1980;41:1919–24.
53. Dodman NH, Williams R, Court MH, et al. Postanesthetic hind limb adductor myopathy in five horses. J Am Vet Med Assoc 1988;193:83–6.
54. Duke T, Filzek U, Read M, et al. Clinical observations surrounding an increased incidence of postanesthetic myopathy in halothane-anesthetized horses. Vet Anaesth Analg 2006;33:122–7.
55. Little D, Redding WR, Blikslager AT. Risk factors for reduced postoperative fecal output in horses: 37 cases (1997–1998). J Am Vet Med Assoc 2001;218:414–20.
56. Mircica E, Clutton RE, Kyles KW, et al. Problems associated with perioperative morphine in horses: a retrospective case analysis. Vet Anaesth Analg 2003;30:147–55.
57. Senior JM, Pinchbeck G, Dugdale AHA, et al. A retrospective study of the risk factors and prevalence of colic in horses after orthopaedic surgery. Vet Rec 2004;155:321–5.
58. Andersen MS, Clark L, Dyson S, et al. Risk factors for colic in horses after general anaesthesia for MRI or nonabdominal surgery: absence of evidence of effect from perianaesthetic morphine. Equine Vet J 2006;38:368–74.
59. Pang DS, Panizzi L, Paterson JM. Successful treatment of hyperkalaemic periodic paralysis in a horse during isoflurane anaesthesia. Vet Anaesth Analg 2011;38:113–20.
60. Kollias-Baker CA, Pipers FS, Heard D, et al. Pulmonary edema associated with transient airway obstruction in three horses. J Am Vet Med Assoc 1993;202:1116–8.
61. Hubbell JA, Muir WW, Robertson JT, et al. Cardiovascular effects of intravenous sodium penicillin, sodium cefazolin, and sodium citrate in awake and anesthetized horses. Vet Surg 1987;16:245–50.
62. Bettschart R, Johnston GM. Confidential enquiry into perioperative equine fatalities: CEPEF 4-a chance to gain new evidence about the risks of equine general anaesthesia. Equine Vet J 2011;44:7.

Drugs for Cardiovascular Support in Anesthetized Horses

Stijn Schauvliege, DVM, PhD*, Frank Gasthuys, DVM, PhD

KEYWORDS

- Cardiovascular support • Anesthesia • Horses • Inotropes • Chronotropes
- Vasopressors

KEY POINTS

- Despite balanced anesthesia and fluid therapy, drugs are often needed for cardiovascular support in anesthetized horses.
- In most cases inotropes are preferred, and dobutamine remains the agent of choice in most horses.
- Treat hypocalcemia with calcium salts.
- Use vasopressors when hypotension is caused by vasodilation while cardiac output and/or HR are high or when hypotension is not responsive to fluids and inotropes.
- Order of decreasing inotropic and increasing vasopressor effect: dobutamine, dopamine, ephedrine, noradrenaline, phenylephrine.
- Phosphodiesterase III inhibitors and vasopressin (analogues) are promising for future research.
- Combinations of drugs for cardiovascular support can be useful.

INTRODUCTION

Reduced tissue oxygenation may contribute to a higher anesthesia-related mortality rate in horses.[1] Tissue oxygen supply depends on oxygen delivery (DO_2), individual tissue perfusion, and oxygen consumption. Oxygen delivery is the product of arterial oxygen content (CaO_2) and cardiac output ($\dot{Q}_t$). Individual tissue perfusion depends on $\dot{Q}_t$, precapillary arteriolar tone (which also determines systemic vascular resistance [SVR]), and vascular transmural pressure. Transmural pressure is the force that maintains vessel patency and represents the difference between intravascular and extravascular pressures, so it is highly influenced by the arterial blood pressure (ABP) and will more likely become insufficient in tissues with high extravascular pressures (eg, dependent muscles in recumbent horses). Inadequate tissue oxygen supply usually results from decreases in one or more of the following:

- CaO_2
- $\dot{Q}_t$ (= heart rate [HR] × stroke volume [SV])

* Department of Surgery and Anaesthesia of Domestic Animals, Faculty of Veterinary Medicine, University of Ghent, Salisburylaan 133, B-9820 Merelbeke, Belgium.
E-mail address: Stijn.Schauvliege@UGent.be

Vet Clin Equine 29 (2013) 19–49
http://dx.doi.org/10.1016/j.cveq.2012.11.011
0749-0739/13/$ – see front matter © 2013 Elsevier Inc. All rights reserved.
vetequine.theclinics.com

- ABP (determined by circulating volume, $\dot{Q}_t$, and SVR)
- Local arteriolar tone in the specific tissue considered

The complicated interplay between these factors is illustrated in **Fig. 1**. Because horses have a high body weight and easily develop ventilation-perfusion mismatching and cardiovascular depression during anesthesia,[2,3] cardiovascular support is extremely important in maintaining tissue oxygenation.

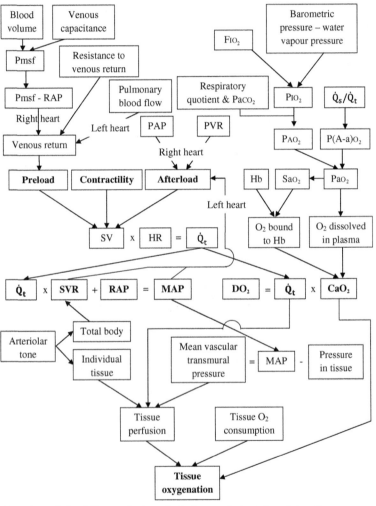

Fig. 1. Overview of the different factors that play a role in determining tissue oxygenation. CaO_2, arterial oxygen content; DO_2, oxygen delivery; FIO_2, inspiratory oxygen fraction; Hb, hemoglobin concentration; HR, heart rate; MAP, mean arterial pressure; P(A-a)o_2, alveolar to arterial oxygen tension difference; Pao_2, alveolar oxygen tension; Pao_2, arterial oxygen tension; PAP, pulmonary artery pressure; PIO_2, inspiratory oxygen tension; Pmsf, mean systemic filling pressure; PVR, pulmonary vascular resistance; $\dot{Q}_s/\dot{Q}_t$, degree of venous admixture; $\dot{Q}_t$, cardiac output; RAP, right atrial pressure; Sao_2, arterial oxygen saturation; SV, stroke volume; SVR, systemic vascular resistance.

CARDIOVASCULAR MONITORING

In daily practice, cardiovascular monitoring in anesthetized horses usually consists of clinical assessment, electrocardiography, pulse-oximetry, and ABP monitoring. Of these, ABP gives the most important information on cardiovascular function. Equine anesthetists normally aim to maintain mean arterial pressure (MAP) above 70 mm Hg, because the intracompartmental pressure in the dependent muscles of adult horses, on an adequately padded surface, reaches values of 30 to 40 mm Hg[4] while vascular transmural pressure needs to be greater than 30 mm Hg for adequate microcirculation.[5]

When hypotension occurs, a distinction should be made between decreases in circulating volume (eg, blood loss), $\dot{Q}_t$, or SVR.

- Changes in circulating volume can be suspected based on the history, pulse quality, mucous-membrane color, capillary refill time, degree of jugular distension on compression, skin turgor, packed cell volume, serum total protein level, and so forth.
- To distinguish between decreases in $\dot{Q}_t$ or SVR, $\dot{Q}_t$ is ideally measured. Decreases in SVR can also be suspected based on signs such as:
  - Low diastolic arterial pressure (DAP) with normal or high pulse pressure
  - Rapid rise and fall of arterial waveform
  - History that suggests vasodilation, for example, administration of vasodilating drugs (eg, acepromazine, isoflurane), endotoxemia, and so forth
- Reductions in $\dot{Q}_t$ that lead to hypotension and that are not caused by bradycardia usually result from a reduced contractility (eg, effect of anesthetics) or preload (hypovolemia, venous vasodilation, increased intrathoracic/right atrial pressure [RAP], and so forth).

TREATMENT STRATEGY

After preoperative preparation of the patient, 3 cornerstones in the prevention and treatment of cardiovascular depression are:

- Reduction of anesthetic depth
- Fluid therapy
- Cardiovascular stimulant drugs

Because volatile anesthetics have only poor analgesic properties,[6,7] reduction of anesthetic depth is best achieved using balanced anesthetic techniques (See articles of Alex Valverde elsewhere in this issue). Fluid therapy is also essential in supporting cardiovascular function (see article of Snyder and Wendt-Hornickle elsewhere in this issue), but appropriate infusion rates are sometimes difficult to achieve in hypovolemic horses, where very large volumes are needed. Despite the use of balanced anesthesia and fluids, cardiovascular stimulant drugs are therefore often needed.

A distinction can be made between:

- Chronotropes
- Inotropes
- Vasopressors

In most species, bradycardia is treated with chronotropes, reduced contractility with inotropes, and vasodilation with vasopressors. In horses, however, some agents may be used under different circumstances. In hypovolemic horses, appropriate fluid administration rates can be difficult to achieve, so inotropes and/or vasopressors are often used in an attempt to quickly improve $\dot{Q}_t$ and ABP until adequate volumes can be administered. Also, anesthetized horses easily develop hypoxemia, which is difficult to prevent or treat, so increasing $\dot{Q}_t$, even to "supranormal" values, can be useful to optimize DO_2. Many equine anesthetists treat hypotension routinely with inotropes, almost regardless of the underlying cause. In a species where tissue perfusion and oxygenation easily become inadequate, this strategy seems fair. Nevertheless, vasopressors can be useful, for example, when hypotension is caused by vasodilation (endotoxemia, drug-induced, and so forth) while contractility and HR are already high. In such cases, β_1-sympathomimetics can increase myocardial oxygen consumption and cause tachycardia and/or arrhythmias. However, when vasopressors are used, possible negative effects, for example, on splanchnic perfusion, have to be taken into account.

CHRONOTROPIC DRUGS

The chronotropes most typically used in practice are the antimuscarinics, which antagonize acetylcholine's muscarinic effects without affecting the nicotinic receptors at the neuromuscular junction. As such, they affect organs innervated by postganglionic parasympathetic fibers, such as the heart, eyes, glandular tissues, and nonvascular smooth muscle.[8] Their main cardiovascular effect is positive chronotropism.

Although HR is an important determinant of $\dot{Q}_t$, chronotropes should not be used to increase $\dot{Q}_t$ unless bradycardia is present. At high HR, myocardial oxygen consumption increases[9] while diastolic time shortens. Because 80% of the coronary blood flow occurs during diastole,[10] tachycardia may compromise myocardial oxygen delivery, especially when tachycardia is severe, cardiac disease is present, or drugs affecting coronary vascular resistance have been administered. In such cases, cardiac oxygen supply can become insufficient, resulting in decreased myocardial contractility[11] or arrhythmias.[12] Atropine also increases the chronotropic effects and arrhythmogenicity of dobutamine.[13] Finally, most antimuscarinics reduce intestinal motility and can induce abdominal discomfort or colic in horses,[14] although this might be avoided by using selective muscarinic type-2 antagonists such as methoctramine.[15]

The antimuscarinic drugs most often used are:

- Atropine (hyoscyamine)
  o Atropine is used for different purposes, for example, during premedication, in conjunction with anticholinesterase drugs, to produce mydriasis, or as an antisialagogue.
  o In awake horses, atropine (0.04 mg/kg intravenously) increased HR 2- to 3-fold.[16]
  o In the past, atropine was widely used to counteract α_2-agonist induced bradycardia and atrioventricular blocks in horses.[17,18] Nowadays this is considered controversial. The bradycardia induced by α_2-agonists is partly attributable to a baroreceptor reflex in response to the initial hypertension. Under such circumstances, atropine may induce even more pronounced hypertension[19] and a substantial increase in cardiac work, because $\dot{Q}_t$ will increase in the presence of a high afterload.
- Glycopyrronium (glycopyrrolate)
  o Glycopyrronium is an ionized quaternary amine
  o Unlike atropine, glycopyrronium does not readily cross the blood-brain barrier or placenta.
  o In humans, it is an effective antisialagogue with long duration of action (± 6 hours). Clear effects on HR and pupillary size occur only at higher doses.[8]
  o In horses its cardiac effects are more comparable with those of atropine.[20,21]

- Hyoscine (scopolamine)
  - In humans hyoscine has a shorter duration of action, less tachycardia, a more powerful antisialagogue effect, and less bronchodilation than atropine.[8]
  - In equids, hyoscine butylbromide, a derivative of scopolamine often used for its spasmolytic properties,[22] can also be used to increase HR.[23–25]

INOTROPES

Available inotropes include digitalis glycosides, sympathomimetics, calcium salts, phosphodiesterase (PDE) inhibitors, and calcium sensitizers. Digitalis glycosides are less effective in healthy patients[26] and have a slow onset[27] but long duration of action,[28] and a narrow therapeutic window.[29] Calcium sensitizers are rather long-acting[30] and quite expensive. Therefore, both classes of drugs are not routinely used for cardiovascular support during anesthesia and are mainly indicated in cardiac patients, and are not discussed further here.

Sympathomimetics

Undoubtedly, sympathomimetics are the agents most widely used to increase $\dot{Q}_t$ in anesthetized horses. Like most inotropes (except calcium sensitizers), they increase myocardial contractility by increasing Ca^{2+} availability to the contractile apparatus.[31] **Fig. 2** represents the series of events that occur when agonists bind on the cardiac β_1-receptor. The final result is phosphorylation of sarcolemmal proteins, phospholamban and troponin-I.[32]

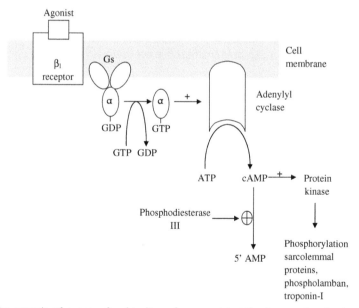

Fig. 2. The cascade of events after binding of an agonist at the β_1 receptor. A stimulatory G protein (Gs) is activated, and the α-subunit–GTP complex dissociates and activates adenylyl cyclase. cAMP is formed, which activates a protein kinase that phosphorylates sarcolemmal proteins, phospholamban and troponin-I, which ultimately leads to positive inotropic effects. cAMP is broken down by phosphodiesterase III. AMP, adenosine monophosphate; ATP, adenosine triphosphate; cAMP, cyclic AMP; GDP, guanosine diphosphate; GTP, guanosine triphosphate.

Phosphorylation of sarcolemmal proteins causes:

- Increased Ca^{2+} influx through slow (L-type) channels in response to membrane depolarization[32]
- Increased intracellular Ca^{2+} levels stimulate release of more Ca^{2+} from the sarcoplasmic reticulum (SR) ('Ca^{2+}-induced Ca^{2+} release'),[33] resulting in increased contractility[34]

Phosphorylation of phospholamban, which regulates the Ca^{2+} pump of the SR, results in an increased:

- Velocity of Ca^{2+} reuptake by SR vesicles
- Affinity of the transport protein for Ca^{2+}
- Turnover of the adenosine triphosphatase reaction[35]

Calcium sequestration by the SR is augmented[36]; this has a lusitropic effect[37] and, because more Ca^{2+} is available for release during the next action potential, the force and rate of contraction are also increased.[38]

Phosphorylation of troponin-I leads to:

- Decreased affinity of troponin C for Ca^{2+}[35]
- Increased rate of Ca^{2+} dissociation from the myofilaments
- Accelerated myocardial relaxation[37]

Possible negative effects of β_1-adrenergics are increases in cardiac work and myocardial oxygen demand,[39] sinus tachycardia, cardiac arrhythmias, and reduced organ perfusion caused by vasoconstriction.[40,41] The increase in HR is related to acceleration of voltage-sensitive sarcolemmal currents ("voltage clock") and Ca^{2+} release from the SR ("calcium clock") in cardiac pacemaker cells.[42]

An overview of some β-sympathomimetics is presented in **Table 1**.

Adrenaline

Adrenaline or epinephrine has powerful α and β_1 effects and moderate β_2 effects.[43] At lower doses (0.04–0.1 μg/kg/min):

- Effects on β-adrenoceptors predominate
- HR, contractility, and conduction velocity are increased (β_1 effect)
- SVR is lowered (β_2 effect) or unchanged[44]
- Systolic arterial pressure (SAP) increases
- DAP may decrease[45]

At higher doses, the α effects become more dominant so that both SVR and ABP increase.[44] The plasma half-life is 10 to 15 seconds.[10] Adrenaline produces many other effects such as mydriasis, bronchodilation, lipolysis, glycogenolysis, hyperglycemia, and sweating.[44,46] The cardiovascular effects are summarized in **Table 1**.

Traditional concerns with adrenaline are:

- Myocardial oxygen supply may become inadequate[43] because:
  - Myocardial oxygen consumption increases because of increases in HR, contractility, and SVR[47]
  - The α effect causes coronary vasoconstriction (though attenuated by the increased work of the heart that causes coronary vasodilation)[8]
- Proarrhythmic activity
  - Ventricular premature contractions (VPCs), ventricular tachycardia, and atrial/ventricular fibrillation observed in horses[48]

Table 1
Dose-dependent effects of β- sympathomimetic agents

Drug	Patients	Dose	Receptor Activity	Cardiovascular Effects	References
Epinephrine	General		Strong α and β1, moderate β2	HR, contractility, and ABP ↑; SVR ↑, ↓, or = (~dose)	43
				May cause tachycardia, arrhythmias, vasoconstriction, myocardial ischemia, myocardial O_2 consumption ↑	174
	Humans	0.04–0.1 µg/kg/min	Mainly β1, β2	β1 effect: HR, contractility and conduction velocity ↑ Moderate β2 effect: SVR ↓ or = SAP ↑, DAP sometimes ↓	8,44,45
		>0.1 µg/kg/min	α effect becomes more important	β1 effect: HR ↑, contractility and conduction velocity α effect: ↑ SVR, ABP ↑	43,44
	Horses	3 µg/kg		Pronounced ↑ ABP, HR initially ↑, but ↓ when pressor response maximal Ventricular arrhythmias	49
		0.25–1.2 µg/kg/min		ABP and HR ↑, VPCs at higher end of dose	48
Dopamine	General		DA_1, DA_2, α1, α2, β1 Part of effect mediated by ↑ release and ↓ uptake of norepinephrine	β1 effect: contractility and HR ↑ DA_1 effect: vascular relaxation, sodium excretion kidney ↑ Postsynaptic α1 and α2 effect: vasoconstriction	53,63
	Humans	<2–4 µg/kg/min	Mainly DA_1 and DA_2	Renal plasma flow, GFR and Na^+ excretion ↑	44,53,63
		3–10 µg/kg/min	Mainly β1	HR and $\dot{Q}_t$ ↑	
		>10 µg/kg/min	Mainly α	Sometimes tachycardia (eg, underhydrated patients) Vasoconstriction, arrhythmias likely	8
		5 µg/kg/min			
	Conscious horses	1–2.5 µg/kg/min		No effect on HR and ABP, but renal blood flow ↑ at 2.5 µg/kg/min	175
				HR ↑ and ABP ↓	176
		5 µg/kg/min		No effect on HR and ABP, but renal blood flow ↑ and arrhythmias	175
	Anesthetized ponies	2.5–5 µg/kg/min		None	40,55
		10–20 µg/kg/min		CI, MAP, and intramuscular blood flow ↑, SVR ↓ Tachyarrhythmias and muscle tremor at highest dose	40
	Anesthetized horses	0.5–3 µg/kg/min		None	41,177
		2.5 µg/kg/min		$\dot{Q}_t$ ↑ and SVR ↓	177
		4 µg/kg/min		ABP ↓ and $\dot{Q}_t$ ↑, minor ↑ HR	178
		5 µg/kg/min		$\dot{Q}_t$ ↑, SVR ↓, ABP =, HR =, arrhythmias	41
		10 µg/kg/min		$\dot{Q}_t$ ↑, SVR =, ABP ↑, HR =, arrhythmias	41
				Variable effect on HR, arrhythmias	179

(continued on next page)

Table 1
(continued)

Drug	Patients	Dose	Receptor Activity	Cardiovascular Effects	References
Dopexamine	General		β_2, DA_1, DA_2, weak β_1 ↓ Norepinephrine reuptake	Renal vascular resistance ↓, neurogenic vasoconstriction ↓	66
				Some positive inotropism	53
				HR and CI ↑, SVR ↓	180
				Sinus tachycardia, tachyarrhythmias	8
	Ponies and horses	0.5–20 μg/kg/min		CI, contractility, MAP and HR ↑, SVR ↓	40,67–69
				Intramuscular blood flow ↑	
				muscle tremor, sweating, excitement, shivering, colic	40,67
				10–20 μg/kg/min tachycardia and arrhythmias	
Fenoldopam	General		DA_1	CI ↑, SVR and ABP ↓	43
				Tachycardia and hypotension	73,74
Dobutamine	General		Mainly β_1, slight α_1 and β_2	SV ↑, $\dot{Q}_t$ ↑, HR ↑ at higher doses	43,181
	Humans	<7.5 μg/kg/min	Mainly β_1	SV ↑, $\dot{Q}_t$ ↑, ABP ↑, HR ↑ at higher doses	44
		>7.5 μg/kg/min	β_1 and β_2 (overshadows α_1)	SVR ↓, but usually ABP still ↑, tachycardia	44,181
	Ponies	1.25–5 μg/kg/min		SVR =, CI, MAP, and SV ↑	55
				At 2.5 and 5 μg/kg/min HR and PCV ↑, some ponies severe tachycardia	
		2.5–10 μg/kg/min		SVR ↓, CI and MAP ↑, highest dose arrhythmias and tachycardia intramuscular blood flow ↑	40
	Horses	0.5–1.0 μg/kg/min		ABP ↑, $\dot{Q}_t$ =, no changes in left ventricular systolic function or SVR	58,182
		3–10 μg/kg/min		ABP ↑, $\dot{Q}_t$ ↑, contractility ↑, variable effect on HR (↑, ↓ or =), effect on SVR small and not significant, PCV ↑	41,161,182,183
				arrhythmias at higher doses (often limited to bradyarrhythmias, AV blocks, AV dissociation, or APCs)	41,60,61

Drug	Group	Mechanism/Dose	Effects	Ref
Xamoterol	General	Partial β$_1$-agonist	Contractility and HR ↑ Effect depends on sympathetic tone: moderate inotropism at rest, but attenuates β-adrenergic response during exercise	75
				8
			SVR and ABP ↑ (through β$_2$ vascular blocking action?)	184
Ephedrine	General	Direct α$_1$ effect and also causes synaptic release of norepinephrine and inhibits its metabolism	Q̇$_t$, SVR, ABP, and HR ↑ Tachyphylaxis with continued use	8
	Horses	0.06 mg/kg	ABP ↑, HR and PCV =, no arrhythmias	57
Isoprenaline	General	Very potent β$_1$ and β$_2$, no α effect	Contractility and Q̇$_t$ ↑, HR ↑↑ (sometimes excessive tachycardia), peripheral and bronchial vasodilation, SVR, DAP and MAP ↓, coronary perfusion may ↓, myocardial O$_2$ consumption ↑, arrhythmias	44,77–79
	Horses	0.85 µg/kg	HR ↑↑, arrhythmias, ABP ↑ slightly	49

↑, increase; ↓, decrease; =, no change.

Abbreviations: ABP, arterial blood pressure; APC, atrial premature contraction; AV, atrioventricular; CI, cardiac index; DA$_1$, dopamine-1 receptor; DA$_2$, dopamine-2 receptor; DAP, diastolic arterial pressure; GFR, glomerular filtration rate; HR, heart rate; MAP, mean arterial pressure; Na$^+$, sodium; O$_2$, oxygen; PCV, packed cell volume; Q̇$_t$, cardiac output; SAP, systolic arterial pressure; SV, stroke volume; SVR, systemic vascular resistance; VPC, ventricular premature contraction.

- 3 μg/kg intravenously: VPCs in 8 of 13 conscious horses[49]
- Arrhythmogenicity influenced by anesthetic protocol, for example:
  - Risk for arrhythmias may be higher during halothane than during isoflurane or sevoflurane anesthesia[49,50]
  - Hypercapnia increases risk for adrenaline-induced ventricular arrhythmias[51]
  - Acepromazine may reduce incidence of adrenaline-induced arrhythmias[52]

Indications for its use are:

- Anaphylaxis
- Cardiopulmonary resuscitation: pulseless electrical activity or asystole[44]
- To coarsen "fine" ventricular fibrillation (high-frequency, low-amplitude waves) before direct current cardioversion[8]
- Patients with life-threatening hypotension irresponsive to dobutamine or dopamine[43,49]

Dobutamine

Dobutamine, a synthetic catecholamine chemically related to dopamine, is one of the most potent inotropes available[44] and undoubtedly the most often used inotrope in anesthetized horses. Dobutamine is marketed as a racemic mixture with the following properties:

- Predominant β_1 activity
- Balanced β_2 and α_1 effect[53]
- Lower dosages mainly β_1 effect, higher dosages (>7.5 μg/kg/min) additional β_2 effects
- α_1 effects (vasoconstriction) usually antagonized by β_2 effects (vasodilation)[44]
- Plasma half-life 2 to 3 minutes, rapid hepatic metabolization[8]
- Time to onset of action 1 to 10 minutes, peak effect within 10 to 20 minutes[44]

Many investigators have described the cardiovascular effects of dobutamine in ponies and horses (see **Table 1**). At rates below 1 to 1.5 μg/kg/min, ABP increases whereas $\dot{Q}_t$ is little affected. At higher rates, ABP and $\dot{Q}_t$ both increase but tachycardia and arrhythmias can occur. However, dobutamine's effect on HR appears to be variable: some investigators reported increases[54–56] and others decreases[41,57] at doses of 2.5 to 5 μg/kg/min. At 10 μg/kg/min, Swanson and colleagues[41] did not find significant differences from baseline, whereas Lee and colleagues[40] reported ventricular arrhythmias and tachycardia at the same dose. Most likely, the actual effect in an individual horse depends on the prevailing autonomic nervous system activity, ABP, and HR before initiating dobutamine administration. Changes in SVR are usually small and often not significant. However, SVR only gives a general impression of the mean arteriolar tone throughout the body and may not accurately reflect the situation in each specific tissue. Lee and colleagues[40] reported that dobutamine increased intramuscular blood flow more consistently than dopamine, dopexamine or phenylephrine, although Raisis and colleagues[58] did not find increases in microvascular muscle perfusion. Based on the available literature (see **Table 1**), dobutamine seems more effective than dopamine at improving ABP and $\dot{Q}_t$.

Dobutamine is a weaker proarrhythmic than most other catecholamines.[59] The arrhythmias observed at 3 to 5 μg/kg/min in horses are usually limited to bradyarrhythmias, second-degree atrioventricular blocks, premature atrial contractions, and isorhythmic atrioventricular dissociation.[41,60,61] Caution is advised when combining parasympatholytics with dobutamine. Atropine increases the risk for tachyarrhythmias in response to dobutamine,[61] while the dose of dobutamine required to induce repeated

VPCs or sustained tachyarrhythmias was almost 3-fold lower.[13] Nevertheless, dobutamine seems to be a relatively safe drug in horses when used with caution.

Dopamine

Dopamine is the precursor of noradrenaline (norepinephrine),[62] and stimulates presynaptic dopamine-2 (DA_2) and α_2 receptors as well as postsynaptic dopamine-1 (DA_1), α_1, α_2, and β_1 receptors.[63] It also causes the release and prevents the reuptake of noradrenaline.[53] Because of the effects at postsynaptic β_1 receptors, mainly by inducing noradrenaline release, dopamine has positive inotropic and chronotropic effects. Postsynaptic DA_1 receptors on vascular smooth muscle mediate vascular relaxation and promote renal sodium excretion. Dopamine causes vasoconstriction by the effects exerted at postsynaptic α_1 and α_2 receptors. Presynaptic α_2 and DA_2 receptors both inhibit noradrenaline release.[63] Dopamine's half-life is 2 minutes, with a time to onset of action of 5 minutes and duration of effect of ± 10 minutes.[44]

In humans, the effects can be described as follows.

Low or 'Renal' Doses (<2–4 µg/kg/min):
- Predominant DA_1 and DA_2 effect
- Increases renal plasma flow, glomerular filtration rate, and sodium excretion[44,63]
- Little convincing evidence that this prevents acute renal failure (ARF) in high-risk patients, or improves renal function or outcome in patients with established ARF[64]

Intermediate Doses (3–10 µg/kg/min):
- Predominant β_1 effect
- Inotropic and chronotropic[63]
- Tachycardia possible, particularly in underhydrated patients[8]
- Used primarily to increase contractility in congestive heart failure (CHF)[44]

Higher Doses (>10 µg/kg/min):
- Mainly α effect
- Vasoconstriction[63]
- Arrhythmias more likely[8]
- Sinus tachycardia or ventricular ectopic activity possible (usually asymptomatic, ventricular tachycardia relatively rare)[65]
- Mainly used to increase ABP during hypotension or shock[44]

The mentioned dose ranges are approximate. Doses at which the different receptors are activated can vary considerably, depending on the patient's clinical status and the preexisting level of sympathetic activity.[63]

The situation in equids is comparable to that in human medicine (see **Table 1**): the cardiovascular effects are dose-dependent, results between various studies are not always consistent, and the response of individual patients to dopamine depends on the degree of sympathetic stimulation and the patient's health status. Rates less than 3 µg/kg/min do not produce clear changes. Higher doses can be used to increase $\dot{Q}_t$ and perhaps also ABP. However, by increasing the dose, the risk of inducing arrhythmias becomes higher.

Dopexamine

This synthetic catecholamine has the following properties in humans[8,53,66]:

- Potency at β_2 receptors ± 60 times higher than dopamine
- Lower activity at dopamine receptors

- Weak β_1-agonist, but some inotropic effect attributable to:
  - Cardiac β_2 activity
  - Inhibition of neuronal reuptake of noradrenaline

In anesthetized ponies and horses, dopexamine (0.5–20 μg/kg/min) reduced SVR and increased cardiac index (CI), MAP, HR, contractility, and intramuscular blood flow.[40,67–69] However, reported side effects included muscular tremor, profuse sweating during administration, excitement and violent shivering during recovery, and signs of colic a few hours after anesthesia.[40,69] At 10 to 20 μg/kg/min, sinus tachycardia, tachyarrhythmias, and ventricular arrhythmias can occur.[40,67]

Ephedrine

This drug has marked chemical and pharmacologic similarity with adrenaline.[70] Its properties in humans can be summarized as follows:

- Increases HR, contractility, and ABP[70]
- Directly stimulates postsynaptic α_1-receptors
- Is actively taken up by sympathetic nerve endings, where it displaces noradrenaline from its storage granules into the synapse and inhibits the intraneuronal metabolism of noradrenaline[8]
- Continued use can cause tachyphylaxis (depletion of noradrenaline stores in sympathetic neurons)[71]
- Similarly, effect may be diminished when sympathetic nervous system is already maximally stimulated
- More prolonged effects than most catecholamines (eg, effect on ABP usually >15 minutes)[70]
- Often administered as a bolus instead of a CRI

In anesthetized horses, ephedrine (0.06 mg/kg intravenously) increased $\dot{Q}_t$, SV, and ABP, without affecting HR or cardiac rhythm.[57,72] In the authors' experience, ephedrine can be useful when dobutamine is less effective at increasing ABP (eg, in endotoxemic horses with low SVR), but occasionally pronounced increases in HR, which last for 10 to 15 minutes, may occur. Caution is advised in compromised patients, especially when HR is already high. Administration of initially low doses, with careful dose titration to reach the desired effect, is recommended.

Other drugs

Fenoldopam, a DA_1 receptor agonist with no α or β effects, increases CI, but reduces SVR[7] and causes hypotension and tachycardia in anesthetized horses[73] and foals.[74]

Xamoterol, a partial agonist of the β_1-adrenoreceptors,[75] has additive effects with released catecholamines and is a moderate inotrope when sympathetic tone is low. When sympathetic drive is high, xamoterol will reduce the effects of endogenous catecholamines and may, for example, cause clinical deterioration in patients with extremely poor left ventricular function.[76] To the authors' knowledge, its use has not been described in horses.

Isoprenaline (isoproterenol) is a synthetic catecholamine with very potent β_1 and β_2 effects, but no α effects.[43] It increases $\dot{Q}_t$, myocardial contractility, and HR,[77,78] and can cause excessive tachycardia.[44] The β_2-mediated vasodilation reduces SVR,[78] DAP,[79] and MAP.[44] In halothane-anesthetized horses, an intravenous dose of 0.85 μg/kg markedly increased HR, with a much slower return to baseline compared with adrenaline, VPCs in all animals, and ventricular or nodal tachycardia in several cases. In most horses, ABP increased slightly.[49]

Calcium Salts

Instead of using inotropes to increase Ca^{2+} availability to the contractile apparatus, an alternative approach is to increase circulatory calcium levels using calcium salts. In dogs and children, equal elemental calcium doses of calcium gluconate and $CaCl_2$ raised ionized calcium levels to a similar degree and produced comparable cardiovascular effects.[80] By contrast, Hempelmann and colleagues[81] found that although the cardiovascular effects of both salts were largely similar, the positive inotropic effects of $CaCl_2$ were more pronounced.

Several researchers have described the cardiovascular effects of calcium salts.

- In man, $CaCl_2$ improved cardiac function that was depressed by anesthesia or cardiac disease.[82]
- Positive inotropic effects have been reported in cats,[83] dogs,[84] calves,[85] and horses.[86,87]
- Calcium gluconate attenuated or reversed the negative lusitropic actions of inhalants in horses.[88]
- $\dot{Q}_t$ and/or SV increased in conscious[87] and anesthetized horses,[86] ponies,[89] hypocalcemic dogs,[90] and humans with cardiac disease.[82]
- In anesthetized ponies[89] and horses,[86] HR decreased and ABP increased.

However, calcium administration significantly increased mortality associated with endotoxic shock[91] and septic peritonitis[92] in rats. Furthermore, significant cardiovascular effects were not always found after calcium administration:

- No effect on ABP in conscious horses[87]
- No effect on $\dot{Q}_t$ in dogs,[93] healthy people,[82,94] or patients recovering from cardiac surgery[95,96]

Possibly these conflicting results may be explained by differences in health status, cardiovascular function, and preexisting serum calcium concentrations. As an example, $\dot{Q}_t$ and SV increased when calcium was administered in hypocalcemic, but not in normocalcemic, dogs.[90] Similarly, Mathru and colleagues[97] found that during normocalcemia the predominant effect of $CaCl_2$ is peripheral vasoconstriction, whereas calcium infusion during hypocalcemia significantly increases left ventricular contractility. It can be concluded that the usefulness of calcium salts for cardiovascular support differs between individual patients. In the authors' opinion, calcium salts are mainly useful when preoperative ionized calcium levels are low.

Phosphodiesterase-III Inhibitors

Whereas β-sympathomimetics increase cyclic adenosine monophosphate (cAMP) synthesis by adenylate cyclase, cAMP is broken down by PDE enzymes (see **Fig. 2**). These enzymes play a role in modulating the amplitude and duration of the effect, the response of cells to prolonged stimulation, and cross-talk between different second-messenger pathways. More than 25 PDEs of 7 different families have been recognized in humans.[98] Some drugs, such as the methylxanthines (theophylline, theobromine, and caffeine),[99] nonselectively inhibit PDEs and can be used as bronchodilators,[100] but also affect the central nervous system, gastrointestinal tract, and cardiovascular system.[101] Other drugs more specifically inhibit a certain family of PDE enzymes. Their effects depend on the type of PDE inhibited: PDE-I inhibition might increase cognitive function,[98] and certain PDE-IV inhibitors may have antidepressant[102] or anti-inflammatory[103] effects. PDE-V inhibitors (eg, sildenafil) have a role in the treatment of pulmonary hypertension.[104] However, the greatest number of available compounds, including, amrinone, milrinone, vesnarinone, enoximone, and pimobendan, among others, primarily inhibit the PDE-III family. These drugs have been developed as antithrombotics,[105] antihypertensives, and/or inotropes.[98]

The inotropic effects of PDE-III inhibitors result from increased cAMP levels in the myocardial cell. However, they also increase cAMP levels in vascular smooth muscle cells, causing a vasorelaxation through 3 different mechanisms:

- Decreased myoplasmic Ca^{2+} concentrations[106] through inhibition of L-type Ca^{2+} channels[107] and enhanced Ca^{2+} pump activity by phosphorylation of phospholamban[108]
- Decreased Ca^{2+} sensitivity of contractile elements[109]
- Phosphorylation of myosin light chain kinase, which interferes with the binding of Ca^{2+}-calmodulin[110]

Three groups of PDE-III inhibitors exist[43]:

- Bipyridines (amrinone, milrinone)
- Imidazole derivatives (enoximone, piroximone)
- Benzimidazole derivatives (sulmazole, pimobendan, adibendan)

Comparative studies failed to show clinically relevant differences between most PDE-III inhibitors.[53] Their effects can be summarized as follows:

- They are "inodilators": combined inotropic and vasodilatory effects[111]
- Vasodilation reduces ventricular wall stress and counteracts the increased oxygen requirement normally needed to support enhanced contractility[112]
- Lesser chronotropic effects than dobutamine[111]
- More pronounced lusitropic effect than β-sympathomimetics[113]
- Long duration of action
- Excessive vasodilation and hypotension possible after rapid bolus[53] or high doses; can be minimized by slow administration, volume expansion, and vasopressors[43]
- In humans, mainly used in CHF and during weaning from cardiopulmonary bypass[30]

Owing to the abundance of information available, only a short overview of 3 well-known drugs is provided here. Because of the inodilator properties, these agents may prove to be useful in horses, for example during α_2-agonist CRIs.

Amrinone

- First PDE-III inhibitor approved for use in humans
- Cardiovascular effects (see above)
- Improved myocardial systolic/diastolic function and reduced systemic inflammatory response syndrome in endotoxemic rabbits[114]
- Side effects: thrombocytopenia, gastrointestinal effects, hypotension, fever, liver-enzyme elevation, anaphylactoid responses[115]
- Accumulation possible in critically ill patients[39]
- Incidence/importance of most side effects limited[115]
- Nowadays used less frequently than milrinone and enoximone

Milrinone

- Derivative of amrinone, 15 times more potent[43]
- Ameliorates contractility, improves diastolic filling, and accelerates isovolumic myocardial relaxation, without altering myocardial oxygen demand[112]

- Lesser proarrhythmic effect than dobutamine[116]
- Possible anti-inflammatory properties[117]
- In halothane-anesthetized horses: increased HR, MAP, $\dot{Q}_t$, ejection fraction, and contractility[118]

Enoximone

- Mainly inhibits PDE-III; PDE-IV inhibition may also contribute to inotropic effects[119]
- Increases coronary blood flow; no significant increases in myocardial oxygen consumption[120,121]
- Increased $\dot{Q}_t$ and decreased SVR, but minimal/no effects on HR and ABP during moderate to severe CHF[122]
- Seems to preferentially reduce limb vascular resistance and augment blood flow to the peripheral musculoskeletal system; little to no effect on renal, hepatic, and splanchnic vascular beds[123]
- In contrast to dobutamine, enoximone improved hepatosplanchnic function and had anti-inflammatory properties in fluid-optimized septic shock[124]
- In patients with severe and prolonged catecholamine and volume refractory endotoxin shock, enoximone restored myocardial contractility and ABP[125]
- In endotoxemic rats, enoximone contributed to systemic hypotension but prevented mucosal hypoperfusion[126]
- Low incidence of side effects with short-term use, for example, in the intensive care unit[127] or following cardiac surgery[128,129]
- In ponies, 0.5 mg/kg enoximone intravenously significantly increased HR, SV, $\dot{Q}_t$, and DO_2, and reduced RAP[130]
- In anesthetized colic horses, similar but less pronounced effects of shorter duration[131]

VASOPRESSORS

Vasopressors can be used to increase ABP through an increase in SVR. Many vasopressors also possess positive inotropic and/or chronotropic properties, but even pure vasopressors can influence $\dot{Q}_t$. When vasoconstriction mainly occurs on the venous side of the circulation, mean systemic filling pressure and venous return increase. This process will tend to augment $\dot{Q}_t$ through an increased preload (see **Fig. 1**). By contrast, arteriolar vasoconstriction increases afterload and may reduce $\dot{Q}_t$, especially when contractility is already compromised, for example, by underlying cardiac disease, sepsis, or anesthetic drugs. With regard to tissue perfusion, the effect of vasopressors depends on the preexisting arteriolar tone. Arteriolar vasoconstriction will increase ABP but reduce perfusion of the tissues distal to constricted arterioles, which may lead to ischemia of vulnerable organs such as the kidneys and the gut. However, arterial hypotension can be associated with a collapse of vessels perfusing tissues with high extravascular pressures, such as the muscles of recumbent horses.[132] Under these circumstances, vasopressors may help to increase transmural pressure, and actually restore patency of blood vessels and tissue perfusion. Vasopressors are best reserved for situations whereby hypotension is caused by a reduction in SVR (eg, drug- or endotoxin-induced), myocardial contractility and $\dot{Q}_t$ are normal or high, and vascular transmural pressure needs to be restored to maintain or reestablish vessel patency.

All vasopressors increase intracellular Ca^{2+} levels in vascular smooth muscle cells. Calcium binds to calmodulin and activates myosin light chain kinase, which phosphorylates myosin, initiating contraction. Calcium also binds directly to myosin and activates protein kinase C, which phosphorylates myosin at a different site than myosin light chain kinase.[133]

Vasopressin Analogues

Endogenous vasopressin (antidiuretic hormone) is released into the bloodstream by the posterior pituitary, in response to increases in plasma osmolarity or large decreases in ABP.[10] Its most important effects are water retention by the kidneys (V_2 receptors) and vasoconstriction (V_1 receptors on vascular smooth muscle).[134] Activation of V_1 receptors stimulates phospholipase C, promoting hydrolysis of phosphatidylinositol 4,5-biphosphate (PIP_2) into inositol triphosphate (IP_3) and diacylglycerol (DAG). IP_3 promotes mobilization of Ca^{2+} from the endoplasmic reticulum, leading to contraction of vascular smooth muscle.[134] Diacylglycerol stimulates protein kinase C, which increases the influx of Ca^{2+} through L-type Ca^{2+} channels.[135] Vasoconstriction mainly occurs in nonvital organ systems such as the skin, skeletal muscles, and intestines, whereas vasodilation occurs in, for example, the cerebral and coronary arteries.[136] Vasopressin may additionally have some inotropic effects after stimulation of myocardial V_1 receptors,[137] but this is usually overshadowed by a baroreflex-mediated reduction in $\dot{Q}_t$. This baroreflex is even facilitated by vasopressin, through both a central and a peripheral effect.[138]

Vasopressin or its analogues may be useful in patients with refractory shock, despite adequate fluid resuscitation and high-dose conventional vasopressors,[139] for the following reasons:

- Vasopressin receptors remain available despite maximal binding of adrenoceptors by catecholamines
- Endogenous vasopressin levels may be low because:
  o Synthesis, transport, and storage of vasopressin in the neurohypophysis takes about 1 to 2 hours[140]
  o The plasma half-life is only 6 to 10 minutes[141]
  o Prolonged stimulation during hemorrhagic[142] or vasodilatory septic shock[143] exhausts the endogenous vasopressin supply in ±1 hour
  o During septic shock baroreflex-mediated secretion of vasopressin may be impaired[143]

Examples of arginine vasopressin (AVP) analogues are terlipressin and F-180. Terlipressin has a somewhat greater preference than vasopressin for vascular V_1 receptors, which has equal affinity for V_1 and V_2 receptors. It is less expensive than vasopressin and has a long half-life, making single-bolus dosing possible.[134] F-180 is a long-acting drug with selective V_1 effects.[144]

Indications for AVP (or analogues) are:

- Advanced vasodilatory or hemorrhagic shock (but influence on final outcome remains uncertain)[145]
- Treatment of cardiac arrest:
  o Effects similar to those of adrenaline in the management of ventricular fibrillation and pulseless electrical activity and superior to those of adrenaline in patients with asystole[146]
  o Vasopressin followed by adrenaline resulted in significantly higher rates of survival to hospital admission and discharge[146]
  o In a porcine cardiac arrest model, with severe hypotension induced by blood loss, vasopressin redirected blood from bleeding sites to more vital organs

and resulted in sustained vital organ perfusion, less metabolic acidosis and prolonged survival, in contrast to large-dose adrenaline or saline administration[147]

Nevertheless, these agents should not be used as the sole vasopressor for the following reasons.

- High doses can reduce $\dot{Q}_t$, DO_2, and mixed venous oxygen saturation, with impaired perfusion and ischemic injury of tissues such as the gut, liver, and skin.[148] During vasodilatory shock, even moderate doses can cause ischemic skin lesions.[149]
- Hyponatremia and tissue edema may occur, as well as decreases in platelet counts and increases in aminotransferase activity and bilirubin concentrations.[148]

To reduce side effects, the following can be recommended:

- Combine with high-volume fluid therapy[148]
- Monitor platelet count, hepatic function, electrolytes, and osmolality[148]
  - CRI of terlipressin appears to be superior to bolus administration in endotoxemic sheep[150]

Literature describing the cardiovascular effects of exogenous AVP or its analogues in equids is scarce. In hypotensive, isoflurane-anesthetized foals, vasopressin (0.3 and 1.0 mU/kg/min) increased SVR and ABP without affecting CI and DO_2, but increased the gastric to arterial CO_2 gap, which is indicative of reduced splanchnic perfusion.[151] In critically ill neonatal foals, AVP increased MAP and urine output, and decreased HR.[152]

Calcium Salts

As already mentioned, $CaCl_2$ or gluconate increased ABP in anesthetized ponies,[89] horses,[86] dogs,[90] and humans.[82,94] This increase was usually due to an increase in SVR rather than $\dot{Q}_t$, illustrating the vasoconstrictive effects of calcium.

Sympathomimetics

Many sympathomimetics cause vasoconstriction by activating α_1-adrenergic receptors on vascular smooth muscle cells, which are linked to a G protein. When activated, the α subunit activates phospholipase C, which hydrolyzes PIP_2 to IP_3 and DAG,[135] with effects on Ca^{2+} transients as already described for vasopressin. Many sympathomimetic vasopressors also have inotropic and/or chronotropic properties. Furthermore, the vasoconstrictive effect of some drugs, such as adrenaline and dopamine, depends on the dose administered. Subdivision of the catecholamines as pure inotropes or pure vasopressors is therefore not always possible.

Noradrenaline (norepinephrine)

This rather potent β_1-agonist and very potent α_1- and α_2-agonist mainly functions as a vasopressor.[43,44] Because a vagally mediated baroreceptor response usually obscures the direct effects of noradrenaline on the heart, noradrenaline tends to cause slight bradycardia.[43] Also, noradrenaline directly increases myocardial contractility,[153] but $\dot{Q}_t$ may in fact decrease owing to the substantial increase in SVR (**Table 2**).[44]

Noradrenaline is used when the importance of increasing perfusion pressure outweighs the disadvantages of lowering $\dot{Q}_t$, or to counterbalance the vasodilatory effects of other agents.[43,53] In addition, the effects of noradrenaline on α- and β_1-receptors in the myocardium may complement the positive inotropic effects of

Table 2
Sympathomimetic agents with primarily a vasopressor action

Drug	Patients	Dose	Receptor Activity	Cardiovascular Effects	References
Norepinephrine	General		Very potent α_1 and α_2 Additional β_1 effect	Mainly vasopressor effect, SVR and ABP ↑	43,44
				Usually slight bradycardia (vagally mediated) Contractility ↑ but Q_t may ↓ due to ↑↑ SVR	44,154
				May cause arrhythmias, ↑ myocardial O_2 consumption, renal, abdominal visceral, and skeletal muscle ischemia	
	Horses	3 µg/kg		MAP ↑ during 6 min but less pronounced than with epinephrine, HR initially ↑ slightly, but pronounced ↓ during maximal pressor response	49
	Foals	0.05–0.40 µg/kg/min		Ventricular arrhythmias in 2 of 4 animals ABP and SVR ↑, HR and CI ↓	155,156,185
		0.3–1 µg/kg/min		During deep isoflurane anesthesia (with hypotension) in neonatal foals: SVR and ABP ↑, CI and DO_2 also ↑ but less pronounced than with dobutamine	151
Phenylephrine	General		Selective α_1-agonist Little effect on β receptors	SVR and ABP ↑, minimal direct effect on HR and contractility, vagally mediated bradycardia may occur	158
	Conscious horses	1–6 µg/kg/min		RAP, SAP, DAP, MAP, and PCV ↑, HR and Q_t ↓, SV =, AV blocks	158
	Anesthetized ponies and horses	0.25–2 µg/kg/min		MAP, CVP, SVR, and PCV ↑, muscle blood flow and CI =	40,186

Methoxamine	General		Selective α_1-agonist	As for phenylephrine	8
	Horses	40 μg/kg before induction		No change in cardiopulmonary function during anesthesia	161
	Ponies	13 μg/kg, then 5 μg/kg/min		SVR and ABP ↑, $\dot{Q}_t$ ↓	162
Metaraminol	General		Direct effect on vascular adrenergic receptors Stimulates norepinephrine release	SVR and ABP ↑	8,157

↑, increase; ↓, decrease; =, no change.

Abbreviations: ABP, arterial blood pressure; AV, atrioventricular; CI, cardiac index; CVP, central venous pressure; DAP, diastolic arterial pressure; DO_2, oxygen delivery; HR, heart rate; MAP, mean arterial pressure; O_2, oxygen; PCV, packed cell volume; $\dot{Q}_t$, cardiac output; RAP, right atrial pressure; SAP, systolic arterial pressure; SV, stroke volume; SVR, systemic vascular resistance.

other drugs. With relatively low doses (0.5–1.5 μg/kg/min), excessive vasoconstriction is less likely and there are no deleterious effects on renal function.[8] Time to onset of action of noradrenaline is 1 to 2 minutes and, because the half-life is very short (20–30 seconds),[10] the duration of the effect is limited to 1 to 2 minutes.[44]

Noradrenaline has arrhythmogenic properties.[154] Myocardial oxygen consumption is invariably increased, ischemia may be exacerbated, and ventricular function can be compromised.[43,44] Because of generalized vasoconstriction, renal, abdominal, visceral, and skeletal muscle ischemia may also occur[44] and, if used in shock patients, the state of shock may actually be worsened.[8]

The available data on the effects of norepinephrine in horses are summarized in **Table 2**. A dose of 0.1 μg/kg/min did not cause significant differences in urine output, creatinine clearance, or fractional electrolyte excretion in Thoroughbred foals,[155] but urine output and creatinine clearance increased with a dose of 0.3 μg/kg/min in pony foals.[156] The latter investigators concluded that noradrenaline may be useful for hypotensive foals, because it increases SVR and ABP without negatively affecting renal function. In neonatal hypotensive foals during deep isoflurane anesthesia, noradrenaline (0.3 and 1.0 μg/kg/min) increased not only SVR and ABP but also CI and DO_2, whereas the oxygen extraction ratio decreased. However, as would be expected, the increases in CI and DO_2 were much less pronounced than after dobutamine administration.[151]

Phenylephrine

This selective α_1-adrenergic agonist, with little effect on β-adrenoceptors of the heart,[157] has minimal direct effects on HR and contractility, but bradycardia can be observed in response to the increase in ABP.[158] In septic shock, hepatosplanchnic blood flow and DO_2 were lower during treatment with phenylephrine when compared with noradrenaline.[159]

The effects of phenylephrine in horses or ponies are summarized in **Table 2**, and consist of increases in ABP, SVR, and PCV, decreases in HR and $\dot{Q}_t$, and a high incidence of second-degree atrioventricular block, without improving femoral arterial or intramuscular blood flow. Phenylephrine is also commonly used in horses during the treatment of nephrosplenic entrapment of the large colon, where splenic contraction is the therapeutic target.[160]

Others

Methoxamine has similar effects to those of phenylephrine. When given before induction of anesthesia, 40 μg/kg methoxamine did not significantly affect cardiopulmonary function during anesthesia in horses.[161] However, when given during anesthesia in ponies, methoxamine 13 μg/kg followed by 5 μg/kg/min was able to maintain normotension, while $\dot{Q}_t$ was lower and SVR higher than in the saline goup.[162]

Metaraminol has a direct effect on vascular adrenergic receptors and also stimulates noradrenaline release.[163] To the authors' knowledge, its use in horses has not been described.

COMBINATIONS

Under certain circumstances, it may be advantageous to combine agents that exert different effects (eg, vasopressors and inotropic drugs) or agents that exert similar effects through a different mechanism of action (eg, sympathomimetic inotropes with PDE inhibitors, sympathomimetic vasopressors with vasopressin analogues). Because extensive research has been performed in this area, it is only possible to give a few examples.

- Sympathomimetic combinations:
  - Low ("renal") dose dopamine with
    - Noradrenaline during vasodilatory shock:
      - Aims: increased myocardial contractility, peripheral vasoconstriction and preserved renal function[164]
      - Uncertain whether this combination is superior to dopamine alone[139]
    - Dobutamine in shock states where $\dot{Q}_t$ is low (eg, septic or cardiogenic shock) in an attempt to improve both renal and cardiac function[8]
  - Noradrenaline (0.1 µg/kg/min) + dobutamine (5 µg/kg/min) in normotensive neonatal foals[155]:
    - Increased ABP and SVR
    - Decreased HR and CI
    - No differences in urine output, creatinine clearance, or fractional electrolyte excretion
  - Dobutamine and phenylephrine in horses
    - Can be used instead of drugs with mixed inotropic and vasopressor effects, such as ephedrine
    - Advantage: dose of each drug can be titrated separately until the desired effect is reached
- Calcium salts
  - Tended to attenuate cardiotonic effects of β-sympathomimetics in man[95,96]
    - Most likely negative effect of free Ca^{2+} ions on the activity of adenylyl cyclase[165]
  - Decreased inotropic effect of milrinone[166]
  - Did not alter effects of enoximone in ponies[167]
- Inotropic β-sympathomimetics and PDE-III inhibitors
  - Increase cAMP concentration through different mechanisms, so may produce more powerful inotropic effects when used in combination
  - Vasopressor action of certain sympathomimetics may be useful in preventing or treating exaggerated decreases in SVR after administration of PDE-III inhibitors.
  - Beneficial effects described of combinations of amrinone with dobutamine,[168] noradrenaline,[169] dopamine,[170] and adrenaline[171]
  - Combination of enoximone and dobutamine
    - Larger increases in CI, left ventricular stroke work index, and HR, and more pronounced vasodilatory effects[172]
    - Similar findings in experimental ponies[173]

SUMMARY

To optimize tissue oxygenation, cardiovascular support is often needed in horses despite the use of balanced anesthetic protocols and fluid therapy. Bradycardia that is not related to hypertension can be treated using antimuscarinics. In most cases, hypotension is best treated using inotropes; more specifically, dobutamine remains the agent of choice in horses. Exceptions are hypocalcemic horses (treated using calcium salts), cases in which hypotension results from vasodilation while HR and $\dot{Q}_t$ are high, or patients with dangerously low ABP that is not responsive to fluids and inotropes (treated using vasopressors). Although the effects often depend on the dose administered, the sympathomimetics most often used in anesthetized horses can broadly be ranked in order of decreasing inotropic and increasing vasopressor effects, as follows: dobutamine, dopamine, ephedrine, norepinephrine, and phenylephrine. In some cases combinations of these can be useful; for example, because of its very limited to absent direct cardiac effects, phenylephrine can be used safely during dobutamine infusions when additional vasoconstriction is needed. PDE inhibitors and vasopressin (or terlipressin) may also have a role during cardiovascular support in horses, but further research is needed in this area. Finally, adrenaline and vasopressin are both useful during cardiopulmonary resuscitation.

REFERENCES

1. Johnston GM, Eastment JK, Wood JL, et al. The confidential enquiry into perioperative equine fatalities (CEPEF): mortality results of phases 1 and 2. Vet Anaesth Analg 2002;29:159–70.
2. Eberly VE, Gillespie JR, Tyler WS, et al. Cardiovascular values in the horse during halothane anaesthesia. Am J Vet Res 1968;29:305–14.
3. Gillespie JR, Tyler WS, Hall LW. Cardiopulmonary dysfunction in anaesthetized laterally recumbent horses. Am J Vet Res 1969;30:61–72.
4. White NA, Suarez M. Change in triceps muscle intracompartmental pressure with repositioning and padding of the lowermost thoracic limb of the horse. Am J Vet Res 1986;47:2257–60.
5. Young SS. Post-anesthetic myopathy. Equine Vet Educ 1993;5:200–3.
6. Petersen-Felix S, Arendt-Nielsen L, Bak P, et al. Analgesic effect in humans of subanaesthetic isoflurane concentrations evaluated by experimentally induced pain. Br J Anaesth 1995;75:55–60.
7. Tomi K, Mahimo T, Tashiro C, et al. Alterations in pain threshold and psychomotor response associated with subanaesthetic concentrations of inhalation anaesthetics in humans. Br J Anaesth 1993;70:684–6.
8. Calvey TN, Williams NE. Principles and practice of pharmacology for anaesthetists. 4th edition. London: Blackwell Science Ltd; 2001. p. 237–70.
9. Van Citters RL, Ruth WE, Reissmann KR. Effect of heart rate on oxygen consumption of isolated dog heart performing no external work. Am J Physiol 1957;191:443–5.
10. Power I, Kam P. Cardiovascular physiology. Principles of physiology for the anaesthetist. 1st edition. London: Arnold; 2001. p. 150, 290–305.
11. Jose AD, Stitt F. Effects of hypoxia and metabolic inhibitors on the intrinsic heart rate and myocardial contractility in dogs. Circ Res 1969;25:53–66.
12. Senges J, Brachmann J, Pelzer D, et al. Effects of some components of ischemia on electrical activity and reentry in the canine ventricular conducting system. Circ Res 1979;44:864–72.
13. Light GS, Hellyer PW. Effects of atropine on the arrhythmogenic dose of dobutamine in xylazine-thiamylal-halothane-anesthetized horses. Am J Vet Res 1993; 54:2099–103.
14. Ducharme NG, Fubini SL. Gastrointestinal complications associated with the use of atropine in horses. J Am Vet Med Assoc 1983;182:229–31.
15. Teixeira Neto FJ, McDonell WN, Black WD, et al. Effects of a muscarinic type-2 antagonist on cardiorespiratory function and intestinal transit in horses anesthetized with halothane and xylazine. Am J Vet Res 2004;65: 464–72.
16. Hamlin RL, Klepinger WL, Gilpin KW, et al. Autonomic control of heart rate in the horse. Am J Physiol 1972;222:976–8.
17. Alitalo I, Vainio O, Kaartinen L, et al. Cardiac effects of atropine premedication in horses sedated with detomidine. Acta Vet Scand Suppl 1986;82:131–6.

18. Brouwer GJ, Hall LW, Kuchel TR. Intravenous anaesthesia in horses after xylazine premedication. Vet Rec 1980;107:241–5.
19. Pimenta EL, Teixeira Neto FJ, Sá PA, et al. Comparative study between atropine and hyoscine-N-butylbromide for reversal of detomidine induced bradycardia in horses. Equine Vet J 2011;43:332–40.
20. Dyson DH, Pascoe PJ, McDonell WN. Effects of intravenously administered glycopyrrolate in anesthetized horses. Can Vet J 1999;40:29–32.
21. Singh S, McDonell WN, Young SS, et al. The effect of glycopyrrolate on heart rate and intestinal motility in conscious horses. J Vet Anaesth 1997;24:14–9.
22. Roelvink ME, Goossens L, Kalsbeek HC, et al. Analgesic and spasmolytic effects of dipyrone, hyoscine-N-butylbromide and a combination of the two in ponies. Vet Rec 1991;129:378–80.
23. Borer KE, Clarke KW. The effect of hyoscine on dobutamine requirement in spontaneously breathing horses anaesthetized with halothane. J Vet Anaesth 2006;33:149–57.
24. Geimer TR, Ekström PM, Ludders JW, et al. Haemodynamic effects of hyoscine-N-butylbromide in ponies. J Vet Pharmacol Ther 1995;18:13–6.
25. Marques JA, Teixeira Neto FJ, Campebell RC, et al. Effects of hyoscine-N-butylbromide given before romifidine in horses. Vet Rec 1998;142:166–8.
26. Braunwald E. Effects of digitalis on the normal and the failing heart. J Am Coll Cardiol 1985;5(5 Suppl A):51A–9A.
27. Hamlin RL, Dutta S, Smith CR. Effects of digoxin and digitoxin on ventricular function in normal dogs and dogs with heart failure. Am J Vet Res 1971;32:1391–8.
28. Button C, Gross DR, Johnston JT, et al. Digoxin pharmacokinetics, bioavailability, efficacy, and dosage regimens in the horse. Am J Vet Res 1980;41:1388–95.
29. Sage AM. Cardiac disease in the geriatric horse. Vet Clin North Am Equine Pract 2002;18:575–89.
30. Lehtonen LA, Antila S, Pentikainen PJ. Pharmacokinetics and pharmacodynamics of intravenous inotropic agents. Clin Pharmacokinet 2004;43:187–203.
31. Choudhury M, Saxena N. Inotropic agents in paediatric cardiac surgical patients: current practice, concerns and controversies. Indian J Anaesth 2003;47:246–53.
32. Evans DB. Modulation of cAMP: mechanism for positive inotropic action. J Cardiovasc Pharmacol 1986;8(Suppl 9):S22–9.
33. Fabiato A. Calcium-induced release of calcium from the cardiac sarcoplasmatic reticulum. Am J Physiol 1983;245:C1–14.
34. Vernon MW, Heel RC, Brogden RN. Enoximone: a review of its pharmacological properties and therapeutic potential. Drugs 1991;42:997–1017.
35. Kranias EG, Solaro RJ. Coordination of cardiac sarcoplasmic reticulum and myofibrillar function by protein phosphorylation. Fed Proc 1983;42:33–8.
36. Tada M, Inui M, Yamada M, et al. Effects of phospholamban phosphorylation catalyzed by adenosine 3′:5′-monophosphate- and calmodulin-dependent protein kinases on calcium transport ATPase of cardiac sarcoplasmic reticulum. J Mol Cell Cardiol 1983;15:335–46.
37. Li L, Desantagio J, Chu G, et al. Phosphorylation of phospholamban and troponin I in beta-adrenergic-induced acceleration of cardiac relaxation. Am J Physiol Heart Circ Physiol 2000;278:H769–79.
38. Luo W, Grupp IL, Harrer J, et al. Targeted ablation of the phospholamban gene is associated with markedly enhanced myocardial contractility and loss of beta-agonist stimulation. Circ Res 1994;74:401–9.

39. Notterman DA. Inotropic agents. catecholamines, digoxin, amrinone. Crit Care Clin 1991;7:583–613.
40. Lee YH, Clarke KW, Alibhai HI, et al. Effects of dopamine, dobutamine, dopexamine, phenylephrine and saline solution on intramuscular blood flow and other cardiopulmonary variables in halothane-anesthetized ponies. Am J Vet Res 1998;59:1463–72.
41. Swanson CR, Muir WW 3rd, Bednarski RM, et al. Hemodynamic responses in halothane-anesthetized horses given infusions of dopamine or dobutamine. Am J Vet Res 1985;46:365–70.
42. Joung B, Tang L, Maruyama M, et al. Intracellular calcium dynamics and acceleration of sinus rhythm by β-adrenergic stimulation. Circulation 2009;119: 788–96.
43. Barnard MJ, Linter SP. Acute circulatory support. BMJ 1993;307:35–41.
44. Morrill P. Pharmacotherapeutics of positive inotropes. AORN J 2000;71:171–85.
45. Sanders EA, Gleed RD, Hackett RP, et al. Action of sympathomimetic drugs on the bronchial circulation of the horse. Exp Physiol 1991;76:301–4.
46. Anderson MG, Aitken MM. Biochemical and physiological effects of catecholamine administration in the horse. Res Vet Sci 1977;22:357–60.
47. Fawaz G, Tutunji B. The effect of adrenaline and noradrenaline on the metabolism and performance of the isolated dog heart. Br J Pharmacol Chemother 1960;15:389–95.
48. Gaynor JS, Bednarski RM, Muir WW 3rd. Effect of xylazine on the arrhythmogenic dose of epinephrine in thiamylal/halothane-anesthetized horses. Am J Vet Res 1992;53:2350–4.
49. Lees P, Tavernor WD. Influence of halothane and catecholamines on heart rate and rhythm in the horse. Br J Pharmacol 1970;39:149–59.
50. Imamura S, Ikeda K. Comparison of the epinephrine-induced arrhythmogenic effect of sevoflurane with isoflurane and halothane. J Anesth 1987; 1:62–8.
51. Gaynor JS, Bednarski RM, Muir WW 3rd. Effect of hypercapnia on the arrhythmogenic dose of epinephrine in horses anaesthetized with guaifenesin, thiamylal sodium and halothane. Am J Vet Res 1993;54:315–21.
52. Muir WW, Werner LL, Hamlin RL. Effects of xylazine and acetylpromazine upon induced ventricular fibrillation in dogs anesthetized with thiamylal and halothane. Am J Vet Res 1975;36:1299–303.
53. Via G, Veronesi R, Maggio G, et al. The need for inotropic drugs in anesthesiology and intensive care. Ital Heart J 2003;4(Suppl 2):50S–60S.
54. De Vries A, Brearley JC, Taylor PM. Effects of dobutamine on cardiac index and arterial blood pressure in isoflurane-anaesthetized horses under clinical conditions. J Vet Pharmacol Ther 2009;32:353–8.
55. Gasthuys F, de Moor A, Parmentier D. Influence of dopamine and dobutamine on the cardiovascular depression during a standard halothane anaesthesia in dorsally recumbent, ventilated ponies. Zentralbl Veterinarmed A 1991;38: 494–500.
56. Gehlen H, Weichler A, Bubeck K, et al. Effects of two different dosages of dobutamine on pulmonary artery wedge pressure, systemic arterial blood pressure and heart rate in anaesthetized horses. J Vet Med A Physiol Pathol Clin Med 2006;53:476–80.
57. Hellyer PW, Wagner AE, Mama KR, et al. The effects of dobutamine and ephedrine on packed cell volume, total protein, heart rate and arterial blood pressure in anaesthetized horses. J Vet Pharmacol Ther 1998;21:497–9.

58. Raisis AL, Young LE, Blissitt KJ, et al. Effect of a 30-minute infusion of dobutamine hydrochloride on hind limb blood flow and hemodynamics in halothane-anesthetized horses. Am J Vet Res 2000;61:1282–8.
59. Ueda M, Matsamura S, Matsuda S, et al. Comparative study between dobutamine and other catecholamines in their effects on the cardiac contraction and rhythm (author's transl). Nippon Yakurigaku Zasshi 1977;73:501–16.
60. Donaldson LL. Retrospective assessment of dobutamine therapy for hypotension in anaesthetized horses. Vet Surg 1988;17:53–7.
61. Light GS, Hellyer PW, Swanson CR. Parasympathetic influence on the arrhythmogenicity of graded dobutamine infusions in halothane-anesthetized horses. Am J Vet Res 1992;53:1154–60.
62. Blaschko H. The specific action of l-dopa decarboxylase. J Physiol 1939;96:50P.
63. Murphy MB, Elliott WJ. Dopamine and dopamine receptor agonists in cardiovascular therapy. Crit Care Med 1990;18:S14–8.
64. Denton MD, Chertow GM, Brady HR. "Renal-dose" dopamine for the treatment of acute renal failure: scientific rationale, experimental studies and clinical trials. Kidney Int 1996;50:4–14.
65. Tisdale JE, Patel R, Webb CR, et al. Electrophysiologic and proarrhythmic effects of intravenous inotropic agents. Prog Cardiovasc Dis 1995;38:167–80.
66. Brown RA, Dixon J, Farmer JB, et al. Dopexamine: a novel agonist at peripheral dopamine receptors and beta 2-adrenoceptors. Br J Pharmacol 1985;85:599–608.
67. Muir WW 3rd. Cardiovascular effects of dopexamine HCl in conscious and halothane-anaesthetized horses. Equine Vet J Suppl 1992;(11):24–9.
68. Muir WW 3rd. Inotropic mechanisms of dopexamine hydrochloride in horses. Am J Vet Res 1992;53:1343–6.
69. Young LE, Blissitt KJ, Clutton RE, et al. Temporal effects of an infusion of dopexamine hydrochloride in horses anesthetized with halothane. Am J Vet Res 1997;58:516–23.
70. Stehle RL. Ephedrine—a new (?) sympathomimetic drug. Can Med Assoc J 1925;15:1158–60.
71. Valette G, Cohen Y, Huidobro H. Effects of perfusion of noradrenaline on the tachyphylaxis from ephedrine in the dog. J Physiol (Paris) 1960;52:238–9.
72. Grandy JL, Hodgson DS, Dunlop CI, et al. Cardiopulmonary effects of ephedrine in halothane-anesthetized horses. J Vet Pharmacol Ther 1989;12:389–96.
73. Clark ES, Moore JN. Effects of fenoldopam on cecal blood flow and mechanical activity in horses. Am J Vet Res 1989;50:1926–30.
74. Hollis AR, Ousey JC, Palmer L, et al. Effects of fenoldopam mesylate on systemic hemodynamics and indices of renal function in normotensive neonatal foals. J Vet Intern Med 2006;20:595–600.
75. Nuttall A, Snow HM. The cardiovascular effects of ICI 118,587: a beta 1-adrenoceptor partial agonist. Br J Pharmacol 1982;77:381–8.
76. Molajo AO, Bennett DH. Effects of xamoterol (ICI 118587), a new beta1 adrenoceptor partial agonist, on resting haemodynamic variables and exercise tolerance in patients with left ventricular dysfunction. Br Heart J 1985;54:17–21.
77. Chamberlain JH, Pepper JR, Yates AK. Dobutamine, isoprenaline and dopamine in patients after open heart surgery. Intensive Care Med 1980;7:5–10.
78. Mueller HS. Effects of dopamine on haemodynamics and myocardial energetic in man: comparison with effects of isoprenaline and L-noradrenaline. Resuscitation 1978;6:179–89.

79. Mansell PI, Fellows IW, Birmingham AT, et al. Metabolic and cardiovascular effects of infusions of low doses of isoprenaline in man. Clin Sci (Lond) 1988; 75:285–91.

80. Cote CJ, Drop LJ, Daniels AL, et al. Calcium chloride versus calcium gluconate: comparison of ionization and cardiovascular effects in children and dogs. Anesthesiology 1987;66:465–70.

81. Hempelmann G, Piepenbrock S, Frerk C, et al. Effects of calcium gluconate and calcium chloride on cardiocirculatory parameters in man. Anaesthesist 1978;27: 516–22 [in German (author's transl)].

82. Eriksen C, Sorensen MB, Bille-Brahe NE, et al. Haemodynamic effects of calcium chloride administered intravenously to patients with and without cardiac disease during neuroleptanaesthesia. Acta Anaesthesiol Scand 1983;27:13–7.

83. Bosnjak ZJ, Kampine JP. Effects of halothane on transmembrane potentials, Ca^{2+} transients and papillary muscle tension in the cat. Am J Physiol 1986; 251:H374–81.

84. Pagel PS, Kampine JP, Schmeling WT, et al. Reversal of volatile anesthetic-induced depression of myocardial contractility by extracellular calcium also enhances left ventricular diastolic function. Anesthesiology 1993;78:141–54.

85. Stanley TH, Isern-Amaral J, Liu WS, et al. Peripheral vascular versus direct cardiac effects of calcium. Anesthesiology 1976;45:46–58.

86. Grubb TL, Benson GJ, Foreman JH, et al. Hemodynamic effects of ionized calcium in horses anesthetized with halothane or isoflurane. Am J Vet Res 1999;60:1430–5.

87. Grubb TL, Foreman JH, Benson GJ, et al. Hemodynamic effects of calcium gluconate administered to conscious horses. J Vet Intern Med 1996;10:401–4.

88. Grubb TL, Constable PD, Benson GJ, et al. Techniques for evaluation of right ventricular relaxation rate in horses and effects of inhalant anesthetics with and without intravenous administration of calcium gluconate. Am J Vet Res 1999;60:872–9.

89. Gasthuys F, De Moor A, Parmentier D. Cardiovascular effects of low dose calcium chloride infusions during halothane anaesthesia in dorsally recumbent ventilated ponies. Zentralbl Veterinarmed A 1991;38:728–36.

90. Drop LJ, Scheidegger D. Plasma ionized calcium concentration: important determinant of the hemodynamic response to calcium infusion. J Thorac Cardiovasc Surg 1980;79:425–31.

91. Malcolm DS, Zaloga GP, Holaday JW. Calcium administration increases the mortality of endotoxic shock in rats. Crit Care Med 1989;17:900–3.

92. Zaloga GP, Sager A, Black KW, et al. Low dose calcium administration increases mortality during septic peritonitis in rats. Circ Shock 1992;37:226–9.

93. Scheidegger D, Drop LJ, Schellenberg JC. Role of the systemic vasculature in the hemodynamic response to changes in plasma ionized calcium. Arch Surg 1980;115:206–11.

94. Marone C, Beretta-Piccoli C, Weidmann P. Acute hypercalcemic hypertension in man: role of hemodynamics, catecholamines and rennin. Kidney Int 1981;20: 92–6.

95. Butterworth JF 4th, Prielipp RC, Royster RL, et al. Dobutamine increases heart rate more than epinephrine in patients recovering from aortocoronary bypass surgery. J Cardiothorac Vasc Anesth 1992;6:535–41.

96. Zaloga GP, Strickland RA, Butterworth JF, et al. Calcium attenuates epinephrine's beta-adrenergic effects in postoperative heart surgery patients. Circulation 1990;81:196–200.

97. Mathru M, Rooney MW, Goldberg SA, et al. Separation of myocardial versus peripheral effects of calcium administration in normocalcemic and hypocalcemic states using pressure-volume (conductance) relationships. Anesth Analg 1993;77:250–5.

98. Beavo JA. Cyclic nucleotide phosphodiesterases: functional implications of multiple isoforms. Physiol Rev 1995;75:725–48.

99. Butcher RW, Sutherland EW. Adenosine 3′,5′-phosphate in biological materials. I. Purification and properties of cyclic 3′,5′-nucleotide phosphodiesterase and use of this enzyme to characterize adenosine 3′,5′-phosphate in human urine. J Biol Chem 1962;237:1244–50.

100. Shenfield GM. Combination bronchodilator therapy. Drugs 1982;24:414–39.

101. Slapke J, Hummel S, Wilke A, et al. Therapy of asthma with theophylline preparations. Z Erkr Atmungsorgane 1988;170:32–48.

102. Bobon D, Breulet M, Gerard-Vandenhove MA, et al. Is phosphodiesterase inhibition a new mechanism of antidepressant action? A double-blind double-dummy study between rolipram and desipramine in hospitalized major and/or endogenous depressives. Eur Arch Psychiatry Neurol Sci 1988;238:2–6.

103. Teixeira MM, Rossi AG, Williams TJ, et al. Effects of phosphodiesterase isoenzyme inhibitors on cutaneous inflammation in the guinea-pig. Br J Pharmacol 1994;112:332–40.

104. Michelakis E, Tymchak W, Lien D, et al. Oral sildenafil is an effective and specific pulmonary vasodilator in patients with pulmonary arterial hypertension: comparison with inhaled nitric oxide. Circulation 2002;105:2398–403.

105. Shintani S, Watanabe K, Kawamura K, et al. General pharmacological properties of cilostazol, a new antithrombotic drug. Part II: Effect on the peripheral organs. Arzneimittelforschung 1985;35:1163–72.

106. McDaniel NL, Rembold CM, Richard HM, et al. Cyclic AMP relaxes arterial smooth muscle predominantly by decreasing cell Ca^{2+} concentration. J Physiol 1991;439:147–60.

107. Sperelakis N, Xiong Z, Haddad G, et al. Regulation of slow calcium channels of myocardial cells and vascular smooth muscle cells by cyclic nucleotides and phosphorylation. Mol Cell Biochem 1994;140:103–17.

108. Kimura Y, Inui M, Kadoma M, et al. Effects of monoclonal antibody against phospholamban on calcium pump ATPase of cardiac sarcoplasmic reticulum. J Mol Cell Cardiol 1991;23:1223–30.

109. Itoh H, Kusagawa M, Shimomura A, et al. Ca^{2+} dependent and Ca^{2+} independent vasorelaxation induced by cardiotonic phosphodiesterase inhibitors. Eur J Pharmacol 1993;240:57–66.

110. Adelstein RS, Pato MD, Sellers JR, et al. Regulation of contractile proteins by reversible phosphorylation of myosin and myosin kinase. Soc Gen Physiol Ser 1982;37:273–81.

111. Baim DS. Effect of phosphodiesterase inhibition on myocardial oxygen consumption and coronary blood flow. Am J Cardiol 1989;63:23A–6A.

112. Colucci WS. Cardiovascular effects of milrinone. Am Heart J 1991;121(6 Pt 2): 1945–7.

113. Lobato EB, Gravenstein N, Martin TD. Milrinone, not epinephrine, improves left ventricular compliance after cardiopulmonary bypass. J Cardiothorac Vasc Anesth 2000;14:374–7.

114. Takeuchi K, del Nido PJ, Ibrahim AE, et al. Vesnarinone and amrinone reduce the systemic inflammatory response syndrome. J Thorac Cardiovasc Surg 1999;117:375–82.

115. Treadway G. Clinical safety of intravenous amrinone—a review. Am J Cardiol 1985;56:39B–40B.
116. Caldicott LD, Hawley K, Heppell R, et al. Intravenous enoximone or dobutamine for severe heart failure after acute myocardial infarction: a randomized double-blind trial. Eur Heart J 1993;14:696–700.
117. Möllhoff T, Loick HM, Van Aken H, et al. Milrinone modulates endotoxemia, systemic inflammation and subsequent acute phase response after cardiopulmonary bypass (CPB). Anesthesiology 1999;90:72–80.
118. Muir WW. The haemodynamic effects of milrinone HCl in halothane anaesthetized horses. Equine Vet J Suppl 1995;(19):108–13.
119. Szilágyi S, Pollesello P, Levijoki J, et al. Two inotropes with different mechanisms of action: contractile, PDE-inhibitory and direct myofibrillar effects of levosimendan and enoximone. J Cardiovasc Pharmacol 2005;46:369–76.
120. Dage RC, Okerholm RA. Pharmacology and pharmacokinetics of enoximone. Cardiology 1990;77(Suppl 3):2–13.
121. Ghio S, Constantin C, Raineri C, et al. Enoximone echocardiography: a novel test to evaluate left ventricular contractile reserve in patients with heart failure on chronic beta-blocker therapy. Cardiovasc Ultrasound 2003;25:1–13.
122. Winkle RA, Smith NA, Ruder MA, et al. Pharmacodynamics of enoximone during intravenous infusion. Int J Cardiol 1990;28(Suppl 1):S1–2.
123. Leier CV, Meiler SE, Matthews S, et al. A preliminary report of the effects of orally administered enoximone on regional hemodynamics in congestive heart failure. Am J Cardiol 1987;60:27C–30C.
124. Kern H, Schröder T, Kaulfuss M, et al. Enoximone in contrast to dobutamine improves hepatosplanchnic function in fluid-optimized septic shock patients. Crit Care Med 2001;29:1519–25.
125. Ringe HI, Varnholt V, Gaedicke G. Cardiac rescue with enoximone in volume and catecholamine refractory septic shock. Pediatr Crit Care Med 2003;4:471–5.
126. Schmidt W, Tinelli M, Secchi A, et al. Enoximone maintains intestinal villus blood flow during endotoxaemia. Int J Surg Investig 2001;2:359–67.
127. Sicignano A, Bellato V, Riboni A, et al. Continuous infusion of enoximone in the treatment of acute myocardial ischemia with low output syndrome. Minerva Anestesiol 1994;60:109–13.
128. Gonzalez M, Desager JP, Jacquemart JL, et al. Efficacy of enoximone in the management of refractory low-output states following cardiac surgery. J Cardiothorac Anesth 1988;2:409–18.
129. Zeplin HE, Dieterich HA, Stegmann T. The effect of enoximone and dobutamine on hemodynamic performance after open heart surgery. A clinical comparison. J Cardiovasc Surg (Torino) 1990;31:574–7.
130. Schauvliege S, Van den Eede A, Duchateau L, et al. Cardiovascular effects of enoximone in isoflurane anaesthetized ponies. Vet Anaesth Analg 2007;34:416–30.
131. Schauvliege S, Gozalo Marcilla M, Duchateau L, et al. Cardiorespiratory effects of enoximone in anaesthetized colic horses. Equine Vet J 2009;41:778–85.
132. Lindsay WA, McDonell W, Bignell W. Equine postanesthetic forelimb lameness: intracompartmental muscle pressure changes and biochemical patterns. Am J Vet Res 1980;41:1919–24.
133. Adelstein RS, Sellers JR. Effects of calcium on vascular smooth muscle contraction. Am J Cardiol 1987;59:4B–10B.
134. Mutlu GM, Factor P. Role of vasopressin in the management of septic shock. Intensive Care Med 2004;30:1276–91.

135. Marshall I, Burt RP, Chapple CR. Signal transduction pathways associated with alpha1-adrenoceptor subtypes in cells and tissues including human prostate. Eur Urol 1999;36(Suppl 1):42–7.

136. Vanhoutte PM, Katusić ZS, Shepherd JT. Vasopressin induces endothelium-dependent relaxations of cerebral and coronary, but not of systemic arteries. J Hypertens Suppl 1984;2(3):S421–2.

137. Fujisawa S, Iijima T. On the inotropic actions of arginine vasopressin in ventricular muscle of the guinea pig heart. Jpn J Pharmacol 1999;81:309–12.

138. Abboud FM, Floras JS, Aylward PE, et al. Role of vasopressin in cardiovascular and blood pressure regulation. Blood Vessels 1990;27:106–15.

139. Beale RJ, Hollenberg SM, Vincent J, et al. Vasopressors and inotropic support in septic shock: an evidence-based review. Crit Care Med 2004;32(Suppl 11): S455–65.

140. Sklar AH, Schrier RW. Central nervous system mediators of vasopressin release. Physiol Rev 1983;63:1243–80.

141. Morelli A, Ertmer C, Pietropaoli P, et al. Terlipressin: a promising vasoactive agent in hemodynamic support of septic shock. Expert Opin Pharmacother 2009;10:2569–75.

142. Rajani RR, Ball CG, Feliciano DV, et al. Vasopressin in hemorrhagic shock: review article. Am Surg 2009;75:1207–12.

143. Landry DW, Levin HR, Gallant EM, et al. Vasopressin deficiency contributes to the vasodilation of septic shock. Circulation 1997;95:1122–5.

144. Bernadich C, Bandi JC, Melin P, et al. Effects of F-180, a new selective vasoconstrictor peptide, compared with terlipressin and vasopressin on systemic and splanchnic hemodynamics in a rat model of portal hypertension. Hepatology 1998;27:351–6.

145. Jochberger S, Wenzel V, Dünser MW. Arginine vasopressin as a rescue vasopressor agent in the operating room. Curr Opin Anaesthesiol 2005;18: 396–404.

146. Krismer AC, Dünser MW, Lindner KH, et al. Vasopressin during cardiopulmonary resuscitation and different shock states: a review of the literature. Am J Cardiovasc Drugs 2006;6:51–68.

147. Voelckel WG, Lurie KG, Lindner KH, et al. Vasopressin improves survival after cardiac arrest in hypovolemic shock. Anesth Analg 2000;91:627–34.

148. Ertmer C, Rehberg S, Westphal M. Vasopressin analogues in the treatment of shock states: potential pitfalls. Best Pract Res Clin Anaesthesiol 2008;22:393–406.

149. Dünser MW, Mayr AJ, Tür A, et al. Ischemic skin lesions as a complication of continuous vasopressin infusion in catecholamine-resistant vasodilatory shock: incidence and risk factors. Crit Care Med 2003;31:1394–8.

150. Lange M, Morelli A, Ertmer C, et al. Continuous versus bolus infusion of terlipressin in ovine endotoxemia. Shock 2007;28:623–9.

151. Valverde A, Giguère S, Sanchez LC, et al. Effects of dobutamine, norepinephrine and vasopressin on cardiovascular function in anesthetized neonatal foals with induced hypotension. Am J Vet Res 2006;67:1730–7.

152. Dickey EJ, McKenzie HC 3rd, Johnson A, et al. Use of pressor therapy in 34 hypotensive critically ill neonatal foals. Aust Vet J 2010;88:472–7.

153. Garb S. Inotropic action of epinephrine, norepinephrine, and N-isopropyl-norepinephrine on heart muscle. Proc Soc Exp Biol Med 1950;73:134.

154. Friedrichs GS, Merrill GF. Adenosine deaminase and adenosine attenuate ventricular arrhythmias caused by norepinephrine. Am J Physiol 1991;260(3 Pt 2): H979–84.

155. Hollis AR, Ousey JC, Palmer L, et al. Effects of norepinephrine and a combined norepinephrine and dobutamine infusion on systemic hemodynamics and indices of renal function in normotensive neonatal thoroughbred foals. J Vet Intern Med 2006;20:1437–42.

156. Hollis AR, Ousey JC, Palmer L, et al. Effects of norepinephrine and combined norepinephrine and fenoldopam infusion on systemic hemodynamics and indices of renal function in normotensive neonatal foals. J Vet Intern Med 2008;22:1210–5.

157. Kee VR. Hemodynamic pharmacology of intravenous vasopressors. Crit Care Nurse 2003;23:79–82.

158. Hardy J, Bednarski RM, Biller DS. Effect of phenylephrine on hemodynamics and splenic dimensions in horses. Am J Vet Res 1994;55:1570–8.

159. Reinelt H, Radermacher P, Kiefer P, et al. Impact of exogenous beta-adrenergic receptor stimulation on hepatosplanchnic oxygen kinetics and metabolic activity in septic shock. Crit Care Med 1999;27:325–31.

160. Hardy J, Minton M, Robertson JT, et al. Nephrosplenic entrapment in the horse: a retrospective study of 174 cases. Equine Vet J Suppl 2000;(32):95–7.

161. Dyson DH, Pascoe PJ. Influence of preinduction methoxamine, lactated Ringer solution or hypertonic saline solution infusion or postinduction dobutamine infusion on anesthetic-induced hypotension in horses. Am J Vet Res 1990;51:17–21.

162. Brodbelt DC, Harris J, Taylor PM. Pituitary-adrenocortical effects of methoxamine infusion on halothane anaesthetised ponies. Res Vet Sci 1998;65:119–23.

163. Holmes CL. Vasoactive drugs in the intensive care unit. Curr Opin Crit Care 2005;11:413–7.

164. Schaer GL, Fink MP, Parillo JE. Norepinephrine alone versus norepinephrine plus low-dose dopamine: enhanced renal blood flow with combination pressor therapy. Crit Care Med 1985;13:492–6.

165. Drummond GI, Duncan L. Adenylyl cyclase in cardiac tissue. J Biol Chem 1970;245:976–83.

166. Goyal RK, McNeill JH. Effects of [Na^+] and [Ca^{2+}] on the responses to milrinone in rat cardiac preparations. Eur J Pharmacol 1986;120:267–74.

167. Schauvliege S, Van den Eede A, Duchateau L, et al. Influence of calcium chloride on the cardiorespiratory effects of a bolus of enoximone in isoflurane anaesthetized ponies. Vet Anaesth Analg 2007;36:101–9.

168. Uretsky BF, Lawless CE, Verbalis JG, et al. Combined therapy with dobutamine and amrinone in severe heart failure. Improved hemodynamics and increased activation of the renin-angiotensin system with combined intravenous therapy. Chest 1987;92:657–62.

169. Robinson RJ, Tchervenkov C. Treatment of low cardiac output after aortocoronary bypass surgery using a combination of norepinephrine and amrinone. J Cardiothorac Anesth 1987;1:229–33.

170. Olsen KH, Kluger J, Fieldman A. Combination high dose amrinone and dopamine in the management of moribund cardiogenic shock after open heart surgery. Chest 1988;94:503–6.

171. Royster RL, Butterworth JF 4th, Prielipp RC, et al. Combined inotropic effects of amrinone and epinephrine after cardiopulmonary bypass in humans. Anesth Analg 1993;77:662–72.

172. Gilbert EM, Hershberger RE, Wiechmann RJ, et al. Pharmacologic and hemodynamic effects of combined ß-agonist stimulation and phosphodiesterase inhibition in the failing human heart. Chest 1995;108:1524–32.

173. Schauvliege S, Van den Eede A, Duchateau L, et al. Cardiorespiratory effects of dobutamine after enoximone in isoflurane anaesthetized ponies. Vet Anaesth Analg 2008;35:306–18.
174. Schechter E, Wilson MF, Kong YS. Physiologic responses to epinephrine infusion: the basis for a new stress test for coronary artery disease. Am Heart J 1983;105:554–60.
175. Trim CM, Moore JN, Clark ES. Renal effects of dopamine infusion in conscious horses. Equine Vet J Suppl 1989;(7):124–8.
176. Clark ES, Moore JN. Effects of dopamine administration on cecal mechanical activity and caecal blood flow in conscious healthy horses. Am J Vet Res 1989;50:1084–8.
177. Trim CM, Moore JN, White NA. Cardiopulmonary effects of dopamine hydrochloride in anaesthetized horses. Equine Vet J 1985;17:41–4.
178. Young LE, Blissitt KJ, Clutton RE, et al. Haemodynamic effects of a sixty minute infusion of dopamine hydrochloride in horses anaesthetized with halothane. Equine Vet J 1998;30:310–6.
179. Robertson SA, Malark JA, Steele CJ, et al. Metabolic, hormonal and hemodynamic changes during dopamine infusions in halothane anesthetized horses. Vet Surg 1996;25:88–97.
180. Leier CV, Binkley PF, Carpenter J, et al. Cardiovascular pharmacology of dopexamine in low output congestive heart failure. Am J Cardiol 1988;62:94–9.
181. Tuttle RR, Mills J. Dobutamine: development of a new catecholamine to selectively increase cardiac contractility. Circ Res 1975;36:185–96.
182. Swanson CR, Muir WW 3rd. Dobutamine-induced augmentation of cardiac output does not enhance respiratory gas exchange in anesthetized recumbent healthy horses. Am J Vet Res 1986;47:1573–6.
183. Young LE, Blissitt KJ, Clutton RE, et al. Temporal effects of an infusion of dobutamine hydrochloride in horses anaesthetized with halothane. Am J Vet Res 1998;59:1027–32.
184. Galiè N, Metalli M, Zannoli R, et al. Myocardial, coronary and peripheral effects of xamoterol (ICI 118,587) in open-chest pigs. Cardiovasc Drugs Ther 1989;3:91–7.
185. Craig CA, Haskins SC, Hildebrand SV. The cardiopulmonary effects of dobutamine and norepinephrine in isoflurane-anesthetized foals. Vet Anaesth Analg 2007;34:377–87.
186. Raisis AL, Young LE, Taylor PM, et al. Doppler ultrasonography and single-fiber laser Doppler flowmetry for measurement of hind limb blood flow in anesthetized horses. Am J Vet Res 2000;61:286–90.

Mechanical Ventilation and Respiratory Mechanics During Equine Anesthesia

Yves Moens, DVM, PhD, Priv Doz

KEYWORDS

- Mechanical ventilation • Horse • Compliance • Monitoring • Recruitment

KEY POINTS

- Although correcting hypoventilation remains the main indication for mechanical ventilation, the effect on oxygenation is unpredictable.
- Early onset of mechanical ventilation (at induction) is advantageous for oxygenation.
- Mechanical ventilation has negative cardiovascular side effects.
- Capnography is well suited to support management of mechanical ventilation.
- Continuous measurement of respiratory volumes and compliance during anesthesia has become practical for horses.
- Changes in compliance of the thoracic compartment influence ventilator performance.

INTRODUCTION

Mechanical ventilation in horses has been documented since the beginning of the nineteenth century. In the first place it was used to sustain ventilation in case of respiratory arrest intentionally caused by the use of curare and using an undefined bellows.[1] Later when general anesthesia was introduced in horses and the respiratory depressant effects of the anesthetic drugs became apparent, different types of foot operated or manually operated bellows-type devices were used and also incorporated in large animal anesthesia circuits.[2–4] Subsequently, different more sophisticated large animal ventilators were designed in the United States and Europe, and the use of mechanical ventilation to provide ventilatory support during equine anesthesia became common.

BASIC TERMINOLOGY AND PHYSIOLOGY

Techniques to provide ventilatory support in horses exclusively use positive pressure to expand the lungs. Positive pressure "breaths" are then delivered manually by

The author has nothing to disclose.
Anaesthesiology and Perioperative Intensive Care, University of Veterinary Medicine, Veterinaerplatz 1, Vienna A-1210, Austria
E-mail address: yves.moens@vetmeduni.ac.at

squeezing the breathing bag of an anesthetic system or are "mechanically" delivered by a large animal ventilator. This technique is commonly referred to as intermittent positive pressure ventilation (IPPV). Sometimes the term "continuous mandatory ventilation" is preferred when IPPV is used continuously at a regular rate. This rate is most commonly controlled by the anesthetist and the procedure called "controlled" ventilation in contrast to "assisted ventilation," where the horse through its own inspiratory effort triggers the mechanical positive pressure breath. Although this modus is available on some ventilators, it is seldom used as standard ventilatory modus in horses. Ventilatory support during inhalant anesthesia using an anesthetic system and a ventilator is typically coupled with provision of elevated concentrations of inspired oxygen usually between 50% and 90%.

Although today mechanical ventilation of horses is a common procedure, its appropriate use needs the recognition of the fact that applying positive pressure in recumbent horses is in a sense an "unphysiologic" challenge. During normal spontaneous breathing, intrapleural pressure cycles between -10 cm H_2O (inspiration) and -3 cm H_2O (rest) and mean intrathoracic pressure is subatmospheric. This subatmospheric pressure and the cycling nature of the pressure swings promote venous return to the heart (the respiratory pump).[5] When spontaneous ventilation is substituted by mechanical ventilation, intrapleural pressures cycles in the positive range, for example from $+3$ cm H_2O (end expiration) to $+30$ cm H_2O (peak inspiration). Mean intrathoracic pressure now becomes positive to an extent, which depends on the particular characteristics of the implemented ventilation mode, and directly influences venous return and cardiac output, which likely decrease. Also, mechanical ventilation during anesthesia is normally applied to horses in lateral or dorsal recumbency. In the standing horse, optimal pulmonary function and gas exchange are favored by the specific anatomic arrangement of lungs, diaphragm, and intestines. However, during recumbency these physiologic advantages are lost and major parts of the lung are now subject to pressure from the abdominal compartment via the dome-shaped diaphragm with direct negative consequences for gas exchange. A positive aspect of mechanical ventilation per se is reduction of the work of breathing. During spontaneous breathing, the inspiration is an active process. Stretching the chest wall and overcoming frictional resistance to airflow during inspiration consumes energy (work of breathing). This work of breathing is reduced with the use of appropriately sized endotracheal tubes because of a reduced frictional resistance when the upper airways are bypassed.[6] However, in case of IPPV the work of breathing during inspiration is now provided by the ventilator. In contrast, expiration is a passive process although in the horse particularly the abdominal muscles contribute actively at end-expiration.

ESSENTIALS ABOUT EQUIPMENT

Large animal ventilators have usually a bag-in-box design whereby a gas flow introduced in the box compresses the rebreathing bag and forces gas from the anesthesia machine into the horse's lung. The bellows contains the respiratory gas mixture from the patient and is separated from the driving gas in the surrounding box. Intermittent introduction from pressurized driving gas replaces manual squeezing of the breathing bag. The driving gas can in principle be oxygen, but usually for economic reasons compressed air is used. The way the bellows is mounted in the box differs: there are hanging bellows (also called descending) and standing bellows types (ascending). The terms "ascending" and "descending" describe the action of the bellows during the expiratory phase. These 2 types behave differently during a preanesthetic leak test and during IPPV in case a leak in the anesthetic system exists. During the test, standing bellows will descend gradually from fully ascended position and during IPPV they will not fully ascend at expiration. Additionally, condensed water is more easily drained from standing bellows. With the hanging bellows it is more difficult to detect leaks. Furthermore, condensed water can accumulate in the bellows. Some ventilators need, in addition to pressurized gas, electrical power to operate the system. One recent ventilator uses a motor-driven piston to deliver the positive pressure breaths and needs only electrical power (see later discussion). A large animal ventilator can be a stand-alone device that can be connected to an anesthetic circle system at the place of the breathing bag. Alternatively, the ventilator is an integral part of a complete anesthetic machine.

To provide IPPV, the anesthetist is able to adjust different variables that differ among ventilators. Apart from the main variables tidal volume (VT) and peak inspiratory pressure (PIP), adjustable variables can include respiratory rate, inspiratory flow rate and time, inspiratory to expiratory ratio (I:E ratio), and expiratory time. Large animal ventilators seldom have the possibility to create positive end-expiratory pressure (PEEP) and if so, the level rarely exceeds 10 cm H_2O. A PEEP is used in an attempt to improve oxygenation when a lot of lung atelectasis is present (see later discussion). Usually the tidal volume is delivered in less than 2 to 3 seconds and the ventilator must be able to generate high inspiratory flows (up to 600 L/min) when tidal volume is large. Both variables inspiratory flow and time together with respiratory rate determine I:E ratio. Alternatively, I:E ratio can be adjusted directly. Generally, it is advised to keep I:E ratio at least at 1:2 to allow sufficient time for lung deflation, create low mean airway pressure, and hence promote good venous return during the expiratory phase.

Basically ventilators can operate in 1 or 2 different modes according to their target variable: this is the primary variable controlled by the anesthetist. In the volume-controlled mode this variable is tidal volume, whereas in the pressure-controlled mode it is peak inspiratory pressure. Whether volume-controlled ventilation or pressure-controlled ventilation is the more advantageous technique for gas exchange remains controversial and likely to be influenced by many factors. In equidae no comparative studies exists. Clinically, it is important to recognize that changes of the compliance of the thoracic compartment will influence ventilator performance differently. In the volume-controlled mode, the preset volume will be delivered regardless of compliance and if for example compliance decreases, higher PIP will be generated when the breath is delivered. In contrast, when the pressure-controlled mode is used a decreased compliance will result in the delivery of a smaller tidal volume, which may remain unnoticed and lead to hypoventilation.

Large animal ventilators all display airway pressure but they do not measure effective tidal volume. A rough visual estimation of the tidal volume delivered is possible when the ventilator has a graduated concertina-type bellows. However, there might be a large discrepancy with the effectively delivered tidal volume in certain circumstances, for example when condensed water accumulates in the concertina. Even if the ventilator allows setting of a precise tidal volume, the real volume delivered to the patient will nevertheless be different. It can be less because of volume loss caused by the compliance of breathing hoses or leaks in the system or it can be more because of the use of a high fresh gas flow. For accurate knowledge of delivered tidal volume, spirometry is mandatory and preferably performed at the level of the connection of circuit and the endotracheal tube (see later discussion). An excellent overview of currently used large animal ventilators, their particular characteristics, and problem solving is seen and published elsewhere.[7]

COMMON INDICATIONS FOR VENTILATORY SUPPORT DURING ANESTHESIA
Hypoventilation and Hypercapnia

Treatment of hypoventilation and the ensuing hypercapnia and respiratory acidosis is the most common indication for providing ventilatory support. When horses are anesthetized and become recumbent, the volume and conformation of the rib cage changes and lung volumes are reduced.[8] This reduction and the accompanying changes of the respiratory mechanics interfere with maintenance of normal ventilation. Moreover, the normal regulatory respiratory compensation mechanisms are depressed by anesthetic drugs. Therefore, respiratory rate and tidal volume do not adapt to the extent necessary so that sufficient minute ventilation is produced to maintain normocapnia (arterial partial pressure of CO_2, $PaCO_2$, of 40–45 mm Hg). This hypoventilation results in hypercapnia and respiratory acidosis, which tends to increase with the duration of anesthesia in particular with inhalation agents, and $Paco_2$ values of 60 to 70 mm Hg are common during spontaneous ventilation.[9,10] When total intravenous anesthesia is used, the degree of respiratory depression depends on the drug combination and the doses used.

The $PaCO_2$ level at which ventilatory support should be provided is discussed controversially in the clinical context. Some anesthetists favor the potentially beneficial effects during anesthesia of horses of moderate hypercapnia (up to $PaCO_2$ of 70 mm Hg). This includes sympathetic stimulation and vasodilatation and thus an increase in cardiac output. However, large increases (>70 mm Hg) may produce myocardial depression, arrhythmias, and impairment of metabolism because of the accompanying respiratory acidosis.[11,12] Therefore, ventilatory support should be provided at least when $PaCO_2$ is greater than 70 mm Hg. This is likely to happen when the respiratory rate of a horse falls below 4 to 5 per minute during anesthesia or when respiration becomes shallow, even with higher rates. However, when blood pH level is low (<7.2), for example because of the presence of a superimposed metabolic acidosis, the start of IPPV at much lower levels of $PaCO_2$ may be mandatory. Once started, the settings of IPPV (delivered minute volume) must not be targeted at reaching eucapnia ($PaCO_2$ 40–50 mm Hg) per se. Cardiovascular stimulation of moderate hypercapnia is considered as well as the fact that IPPV settings that target higher minute volumes inevitably increase intrathoracic pressure and exacerbate the negative cardiovascular impact of mechanical ventilation (decreased venous return).[13] Therefore, clinical or instrumental monitoring of hemodynamic performance is important. This will guide decisions as whether to change IPPV settings or to provide hemodynamic support (eg, with fluid loading and/or inotropes) or both.

The ratio of metabolic CO_2 production and alveolar ventilation determines $PaCO_2$. Therefore, $PaCO_2$ levels can be well managed by setting the ventilator to deliver the appropriate minute volume. In human anesthesia, nomograms have been used to predict the necessary minute volume for normocapnic ventilation for a certain body mass.[14] A simple nomogram for the horse exists (**Fig. 1**).[15] However, these nomograms are only guidelines and ideally should be confirmed by the results of blood gas analysis. Typically, a respiratory rate of 6 to 8 breaths/min and a tidal volume of 10 to 12 mL/kg should result in $PaCO_2$ of 50 to 60 mm Hg. However, in practice a discrepancy between expected (nomogram) and effectively measured $PaCO_2$ is often seen. This is because the part of minute ventilation, which is called dead space ventilation (VD) and is wasted for gas exchange and CO_2 elimination is not fixed but variable. This physiologic dead space is often expressed as a fraction of tidal volume (VD/VT). In mammals, approximately one-third of minute ventilation is dead space when tidal volume is physiologic. In horses, VD/VT is greater and about 0.5 to 0.6,

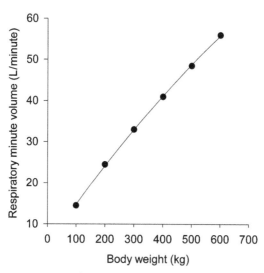

Fig. 1. A simple nomogram provides a rough estimate for the respiratory minute volume required to realize normocapnia during anesthesia of a horse. (*Data from* Smith M. Nomogram. In: Manual smith respirator LA-2100. 2012. p. 15. Available at: http://www. veterinarytechnics.com. Accessed December 10, 2012.)

but this can increase during anesthesia and recumbency.[10] This physiologic dead space is essentially made up of a relatively fixed anatomic dead space (nasal cavity, pharynx, trachea, bronchi) and a variable alveolar dead space (physiologic dead space = anatomic + alveolar dead space). Added apparatus dead space (eg spirometry sensor) is seldom important considering the usual large size of equidae and the relatively small added volumes. Because anatomic dead space is constant, the proportion of wasted ventilation will decrease with large tidal volumes (minute volume is more efficient) and increase with small tidal volumes (minute volume is less efficient). For a defined tidal volume, the variability of dead space is mainly caused by variation in alveolar dead space. Alveolar dead space is, for a great part, generated by a deficit in gas exchange caused by the group of nonperfused or relatively underperfused alveoli (see later discussion).[16] Unfortunately, without additional technical methods, it is difficult to estimate the different fractions of dead space and thus the "efficient" parts of minute and alveolar ventilation.

An attractive alternative to intermittent $PaCO_2$ measurement to fine tune minute ventilation is the use of capnography.[17] By means of this monitoring technique, CO_2 concentrations in the respiratory gas are continuously measured. The rationale is that end-tidal PCO_2 ($ETPCO_2$) closely resembles $PaCO_2$. In this way, the efficiency of minute ventilation is indicated by $ETPCO_2$. However, in the anesthetized horse $PaCO_2$ is, in general, substantially higher than $ETPCO_2$. This difference (described as arterial-to-alveolar PCO_2 difference, $(a-A)PCO_2$, with A standing for the ideal alveolar PCO_2) is, for an important part, generated by the relatively poor or nonperfused alveoli (alveolar dead space). A part of this difference is also generated by right-to-left pulmonary shunting but this is noticeable only with large shunts (virtual alveolar dead space). The normal difference in the anesthetized horse is in the magnitude of 10 mm Hg, but this can increase 3-fold if IPPV with high airway pressures are used or when cardiac output is low. As long as body position, IPPV settings, and cardiovascular status do not change, the (a-A)PCO$_2$ remains stable.[18–20] A special situation can occur during IPPV in which increasing minute ventilation with the goal of decreasing PaCO$_2$ (eg by increasing tidal volume) has unexpectedly little effect on PaCO$_2$, because increased airway pressure by interference with pulmonary capillary circulation concomitantly increases alveolar dead space especially when pulmonary perfusion pressure is low.

Hypoxemia

Where hypercapnia is relatively well controlled by IPPV, the effect on low PaO$_2$ is much less predictable, which ranges from improvement, no change, or even a decrease.[21–23] It is recognized that atelectasis formation in dependent lung regions and the ensuing right-to-left shunt contribute to large alveolar-to-arterial (A-a)PO$_2$ differences and hence low PaO$_2$.[24] It is likely that once important atelectasis has developed, classical IPPV is not able to reopen a substantial amount of alveoli to turn them again into gas exchanging units. Moreover, the accompanying increase in intrathoracic pressure may force more pulmonary blood into these atelectatic regions and so increase the pulmonary shunt fraction and ultimately decrease PaO$_2$.

In this context, 2 different clinical approaches for the timing of IPPV that are commonly used need consideration. One approach is to start IPPV soon after induction and intubation, whereas another approach consists in allowing the horses to breathe spontaneously and only apply IPPV when a defined maximum level of PaCO$_2$ or ETPCO$_2$ is reached. It is now well documented that the option to substitute spontaneous breathing by IPPV soon after induction or even immediately after intubation will result in smaller (A-a)PO$_2$ and higher PaO$_2$.[9,25] Very likely this approach to a certain extent limits atelectasis and shunt formation. However, whenever early IPPV is considered the actual cardiovascular status of the horse must be checked. The negative hemodynamic effects of IPPV in combination with the sudden adoption of recumbency, the hemodynamic effects of anesthetic drugs, and a low cardiac output may be detrimental in certain cases.

In an attempt to improve low PaO$_2$, PEEP during IPPV is used. The rationale is that PEEP prevents alveoli from collapsing. However, the results have been inconsistent and in some cases PaO$_2$ even decreases.[26–29] There are several reasons why the sole application of PEEP can fail to improve PaO$_2$. First, PEEP will not necessarily reopen alveoli that are already collapsed but rather cause overexpansion of remaining well-ventilated alveoli and compress alveolar capillaries.[30] This is supported by the documentation of increased alveolar dead space with PEEP in human patients.[31] Second, at the same time PEEP can force blood preferentially to dependent poorly ventilated but perfused areas and so increase right-to-left pulmonary shunt of venous blood. Also, PEEP increases mean intrathoracic pressure and this impedes venous return and in the horse, decreases cardiac output.[29,32] Important decreases in cardiac output through decreased mixed venous oxygen content also contribute to a decrease of PaO$_2$. Evidence exists in humans and some animal species that PEEP applied before atelectasis has formed is efficient in limiting the decrease in PaO$_2$. There is limited but convincing information that this is also the case for horses. When IPPV was combined with modest PEEP (10 cm H$_2$O) from the beginning of anesthesia, oxygenation was better compared with IPPV without PEEP.[33] This case matches well with the documented improvement of gas exchange when horses receive IPPV immediately after induction compared with a delayed start.[25] Together these findings suggest that immediate start of IPPV combined with modest PEEP can limit atelectasis formation and thus represent a beneficial strategy to optimize gas exchange in hemodynamically stable horses.

Facilitating Inhalation Anesthesia

The fact that IPPV can facilitate maintenance of inhalation anesthesia is often over-looked. Inhalation agents are administered via the lungs and a defined concentration of the agent in the blood must be reached to realize the desired anesthetic effect. In this process, the pharmacokinetics are important and strongly influenced by alveolar ventilation especially for the modern, relatively less soluble agents like isoflurane and sevoflurane. Generally speaking, the alveolar concentration of an agent resembles the concentration of the agent in arterial blood, which in turn resembles the concentration in the brain. Some anesthetic monitors measure the concentration of volatile agents in the respiratory gas, and end-tidal concentration is a useful approximation of the alveolar concentration. The time needed for the alveolar concentration of an agent to approach the inspired concentration will be shorter when minute ventilation increases and hence induction time will be shorter (**Fig. 2**). Similarly, when changes of anesthetic depth are desired and the inspired fraction of the agent is changed, these changes accordingly will occur rapidly. During spontaneous breathing, alveolar ventilation is generally lower and more irregular than during IPPV. In this way, by providing sufficient and stable alveolar ventilation, IPPV facilitates keeping a stable and steerable plane of anesthesia.

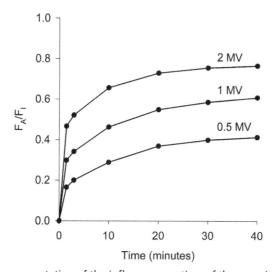

Fig. 2. Schematic representation of the influence over time of the magnitude of respiratory minute volume (MV) on the ratio of alveolar fraction/inspired fraction [F_A/F_I] of an inhalation agent (example halothane). (*Data from* Eger EI II. Anesthetic uptake and action. Baltimore: Williams and Wilkins; 1974.)

RECENT EVOLUTIONS
Monitoring of Respiratory Mechanics During Mechanical Ventilation

Principles and equipment
Monitoring the efficacy of IPPV is an important aspect of anesthetic management. Clinical observation of chest excursions and appreciation of the level of airway pressure generated are a minimum but ultimately blood gas analysis will be most informative. However, this is not always available and also not a continuous method. In the past decades, 2 noninvasive and continuous monitoring techniques made their way

to veterinary anesthetic practice: capnography and pulse oximetry provide information on carbon dioxide elimination and oxygenation, respectively. Pulse oximetry measures the saturation of hemoglobin with oxygen in arterial blood (SpO_2) via a sensor most commonly applied to the tongue. Its portability makes it particularly useful for field anesthesia but peripheral vasoconstriction often interferes with the measurement. During general anesthesia, SpO_2 should preferably not decrease below 90%. This can occur, for example, when a horse is hypoventilating and breathing room air. However, in the presence of a high inspired oxygen fraction and because of the specific sigmoid shape of the oxyhemoglobin dissociation curve, SpO_2 is not a sensitive index for changes in ventilation. Capnography has been proved to be a more versatile monitor for equine anesthesia providing practical information not only on ventilation but also on circulation, metabolism, as well as on different technical aspects.[17] It is an affordable and robust technology well suited to support management of IPPV.

The contribution of capnography to the noninvasive monitoring of ventilation and the management of IPPV in particular is valuable but incomplete. When a horse is ventilated, the moving of gas to and from the alveoli and the pressures and flows generated in the airways by this process are not routinely monitored. Nevertheless, these parameters characterize the particular ventilatory dynamics and give important information needed to optimize mechanical ventilation for each patient and for each particular circumstance. Moreover, with the simultaneous measurement of respiratory volumes (spirometry) and airway pressures, the main components of respiratory mechanics, "compliance" and "resistance" of the respiratory system, are calculated or visualized. The measurement of tidal and minute volume during anesthesia and IPPV is not routine in horses because of the lack of a practical method. Today, modern spirometry is in the reach of the equine practitioner as a pitot tube–based flow sensor, now common in human anesthesia,[34] was remodeled on a larger scale to enable its use in large animals in combination with dedicated monitoring technology (Side Stream Spirometry, Datex-Ohmeda GE Health Care, USA). Details have been published elsewhere.[35] The sensor has no moving parts (unlike mechanical spirometers for human use) and combines the measurement of gas velocity by pitot tubes with the principle of a fixed resistance. The pressure difference that is generated is converted to flow and volume. The flow sensor that is placed between the endotracheal tube and the breathing circuit has also a respiratory gas sample port, which allows in combination with a dedicated host monitor to perform respiratory gas analysis including CO_2, O_2, and volatile agents (**Fig. 3**). Therefore, the spirometric values are automatically corrected for the effect of changing gas concentrations. Such a system fulfills the conditions to monitor important aspects of respiratory mechanics during equine anesthesia.

Compliance is a measure of how well the respiratory system (lungs-thorax) can change its total volume as the inspired airway pressure changes. Although the lungs and thorax each have their own compliance, their combined compliance is clinically relevant and equals tidal volume divided by end-inspiratory pressure minus end-expiratory pressure. Compliance, expressed in ml/cm H_2O, depends also on lung volume and age and normal values in healthy standing horses are 2 to 4 mL/cm H_2O/kg bodyweight. Compliance ideally is calculated when flow is zero in the airways. This is because when air flow is still present, a pressure difference is created because of resistance encountered by this flow in the airways. Such an ideal measurement of compliance is referred to as "static compliance," but it is not commonly performed in clinical conditions. However, it can also be assumed that at end-inspiration and at end-expiration flow is zero for an infinite short moment and compliance is calculated at that moment. This is called "dynamic compliance" (Cdyn) and is the common

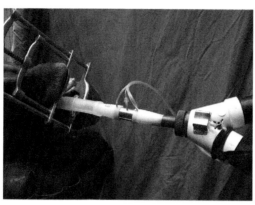

Fig. 3. A pitot-based spirometer for large animals interposed between endotracheal tube and the Y-piece of a circle system during equine anesthesia. The pressure sensing and gas sampling line are facing upwards. (*From* Moens YP. Clinical application of continuous spirometry with a pitot-based flow meter during equine anaesthesia. Equine Vet Educ 2010;22(7):354–60.)

measurement in clinical anesthesia. In its most simple form Cdyn could be calculated using the displacement of a graduated concertina bag of the ventilator and the peak airway pressure from the pressure gauge in the anesthetic circuit. However, modern spirometry using the dedicated monitor system does this more accurately and continuously. Additionally, Cdyn is visualized by a continuously updated display of the pressure-volume (PV, "compliance")-loop of each breath. Frictional resistance opposes or retards air flow in the airways. The variable "airway resistance" quantifies this force through the relationship between the pressure difference that is generated across the airway and the rate at which gas is flowing through the airways. Resistance is expressed in $cmH_2O/L/min$ and values less than 1.2 cm $H_2O/L/s$ were recorded in healthy standing horses[5] and also in intubated horses during short intravenous anesthesia.[6] Resistance is calculated but in the system described earlier resistance is mainly reflected visually in the flow-volume (FV, "resistance")-loop.

Clinical use of spirometry and monitoring of compliance and resistance
For the clinical anesthetist, disposing of visual information on respiratory mechanics in the form of loops has distinct clinical advantages. Similarly, to the interpretation of other waveforms (electrocardiogram, capnogram, blood pressure), quicker and easier recognition of abnormalities is possible and thus corrective action can be taken early. This process is enhanced by the possibility to store a loop in the memory of the monitor screen and have the new loops permanently superimposed on this saved loop. Examples of the use and interpretation of such loops in the management of equine anesthesia have been published elsewhere.[36] The normal PV loop is elliptical in shape and during spontaneous respiration arranged around the y-axis but compliance is not calculated. During IPPV, the loop is plotted at about a 45° angle on an X/Y graph, the slope represents Cdyn and the numerical value is displayed on the monitor (**Fig. 4**). When Cdyn decreases, the angle of the slope diminishes. The pattern of the FV loop is determined by the mechanical properties of the total respiratory system and thus by changes of airway resistance and elastic recoil of the lungs. The FV loop during spontaneous ventilation consists of a smoothly curved inspiratory limb and a triangular expiratory limb, with the apex of the triangle representing peak expiratory flow. Note that inspiration is essentially an active process (from the patient or from the ventilator)

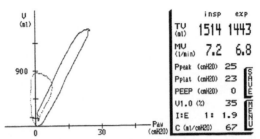

Fig. 4. Spirometric data and loops recorded following induction of inhalation anesthesia of a 700 kg bwt horse. Printout of the complete display of the Capnomac Ultima monitor, flow-derived data to be multiplied by 5. Hypoventilation during spontaneous respiration because of an insufficient tidal volume (stored FV loop, dotted) was diagnosed. IPPV with an adequate tidal volume (actual PV loop) restored normoventilation with normal end-tidal CO_2. The ascending lower limb of the PV curve represents the increasing inspiratory pressure to inflate the lung, and the descending upper limb represents the decreasing pressure during deflation of the lungs. The slope of the PV curve represents the dynamic compliance and the value is indicated. (*From* Moens YP. Clinical application of continuous spirometry with a pitot-based flow meter during equine anaesthesia. Equine Vet Educ 2010;22(7):354–60.)

and expiration a passive one. What a typical loop looks like depends also on the type and size of the endotracheal tube, the characteristics of the ventilator, and its operation mode (pressure-controlled/volume-controlled, accelerating flow/decelerating flow, etc.) (**Fig. 5**).

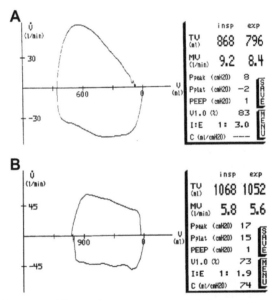

Fig. 5. Spirometric data and flow-volume loops recorded during inhalation anesthesia of a 550 kg bwt horse. Printout of the complete display of the Capnomac Ultima monitor, flow-derived data to be multiplied by 5. (*A*) During spontaneous ventilation. (*B*) During volume-controlled IPPV with constant inspiratory flow. The inspiratory flow is the lower part of the curve, and the upper part represents expiratory flow. The shape of the FV loops is influenced by the characteristics of the anesthetic system and operation modus of the ventilator in use. (*From* Moens YP. Clinical application of continuous spirometry with a pitot-based flow meter during equine anaesthesia. Equine Vet Educ 2010;22(7):354–60.)

The functional result of pulmonary ventilation can to a certain extent be noninvasively monitored in horses with pulse oximetry and capnography. Spirometry does not replace these monitoring techniques but provides several complementary informations. As an example, proper interpretation of abnormal end-tidal CO_2 values provided by capnography is only possible when the contribution of minute volume of ventilation is recognized. Moreover, spirometric information, such as changes in respiratory volumes, Cdyn, or resistance (numerical values or loops), often precedes changes in other parameters and thus action can be taken early. During spontaneous breathing, the respiratory frequency and/or volumes are indicators of the balance of anesthetic depth and surgical stimulus. The quick recognition of respiratory changes helps to maintain a smooth anesthetic plane. The persistence or return of spontaneous respiratory efforts during IPPV because of insufficient anesthetic depth or the wearing-off of the effect of neuromuscular blockade is easily detected by observing typically distorted PV loops.

The effective compliance of the respiratory system and possible changes that occur during anesthesia has a direct impact on anesthetic management during IPPV. Delivery of an adequate minute volume in presence of low compliance will cause higher airway and intrathoracic pressures, which in turn will impede venous return to the heart, decrease the cardiac output, and thus potentially decrease oxygen delivery to the tissues. Low Cdyn (eg, <1 mL/cm H_2O/kg) and changes during anesthesia are often seen in colic horses with tympanic abdomen and horses undergoing laparoscopic surgery with abdominal insufflation of gas. Similar to humans, the increased intra-abdominal pressure in these horses is likely to affect the mechanical properties of the whole respiratory system and decrease Cdyn through cranial displacement of the diaphragm and reduction of lung volume;[37,38] this is amplified when the horses for surgical reasons are positioned head-down and abdominal contents exert more pressure on the diaphragm.[37,39] After surgical exteriorisation and decompression of distended intestinal organs or when the pressurizing gas is evacuated from the abdomen, Cdyn will return toward initial values. These changes in Cdyn are accompanied by changes in delivered tidal volume or airway pressures according to the type of ventilation mode that is used. In severely tympanic horses, it is not unusual to need very high PIP (>50 cm H_2O) to deliver a standard tidal volume (10–12 mL/kg). Therefore, it can be preferred to postpone IPPV until acceptable Cdyn and hemodynamic performance are restored and meanwhile accept a limited period of hypercapnia and possibly hypoxemia. Compliance can also be low or become low with intrathoracic space-occupying processes such as diaphragmatic hernia, pneumothorax, liquidothorax, or tumors. Further causes of decreased compliance are extreme obesity, inadequate muscle relaxation, external pressure on chest and abdomen, and bronchoconstriction. Compliance is best monitored observing the PV loop, but compliance changes will also affect the FV loop. A decrease in compliance causes a higher expiratory peak flow and a steeper slope of expiratory flow. Marked changes in the FV loop are directly linked with increase in resistance because of bronchoconstriction, obstruction or collapse of airways, or with the use of too small bore endotracheal tubes. Furthermore, a range of technical mishaps influencing respiratory volumes and airway pressures can also be detected with spirometry/compliance-resistance monitoring. The immediate detection of sudden changes often before other monitored parameters changed have been useful in detecting inadvertently closed APL valves, obstructing endotracheal tubes, or iatrogenic pneumothorax. Also leaks in the anesthetic circuit can be easily detected by a discrepancy between inspired and expired tidal volumes. Detection, correction, and control hereof is facilitated when the PV or FV loops display are used. A possible special indication for compliance monitoring is the evaluation and fine tuning of alveolar recruitment maneuvers (ARM) during IPPV of horses (see later discussion).

Alveolar Recruitment Strategies During Mechanical Ventilation

Atelectasis formation in dependent lung regions and impaired gas exchange also occur in human patients undergoing general anesthesia[40] albeit to a lesser extent than in anesthetized horses. Therefore, new ventilatory strategies have been introduced that were originally developed for the treatment of deficient gas exchange in people suffering from acute respiratory deficiency syndrome. The aim of the 'Open Lung Concept' is to improve gas exchange with a special intervention ARM (the alveolar recruitment maneuver) consisting in actively "opening" collapsed alveoli with high inspiratory pressures and then "keep them open" by applying sufficient levels of PEEP.[41,42] Different types of ARM are used during IPPV in anesthetized patients[43,44] and are now also under clinical investigation in horses with promising results. As an example, Hopster and colleagues[33] used repeated sustained inflations with PIP of 60 to 80 cm H_2O followed by an arbitrarily chosen PEEP between 10 and 15 cm H_2O in horses suffering from colic and undergoing exploratory laparotomy in dorsal recumbency. As a result, PaO_2 was 2-fold to 3-fold higher than in a control group with classic IPPV without ARM. Similar results were obtained during total intravenous anesthesia.[45] Selecting an optimal post-ARM PEEP remains challenging in the clinical situation. This PEEP should be the minimal PEEP needed to keep the newly recruited alveoli open and causing the least cardiovascular side effects. Schürmann and colleagues[46] for this purpose applied in similar circumstances a special sequence for ARM using ascending/descending titration of airway pressures. They needed similar PIP levels to fully recruit the lungs (PaO_2>400 mm Hg at FiO_2>0.9) but optimal post-ARM PEEP varied from 15 to 28 cm H_2O. These investigators found marked variability in response (a substantial increase in PaO_2) and some horses did not respond. Interestingly, the nonresponders were preferentially horses suffering from extreme intestinal distension suggesting that a high intra-abdominal pressure counteracts the effects of increased airway pressure. In the conditions of both studies, cardiovascular side effects were limited despite the use of high airway pressures but cardiac output was not measured. In human anesthesia, besides PaO_2, measurement of Cdyn is also used to monitor the efficiency of ARM and to identify a best PEEP.[47] Compliance increases when lung tissue is successfully recruited but falls clearly when the post-ARM PEEP is too low to keep the recruited alveoli open (**Fig. 6**). Clearly the concept of opening the lung and applying a post-ARM PEEP has potential to increase oxygenation in horses but much more research into the exact modalities is needed. At the same time, it must be emphasized that ultimately oxygen delivery depends not only on PaO_2 but also on the amount of hemoglobin and the cardiac output.

NEW TRENDS IN VENTILATORS AND MONITORING OF VENTILATION

Commonly used commercial equine ventilators are generally incapable of delivering the pressures and PEEP levels that seem to be needed to apply recruitment strategies in horses. In theory when the anesthetic system and the connection with the patient are airtight hand bagging can be done to generate high PIP. However if recruitment is successfully achieved PEEP needs to follow. Ad hoc modifications in the anesthetic system and ventilator are possible measures to create the necessary PEEP levels in existing combinations. This is for example using a controllable water trap in the expiratory limb of the anesthetic system or at the exhaust port of the ventilator, which allows creation of PEEP up to 30 cm H_2O.[48,49] Alternatively, a commercial graduated spring loaded resistor can be mounted on the exhaust of some ventilators to create different levels of PEEP.[33] Clearly modern versatile ventilators are needed to make ARM easier and more reproducible. Until now the bag-in-box principle was the common design used. A new concept of large animal anesthetic machine has been introduced recently.[50] The "Tafonius" machine uses an electrically powered linear accelerator to drive a piston sealed by a rolling diaphragm (no bellows) and so no driving gas is required. In this new approach, piston movements (and hence ventilation) are entirely microprocessor-controlled and can be changed 200 times/s. The ventilator comes as an integral part of the anesthetic machine with Windows-supported monitoring or as a stand-alone device. Currently the anesthetic machine is set up to furthermore variety of ventilation modes including spontaneous ventilation; IPPV, assisted ventilation with continuous positive airway pressure and PEEP are provided with this system is open for further developments and virtually any breathing pattern desired can be programed.

New emerging technologies in lung function monitoring are likely to become useful tools for veterinary management of IPPV in the future. First, recently ultrasonic plethysmography has been introduced for use in veterinary medicine.[51] This system measures continuously the circumference changes of thorax and abdomen using special belts. Used during anesthesia, this technology allows monitoring of respiratory rate and semi quantitatively also tidal volumes and changes in end expiratory lung volume, for example induced by PEEP.[52] Second, the technical set up to perform volumetric capnograpy during human anesthesia has recently been adapted to allow measurement and analysis of the flows encountered in large animals.[53] This technology combines the spirometric flow signal with the capnographic signal to construct a CO_2-volume plot. Dedicated algorithms allow continuous monitoring of the different fractions of physiologic dead space.[54] Especially noninvasive breath-to-breath quantification of alveolar dead space together with Cdyn is likely to be useful in fine tuning the settings of IPPV and ARM in the horse like it is the case in human.[55] Finally,

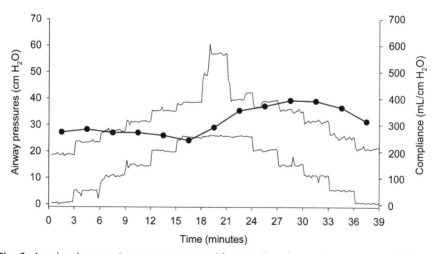

Fig. 6. An alveolar recruitment maneuver with ascending-descending sequence of airway pressures during intermittent positive pressure ventilation showing peak inspiratory pressure and positive end-expiratory pressure over time in an isoflurane anesthetized 500 kg bwt horse in lateral recumbency. The accompanying changes in dynamic compliance are indicated.

management of mechanical ventilation could also profit from the possibilities of an emerging methodology, electrical impedance tomography, which has been recently introduced for monitoring of lung ventilation in human intensive care and anesthesia.[56] This radiation-free technology, the use of which has been preliminary verified in standing ponies,[57] provides with a dedicated electrode belt strapped around the thorax continuous dynamic images of the aeration changes in both lungs. It is expected that continuous monitoring of the influence of ventilator settings on the regional distribution of ventilation in the equine lungs of adult horses (Moens Y, personal communication, 2012) can contribute positively to management of IPPV and the improvement of gas exchange.

SUMMARY

The mechanical ventilation of horses during anesthesia remains a crucial option for optimal anesthetic management in these species prone to hypercapnia and hypoxemia if the possible negative cardiovascular side effects are managed. The combined use of capnography and pitot-based spirometry provide complementary information on ventilation and respiratory mechanics, respectively. This facilitates management of mechanical ventilation in conditions of changing respiratory system compliance and whenever investigating new ventilatory strategies.

REFERENCES

1. Clanny WR. The Wourali poison: experiments with the Wourali poison. Lancet 1839;2:285–6.
2. Rankin AD, Booth N, Sullivan J. Artificial respiration in large animals. J Am Vet Med Assoc 1952;120:196–8.
3. Schebitz H. Zur Narkose beim Pferd unter besonderer Berücksichtigung der Narkose im geschlossenen System. [Anesthesia in the horse using the closed system]. Mh Vet Med 1955;19/20:503–9.
4. Überreiter O. Anästhesie und Muskelrelaxation bei Pferd und Hund. [Anesthesia and muscle relaxation in the horse and the dog]. Wien Tierarztl Monatsschr 1958; 6:338–49.
5. Robinson NE. The respiratory system. In: Muir WW, Hubbell JA, editors. Equine anesthesia-monitoring and emergency therapy. 2nd edition. Saunders-Elsevier; 2009. p. 20–5.
6. Tomasic M, Mann LS, Soma LR. Effects of sedation, anesthesia, and endotracheal intubation on respiratory mechanics in adult horses. Am J Vet Res 1997; 58:641–6.
7. Kerr CL, Mc Donell W. Oxygen supplementation and ventilatory support. In: Muir WW, Hubbell JA, editors. Equine anesthesia-monitoring and emergency therapy. 2nd edition. Saunders-Elsevier; 2009. p. 337–50.
8. Sorenson PR, Robinson NE. Postural effects on lung volumes and asynchronous ventilation in anaesthetized horses. J Appl Phys 1980;48:97–103.
9. Day TK, Gaynor JS, Muir WW, et al. Blood gas values during intermittent positive pressure ventilation and spontaneous ventilation in 160 anesthetized horses positioned in lateral or dorsal recumbency. Vet Surg 1995;24:76–266.
10. Hall LW. Disturbances of cardiopulmonary function in anesthetized horses. Equine Vet J 1971;3:95–8.
11. Khanna AK, McDonell WN, Dyson DH, et al. Cardiopulmonary effects of hypercapnia during controlled intermittent positive pressure ventilation in the horse. Can J Vet Res 1995;59:213–21.

12. Wagner AE, Bednarski RM, Muir WW III. Hemodynamic effects of carbon dioxide during intermittent positive-pressure ventilation in horses. Am J Vet Res 1990;51: 1922–9.
13. Mizuno Y, Aida H, Hara H, et al. Cardiovascular effects of intermittent positive pressure ventilation in the anesthetized horse. J Vet Med Sci 1994;56:39–44.
14. Puri GD, Singh H, Kaushik S, et al. Determination of ventilator minute volumes for normocapnic ventilation under anesthesia in healthy adults. Natl Med J India 1999;12:6–11.
15. Smith M. Nomogram. In: Manual Smith Respirator LA-2100. 2012. p. 15. Available at: http://www.veterinarytechnics.com. Accessed December 10, 2012.
16. Hedenstierna G, McCarthy G. The effect of anaesthesia and intermittent positive pressure ventilation with different frequencies on the anatomical and alveolar dead space. Br J Anaesth 1975;47:847–51.
17. Moens Y. Use of infra-red carbon dioxide analysis during general anaesthesia in the horse. Equine Vet J 1981;13:229–34.
18. Meyer RE, Short CE. Arterial to end-tidal CO_2 tension and alveolar dead space in halothane- or isoflurane anesthetized ponies. Am J Vet Res 1985;46:597–9.
19. Moens Y. Arterial-alveolar carbon dioxide tension difference and alveolar dead space in halothane anaesthetised horses. Equine Vet J 1989;21:282–4.
20. Teixeira Neto FJ, Luna SP, Massone F, et al. The effect of changing the mode of ventilation on the arterial-to-end-tidal CO_2 difference and physiologic dead space in laterally and dorsally recumbent horses during halothane anesthesia. Vet Surg 2000;29:200–5.
21. Hall LW, Gillespie JR, Tyler WS. Alveolar- arterial oxygen tension differences in anaesthetised horses. Br J Anaesth 1968;40:560–8.
22. Weaver BM, Walley RV. Ventilation and cardiovascular studies during mechanical control of ventilation in horses. Equine Vet J 1975;7:9–15.
23. Whitehair K, Willits N. Predictors of arterial oxygen tension in anesthetized horses:1610 cases (1192-1994). J Am Vet Med Assoc 1999;215:978–81.
24. Nyman G, Funkquist B, Kvart C, et al. Atelectasis causes gas exchange impairment in the anaesthetised horse. Equine Vet J 1990;22:317–24.
25. Wolff K, Moens Y. Gas exchange during inhalation anaesthesia of horses: a comparison between immediate versus delayed start of intermittent positive pressure ventilation – a clinical study. Pferdeheilkunde 2010;26:706–11, 24.
26. Nymann G, Hedenstierna G. Ventilation-Perfusion relationships in the anesthetized horse. Equine Vet J 1989;21:274–81.
27. Swanson CR, Muir WW. Dobutamine-induced augmentation of cardiac output does not enhance respiratory gas exchange in anesthetized recumbent healthy horses. Am J Vet Res 1988;47:1573–6.
28. Wilson DV, Mc Feely AM. Positive end-expiratory pressure during colic surgery in horses: 74 cases (1986-1988). J Am Vet Med Assoc 1991;199:917–21.
29. Wilson DV, Soma LR. Cardiopulmonary effects of positive end-expiratory pressure in anesthetized, mechanically ventilated ponies. Am J Vet Res 1990;51:734–9.
30. Niemann GF, Paskanik AM, Bredenberg CE. Effect of positive end-expiratory pressure on alveolar capillary perfusion. J Thorac Cardiovasc Surg 1988;95:712–6.
31. Tusman G, Suarez-Sipmann F, Böhm SH, et al. Monitoring dead space during recruitment and PEEP titration in an experimental model. Intensive Care Med 2006;32:1863–71.
32. Swanson CR, Muir WW. Hemodynamic and respiratory responses in halothane anesthetized horses exposed to positive end-expiratoty pressure alne and with dobutamine. Am J Vet Res 1988;49:539–42.

33. Hopster K, Kästner SB, Rohn K, et al. Intermittent positive pressure ventilation with constant positive end-expiratory pressure and alveolar recruitment manoeuvre during inhalation anaesthesia in horses undergoing surgery for colic, and its influence on the early recovery period. Vet Anaesth Analg 2011;38:169–77.

34. Bardoczky G, Engelman E, D'Hollander A. Continuous spirometry: an aid to monitoring ventilation during operation. Br J Anaesth 1993;71:747–51.

35. Moens Y, Gootjes P, Ionita JC, et al. In vitro validation of a pitot-based flow meter for the measurement of respiratory volume and flow in large animals. Vet Anaesth Analg 2009;36:209–19.

36. Moens Y. Clinical application of continuous spirometry with a pitot-based flow meter during equine anaesthesia. Equine Vet Educ 2010;22:354–60.

37. Filzek U, Fisher U, Scharner D, et al. Auswirkungen laparoskopischer Eingriffe unter Allgemeinanästhesie auf Lungenfunktionen. [Effects on pulmonary functions during laparascopic manipulations under general anesthesia]. Pferdeheilkunde 2001;17:482–6.

38. Oikkonen M, Tallgren M. Changes in respiratory compliance at laparascopy: measurements using side stream spirometry. Can J Anaesth 1995;42:495–7.

39. Tanskanen P, Kytta J, Randell T. The effect of patient positioning on dynamic lung compliance. Acta Anaesthesiol Scand 1997;41:602–6.

40. Rothen HU, Sporre B, Engeberg G. Prevention of atelectasis during general anaesthesia. Lancet 1995;345:1387–91.

41. Lachmann B. Open the lung and keep the lung open. Intensive Care Med 1992;18:319–21.

42. Amato MB, Barbas CS, Medeiros DM, et al. Beneficial effects of the "open lung approach" with low distending pressures in acute respiratory distress syndrome. A prospective randomized study on mechanical ventilation. Am J Respir Crit Care Med 1995;152:1835–46.

43. Tusman G, Belda JF. Treatment of anesthesia-induced lung collapse with lung recruitment maneuvers. Curr Anaesth Crit Care 2010;21:224–49.

44. Tusman G, Böhm SH, Vazquez daAnda G, et al. "Alveolar recruitment strategy" improves arterial oxygenation during general anaesthesia. Br J Anaesth 1999;82:8–13.

45. Bringewatt T, Hopster K, Kästner BR, et al. Influence of modified open lung concept ventilation on the cardiovascular and pulmonary function of horses during total intravenous anaesthesia. Vet Rec 2010;26:1002–6.

46. Schürmann P, Hopster K, Rohn K, et al. Optimierung des pulmonalen Gasaustausches während der Pferdenarkose durch Beatmung nach dem "Open Lung Concept" (Optimized gas exchange during inhalant anaesthesia in horses using "open lung concept" ventilation). Pferdeheilkunde 2008;24:236–42.

47. Suarez-Sipmann F, Böhm SH, Tusman G, et al. Use of dynamic compliance for open lung PEEP-titration in an experimental study. Crit Care Med 2007;35:214–21.

48. Iff I, Levionnois O, Moens Y. Alveolar recruitment manoeuvre in a Shetland pony anaesthetized for laparoscopic castration. Vet Med Austria/Wien Tierarztl Monatsschr 2007;94:264–8.

49. Levionnois O, Iff I, Moens Y. Successful treatment of hypoxemia by an alveolar recruitment maneuver in a horse during general anaesthesia for colic surgery. Pferdeheilkunde 2006;22:1–3.

50. Hallowell S, Sykes K. Tafonius. 2012. Available at: http://www.hallowell.com. Accessed August 03, 2012.

51. Schramel J, Van den Hoven R, Moens Y. In vitro validation of a new respiratory ultrasonic plethysmograph. Vet Anaesth Analg 2012;39:366–72.

52. Russold E, Ambrisko TD, Schramel J, et al. Measurement of tidal volume using respiratory ultrasonic plethysmography in anaesthetised, mechanically ventilated horses. Vet Anaesth Analg 2012. http://dx.doi.org/10.1111/j.1467-2995.2012.00751.

53. Lammer V, Ambrisko TD, Schramel JP, et al. In vitro validation of a new large animal spirometry device. In: Abstracts presented at the Association of Veterinary Anaesthetists Spring Meeting, Bari, Italy, 13-16 April 2011. Vet Anaesth Analg 2011;38:34–5.

54. Tusman G, Sipmann FS, Bohm SH. Rationale of dead space measurement by volumetric capnography. Anesth Analg 2012;114:866–74.

55. Maisch S, Reismann H, Fuellekrug B, et al. Compliance and dead space fraction indicate an optimal level of positive end-expiratory pressure after recruitment in anesthetized patients. Anesth Analg 2008;106:175–81.

56. Canet J, Gallart L. The dark side of the lung: unveiling regional lung ventilation with electrical impedance tomography. Anesthesiology 2012;116:1186–8.

57. Schramel J, Nagel C, Auer U, et al. Distribution of ventilation in pregnant Shetland ponies measured by electrical impedance tomography. Respir Physiol Neurobiol 2012;180:258–62.

Inhaled Anesthetics in Horses

Robert J. Brosnan, DVM, PhD, DACVA

KEYWORDS

• Isoflurane • Sevoflurane • Desflurane • MAC • Immobility • Amnesia • Horse

KEY POINTS

- The median effective concentration for inhaled anesthetics is commonly expressed as the minimum alveolar concentration (MAC).
- Volatile anesthetics with lower blood:gas partition coefficients (such as desflurane) equilibrate partial pressures between the alveoli and central nervous system (CNS) more quickly (resulting in a faster drug onset) than anesthetics with higher blood:gas partition coefficients (such as isoflurane).
- Inhaled anesthetics primarily act within the spinal cord (ventral horn) to produce immobility and within the brain (hippocampus and amygdala) to produce amnesia.
- Inhaled agents likely mediate CNS depression through inhibition of multiple excitatory cell receptors and potentiation of multiple inhibitory cell receptors.
- Different anesthetic end points (immobility, amnesia, muscle relaxation, autonomic quiescence, analgesia/hyperalgesia) occur at different anesthetic concentrations (MAC multiples).
- All volatile anesthetics cause dose-dependent respiratory depression (hypoventilation) and dose-dependent cardiovascular depression (hypotension).

Within 6 months after William T.G. Morton's seminal demonstration in 1846 that diethyl ether could be used to produce insensibility during surgery in people, veterinarians were actively experimenting with inhaled anesthesia in animals. Initial anecdotes regarding anesthesia in horses suggested that "a common soap-dish, filled with ether, and held to the animal's nose, was all that was required, and that the sensation was so delightful that it was eagerly inhaled, and that when sufficiently affected, the animal quietly laid down and submitted to whatever was requisite to be done." However, scientific study quickly revealed a different story; inhaled anesthetics were associated with violent and traumatic anesthetic inductions and recoveries as well as a high incidence of cardiovascular and respiratory system depression or arrest.[1] Inhaled agents comprise a useful class of anesthetic drugs, but equid size, behavior, and

Funding: This work was supported by a grant from the National Institutes of Health (GM092821-02).
Department of Surgical and Radiological Sciences, School of Veterinary Medicine, University of California, Davis, One Shields Avenue, Davis, CA 95616, USA
E-mail address: rjbrosnan@ucdavis.edu

Vet Clin Equine 29 (2013) 69–87
http://dx.doi.org/10.1016/j.cveq.2012.11.006
0749-0739/13/$ – see front matter © 2013 Elsevier Inc. All rights reserved.

physiology continue to contribute significant risks and challenges to inhalation anesthesia in horses relative to other species.[2]

INHALED ANESTHETIC AGENTS

Historically, a diverse array of volatile hydrocarbons have been used to produce general anesthesia in horses, including alkanes, alkenes, and ethers. Because of concerns about flammability, metabolic byproducts, toxicity, or arrhythmogenic side effects from older agents, modern inhalation anesthetic practice in North America principally uses 3 halogenated ether anesthetic derivatives: isoflurane, sevoflurane, and to a lesser degree, desflurane (**Fig. 1**).

There are several commonalities to all 3 modern agents (**Table 1**). All are clear, colorless, and liquid (desflurane scarcely so) at a room temperature of 20°C with a sweet to mildly pungent odor that is reminiscent of ether. Agents are also sufficiently halogenated such that flammability is restricted to a concentration range that is approximately 3 to 6 times the minimum alveolar concentration (MAC, a measure of the anesthetic median effective concentration [EC_{50}]); hence, they are nonflammable under clinical conditions. Administration in horses typically uses an agent-specific, out-of-circuit vaporizer that achieves desired drug concentrations through dilution of a saturated anesthetic vapor within a carrier gas comprising oxygen or a mixture of air-oxygen or helium-oxygen. Anesthetic gas mixtures are delivered via a common gas outlet to a standard large animal (>150-kg horses) or small animal (<150-kg horses) circle breathing circuit, and excess volume is relieved through an adjustable pressure-limiting valve. To minimize personnel exposure in the operating room, waste anesthetic gases are scavenged using an activated charcoal canister or exhausted to the outside environment, where they may act (albeit trivially) as greenhouse gases and contribute to global warming.[3]

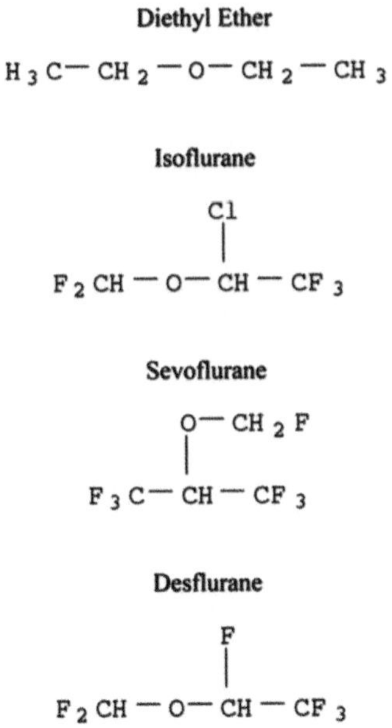

Diethyl Ether

$$H_3C-CH_2-O-CH_2-CH_3$$

Isoflurane

$$F_2CH-O-\overset{\overset{\textstyle Cl}{|}}{CH}-CF_3$$

Sevoflurane

$$F_3C-\overset{\overset{\textstyle O-CH_2F}{|}}{CH}-CF_3$$

Desflurane

$$F_2CH-O-\overset{\overset{\textstyle F}{|}}{CH}-CF_3$$

Fig. 1. Chemical structures of diethyl ether and modern haloether anesthetics.

Table 1
Summary of physical, chemical, and pharmacologic properties of contemporary inhaled ether anesthetics in horses

Property	Isoflurane	Sevoflurane	Desflurane
Molecular weight (amu)	184.49	200.05	168.04
Specific gravity (g/mL, 20°C)[92]	1.5019	1.5203	1.4651
Vapor pressure (mm Hg, 20°C)	240	160	664
Boiling point (°C)	48.5	58.5	23.5
Preservative	None	H_2O[7]	None
Stability in CO_2 absorbents[93] (breakdown product)	Excellent (carbon monoxide)	Good (compound A)	Excellent (carbon monoxide)
Partition coefficients (λ)[77]			
$\lambda_{oil:gas}$	98.9	51.3	19.2
$\lambda_{saline:gas}$	0.517	0.329	0.287
$\lambda_{blood:gas}$	1.13	0.648	0.537
MAC (% atm)	1.31[94]	2.84[74]	8.06[75]

Isoflurane (Aerrane, Attane, Forane, Isoflo)

Isoflurane is the most widely used volatile inhaled anesthetic in equine anesthesia, in part because it is also the least expensive. Isoflurane is the most potent of the 3 agents, as shown by the lowest MAC value of 1.3%, but its greater blood solubility both delays anesthetic equilibration between the alveoli and central nervous system (CNS) and delays anesthetic elimination during recovery. The vapor pressure-temperature relationship for isoflurane is almost colinear with that for halothane; therefore, although use of isoflurane-specific vaporizers is recommended, isoflurane can be safely used in clean, empty, and functional halothane vaporizers.[4]

Sevoflurane (Sevoflo, Ultane)

Sevoflurane is approximately half as potent as isoflurane and correspondingly has a MAC value that is about twice that for isoflurane. Its substantially lower blood solubility predicts faster elimination kinetics compared with isoflurane, although faster anesthetic recovery from sevoflurane may not always be realized in horses because of greater respiratory depression, which delays drug washout.[5]

Approximately 2% to 5% of sevoflurane undergoes hepatic metabolism, more than its comparatives, to hexafluoroisopropanol and free fluoride ions; the latter is a potential nephrotoxin. Sevoflurane reacts with certain carbon dioxide absorbents (either with the monovalent bases sodium hydroxide or potassium hydroxide found in classic soda lime formulations or with barium hydroxide found in Baralyme) to form a second nephrotoxin, compound A. Evidence of possible mild renal injury from sevoflurane in horses has been documented only during prolonged (>10 hours) low-flow techniques,[6] yet a potential nephrotoxic effect in horses cannot be excluded. Nonetheless, this potential risk can be easily reduced by avoiding carbon dioxide absorbents that contain more reactive bases (NaOH, KOH, Ba[OH]$_2$) or by using higher fresh gas flows to decrease compound A concentrations within the circuit.

Sevoflurane also reacts with Lewis acids (such as metal surfaces in anesthetic vaporizers, which may contain metal oxides) to produce hydrofluoric acid, which can corrode the vaporizer filling port and etch the vaporizer sight glass. A small amount of water (>150 ppm) is added as a preservative to some formulations to quench this reaction.[7] The vapor pressure-temperature relationship for sevoflurane is almost colinear with that for enflurane; therefore, although use of sevoflurane-specific vaporizers is recommended, sevoflurane can be safely used in clean, empty, and functional enflurane vaporizers.

Desflurane (Suprane)

Desflurane is the least potent of the 3 modern volatile anesthetics and has a MAC value that is about 6 times higher than that of isoflurane. Desflurane is also the least soluble agent in blood; consequently, horses rapidly awake even after a long 4-hour maintenance period.[8] Taken in combination with low lipid (oil) solubility, there is diminished total tissue capacitance for desflurane. Hence, total body drug uptake as ratio of drug potency (MAC) is less for desflurane compared with equipotent doses of either sevoflurane or isoflurane, and these differences are magnified further over time.[9] From a pharmacokinetic standpoint, desflurane could be the ideal inhalation anesthetic to facilitate rapid recoveries in large horses after long surgical procedures.

Desflurane (and, to a far lesser degree, isoflurane) can degrade in desiccated soda lime containing monovalent bases (NaOH or KOH) to produce carbon monoxide. In practice, it is unknown whether this degradation poses any real risks to desflurane-anesthetized horses connected to a breathing circuit with low fresh gas flows and dry classic soda lime. Partial hydration of the absorbent (as little as 4.8% water in soda lime or 9.7% water in Baralyme) is sufficient to prevent carbon monoxide production.[10] With a horse attached to an anesthetic circle system, large amounts of water condensation from expired gas may be more than adequate to ensure hydration of the CO_2 absorbent.

The boiling point of desflurane is only slightly higher than room temperature, and so it is not possible to achieve thermocompensation using a flow-over-the-wick variable bypass vaporizer, such as with the Tec 3, Tec 4, Tec 5, and Tec 7 isoflurane (GE Healthcare, Little Chalfont, UK) or sevoflurane vaporizers. Instead an electronic vaporizer (Tec 6 or Tec 6 Plus) is used to heat desflurane above its boiling point, and the resulting desflurane gas is injected through a variable resistor to achieve a precise and temperature-compensated anesthetic concentration.[11] Desflurane must be used only in desflurane-specific vaporizers; misfiling desflurane into conventional vaporizers intended for other agents produces a lethal anesthetic concentration.[12]

PHARMACOKINETICS

Pharmacokinetics describes the rates of drug delivery to the anesthetic circuit, pulmonary washin and uptake by the horse, distribution to active sites and other tissues, and metabolism and pulmonary washout. Pharmacokinetics describes what the animal does to the drug.

Drug Delivery to the Anesthetic Circuit

An adequate inspired anesthetic concentration requires an adequate circuit anesthetic concentration. Using a semiclosed circle breathing system with an out-of-circuit vaporizer, the rate of anesthetic concentration change in the circuit is a function of the anesthetic concentration and flow rate in the common gas outlet entering the circuit, the rate of anesthetic uptake from the circuit by the patient, and anesthetic dissolution or destruction within the anesthetic circuit itself. Setting aside drug uptake and distribution, the anesthetic concentration of an unprimed circuit as a function of time, C(t), during washin is described by the relationship:

$$C(t) = C_v \left(1 - e^{-t/\tau}\right)$$

where C_v is the vaporizer concentration, t is the washin time, and τ is the time constant.[13] The time constant is defined as the time required for the circuit concentration to change by about 63.2% of the difference between the starting concentration and the common gas outlet concentration. For example, when a sevoflurane vaporizer is turned to 3% in a circuit initially containing no anesthetic, the sevoflurane concentration after 1 time constant is 0.63 × (3%–0%) and equals 1.90% (**Table 2**). The duration of the time constant reflects the speed with which the circuit anesthetic concentrations can be changed; it is calculated as follows:

$$\tau = \frac{\text{circuit volume}}{\text{fresh gas flow rate}}$$

The volume contained in a large animal breathing circuit is about 50 L, about 7 times larger than a small animal circle system.[14] Large circuit volumes increase τ; this buffers against and delays changes to the circuit anesthetic concentration (see **Table 2**). From a practical standpoint, this situation means that a large animal circuit using control settings typical of a small animal circuit does not achieve sufficient anesthetic concentrations for sometimes an hour or longer (see **Table 2**). Two solutions

Table 2
The effect of circuit size, fresh gas flow rate, and vaporizer dial setting on the circuit time constant (τ) and the rate of increase of sevoflurane in an unprimed anesthetic circle breathing system connected to a 150-kg foal with a functional residual capacity (FRC) of 6 L. The time constant is defined as the total volume (circuit + FRC) divided by the fresh gas flow rate. The number of time constants (no. × τ) and the time in minutes to reach a circuit sevoflurane concentration equal to MAC (2.84%) are calculated. For this example, patient anesthetic uptake is not considered. The time to reach a desired anesthetic concentration can be hastened by decreasing circuit volume (using the smallest circuit and breathing bag or ventilator bellows that accommodates the horse's vital capacity), increasing the fresh gas flow rate, and increasing the vaporizer dial setting. Note that the vaporizer dial setting differs greatly from the circuit anesthetic concentration before the third time constant

Circuit volume (L)	7	7	7	7	50	50	50	50
Circuit + FRC (L)	13	13	13	13	56	56	56	56
Fresh gas flow (L/min)	2	2	6	6	2	2	6	6
Vaporizer setting (%)	3	6	3	6	3	6	3	6
Time constant (τ) (min)	6.5	6.5	1.2	1.2	28	28	9.3	9.3
$0 \times \tau$ (%)	0.00	0.00	0.00	0.00	0.00	0.00	0.00	0.00
$1 \times \tau$ (%)	1.90	3.79	1.90	3.79	1.90	3.79	1.90	3.79
$2 \times \tau$ (%)	2.59	5.19	2.59	5.19	2.59	5.19	2.59	5.19
$3 \times \tau$ (%)	2.85	5.70	2.85	5.70	2.85	5.70	2.85	5.70
$4 \times \tau$ (%)	2.95	5.89	2.95	5.89	2.95	5.89	2.95	5.89
No. × τ @ 2.84% sevoflurane	2.9 × τ	0.6 × τ	2.9 × τ	0.6 × τ	2.9 × τ	0.6 × τ	2.9 × τ	0.6 × τ
Time to 2.84% sevoflurane (min)	19	4	3	1	82	18	27	6

(often in combination) are used with large animal circuits to address this problem. First, higher fresh gas flows decrease τ and hasten the rate of increase in the circuit anesthetic concentration. Second, the vaporizer is set higher than the targeted circuit anesthetic concentration, a technique called overpressuring, so that this concentration target is reached in fewer time constants (see **Table 2**). An unavoidable consequence of overpressuring is that the concentration of anesthetic indicated by the vaporizer dial may bear little resemblance to (and thus cannot be used to approximate) the concentration of anesthetic within the breathing circuit.

Pulmonary Washin and Uptake

Volatile anesthetics are delivered to the alveoli via the inspired breath. Factors that increase alveolar minute ventilation (such as controlled ventilation) or increase the inspired anesthetic partial pressure (by increasing circuit anesthetic concentration) increase the alveolar anesthetic partial pressure and the alveolar-to-venous gradient that drives drug diffusion into the blood.

Anesthetic uptake from the lung (U_L) is described by the equation:

$$U_L = \lambda_{B:G}\, Q\, \frac{P_A - P_v}{P_B}$$

where P_A and P_v are the anesthetic partial pressures in the alveoli and blood, respectively, P_B is barometric pressure (equal to 760 mm Hg at sea level), Q is cardiac output, and $\lambda_{B:G}$ is the anesthetic blood:gas partition coefficient.[15] The Ostwald partition coefficient is a distribution constant that describes the ratio of gas molecules between a solvent and gas phase (or between 2 solvents) at a defined temperature at equilibrium (**Fig. 2**). When $\lambda_{B:G} = 1$, equal volumes of blood and gas contain the same

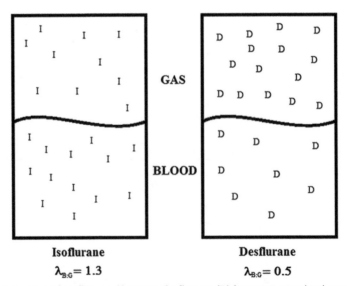

Fig. 2. Distribution of isoflurane (I) versus desflurane (D) between equal volumes of blood and gas phases within a closed container. Each container has the same number of anesthetic molecules, but there are more isoflurane molecules in the blood than the gas phase compared with desflurane, because isoflurane has a higher Ostwald blood:gas partition coefficient ($\lambda_{B:G}$). Isoflurane is more soluble in blood than desflurane.

number of anesthetic molecules. Higher $\lambda_{B:G}$ values indicate greater blood solubility; hence many more anesthetic molecules can move into the blood phase without causing as much of an increase in anesthetic concentration (or partial pressure) in the gas phase. Because anesthetics diffuse according to their gas phase partial pressure gradients (not according to liquid phase concentrations), highly blood-soluble agents maintain a high alveolar-to-venous partial pressure gradient (P_A–P_v), which promotes greater drug uptake. Likewise, greater cardiac output (Q) increases the volume of the blood into which anesthetic can diffuse, resulting in greater drug uptake.

Ventilation-perfusion (V/Q) mismatch and physiologic right-to-left shunts commonly occur in recumbent anesthetized horses, resulting in an increased alveolar-to-arterial oxygen gradient, which reflects impaired pulmonary gas exchange function. As with oxygen, physiologic pulmonary shunts also impede anesthetic uptake and cause an alveolar-to-arterial anesthetic gradient; this effect is greater at the beginning of anesthesia (when uptake is normally high) and greater with poorly soluble agents (because of limited capacity of high V/Q lung regions to make up for poor uptake from low V/Q lung regions).[16,17] Because modern inhaled agents all have low blood solubility, venous admixture in horses at the beginning of anesthesia likely results in an as yet undefined anesthetic gradient, in which the alveolar (or end-tidal) anesthetic partial pressure overestimates the arterial and CNS anesthetic partial pressures.

Anesthetic Distribution

Although it is perhaps counterintuitive, faster anesthetic uptake does not translate into faster anesthetic onset. The vessel-rich group (VRG) of tissues that receive high mass-specific blood flow include sites within the CNS responsible for anesthetic actions.[18] As a result, the partial pressure of anesthetic within the VRG is in delayed equilibrium with the partial pressure of anesthetic in the alveoli. Factors that promote increased anesthetic uptake from the alveoli, namely high cardiac output and high $\lambda_{B:G}$, oppose the rate of partial pressure increase of anesthetic in the alveoli, and thus delay the partial pressure increase in the CNS.

Volatile anesthetics are taken up by all body tissues at rates proportional to the arterial-to-tissue partial pressure gradient, tissue specific blood flow, and blood:tissue partition coefficient. Equilibration between the alveolar and VRG partial pressures is rapid with modern agents. However, tissues with poor blood flow, such as adipose, may take up drug throughout anesthesia without ever achieving equilibrium with the VRG or alveolar partial pressures. Because these agents are all more soluble in lipid than in water (see **Table 1**, $\lambda_{oil:gas} \gg \lambda_{saline:gas}$), adipose acts as a tremendous anesthetic reservoir. Restated, adipose has a high capacity to dissolve anesthetic and maintain a high anesthetic partial pressure gradient, which promotes further uptake and intertissue diffusion away from areas with lower partition coefficients (such as from the heart to the pericardial fat or from the intestine to the omental fat).[19] The amount of anesthetic contained in the adipose reservoir increases with obesity, anesthetic duration, and agents with a high $\lambda_{oil:gas}$. These same factors, in turn, prolong anesthetic washout and recovery time.

Anesthetic Washout and Recovery

Recovery occurs when anesthetic within active sites in the CNS is either eliminated or redistributed to other tissues. Although modern volatile anesthetics are subject to hepatic metabolism to varying extents, this is a comparatively minor route of elimination (even for sevoflurane). The MAC at which (human) patients awake from anesthesia (MAC-awake or MAC_{AW}) occurs at about 35% of MAC for isoflurane, sevoflurane, or desflurane.[20] Thus, even as horses are able to sense and react to their environment, a substantial amount of anesthetic remains and can affect neurologic and motor function during recovery.[5]

The percent clearance (%Cl) of an inhaled anesthetic can be expressed as follows:

$$\%Cl = \frac{V_A}{(\lambda_{B:G} \times Q) + V_A}$$

where $\lambda_{B:G}$ is the anesthetic blood:gas partition coefficient, Q is cardiac output, and V_A is alveolar minute ventilation.[19] Consequently, washout is hastened by increasing minute ventilation (such as with an oxygen demand valve) in the apneic or hypoventilating horse, although hyperventilation should be avoided, because the resulting cerebral vasoconstriction and reduced cerebral blood flow are counterproductive to anesthetic washout from the CNS. The second method to increase pulmonary clearance is to use anesthetic agents that are more insoluble in blood (such as desflurane vs isoflurane). In addition, for the 3 contemporary haloethers, the agents that are less soluble in blood are also less soluble in oil (fat). This finding means that anesthetic washout and recovery from desflurane are less affected by obesity or anesthetic time (context sensitivity) compared with isoflurane, because adipose capacitance, intertissue redistribution, and recirculation are also less.

PHARMACODYNAMICS

Pharmacodynamics addresses mechanisms of drug action, potency, and biologic effects (both desirable and adverse). Pharmacodynamics describes what the drug does to the animal.

Mechanisms of Action

How inhaled anesthetics act to produce anesthesia is a mystery.[21] This drug class has unusual pharmacologic properties. First, inhaled agents can reversibly immobilize not just humans and horses, but all vertebrate and invertebrate animals in which they have been studied. Efficacy is not limited to the animal kingdom, because inhaled anesthetics can even prevent movement in protozoa[22] and plants (those with touch-sensitive contractile leaves).[23] Second, most drugs require a specific shape, size, or polarity in order to interact with specific cell ligands and produce a pharmacologic effect. Yet there is no conserved structural motif among inhaled anesthetics, which include compounds as diverse as single atoms (xenon),[24] short-chain and long-chain alcohols,[25,26] and endogenous byproducts of metabolism (CO_2,[27] ammonia,[28] and ketones[29]), in addition to the contemporary and historical conventional agents.

Molecular sites of action

Around the turn of the twentieth century, Meyer and Overton empirically related increasing oil:gas partition coefficients ($\lambda_{oil:gas}$) to increasing anesthetic potency (**Fig. 3**). They hypothesized that anesthetics acted in the fatty substances in nerve cells: the lipid membrane.[30] This was an appealing hypothesis in part because it provided a unitary mechanism that could explain both the diversity in species affected by anesthetics and the diversity of drugs that could produce it. But was it correct? Volatile anesthetics dissolve in lipid bilayers and increase the fluidity or disorder in cell membrane, by which it was postulated that anesthesia might ensue.[31] However, temperature effects on lipid membrane fluidity exceed those produced by dissolution of inhaled agents, and temperature effects on MAC completely contradict those predicted by a membrane fluidity mechanism of action. Increasing body temperature increases membrane fluidity and anesthetic requirement, whereas decreasing body

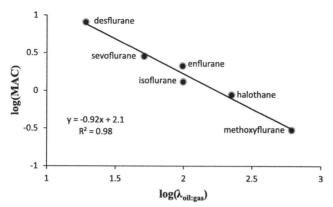

Fig. 3. Log-log plot of the anesthetic MAC in horses versus the Ostwald oil:gas partition coefficient ($\lambda_{oil:gas}$) at 37°C for 6 agents.[15,74,75,77,94,95] The Meyer-Overton hypothesis states that as lipid solubility increases (as reflected by an increased $\lambda_{oil:gas}$), the anesthetic potency also increases (as reflected by a decreased MAC).

temperature decreases membrane fluidity and MAC.[26,32] Moreover, some extremely hydrophobic compounds that should show anesthetic potency based on their lipid solubility are unable to produce immobility, and are appropriately named nonimmobilizers.[21]

These observations do not necessarily exclude a lipid site of anesthetic action. It is possible that distribution within the lipid bilayer is different between compounds that are very hydrophobic and ones that are less so.[33] Anesthetics with greater aqueous affinity concentrate closer to the membrane lipid-water interface and might alter the bilayer pressure profile that proteins must act against as they undergo conformational changes during cell excitation.[34] However, the most compelling argument against a lipid molecular mechanism of anesthetic action is that a lipid membrane need not be present to observe anesthetic-like effects. General anesthetics can inhibit enzyme activity of a purified protein, firefly luciferase, in concentrations that parallel in vivo anesthetic potency.[35] This finding suggests that proteins, not lipids, are the molecular targets for anesthetic action.

Anesthetics affect the function of many protein ion channels and receptors that in turn modulate neuronal excitability. In general, volatile anesthetics potentiate inhibitory cell targets such as γ-aminobutyric acid type A ($GABA_A$) receptors, glycine receptors, and 2-pore domain potassium channels; and these same agents also inhibit excitatory cell targets such as N-methyl-D-aspartate (NMDA) receptors, α-amino-3-hydroxy-5-methyl-4-isoxazole-propionic acid receptors, nicotinic receptors, and voltage-gated sodium channels.[21,25] In many of these proteins, specific mutations at putative anesthetic-binding sites alter anesthetic effects on receptor kinetics or ion conductance, and can sometimes render the receptor insensitive to 1 or more anesthetics altogether. Yet, this evidence for specific protein-receptor ligand interactions is inconsistent with the ability for so many chemically unrelated substances to modulate so many phylogenetically unrelated proteins. It is also unclear why the type of pharmacologic effect on a receptor or channel (either potentiation or inhibition) should vary depending on whether the receptor or channel itself is inhibitory or excitatory. How does the anesthetic know whether the receptor is inhibitory or excitatory? The creation of several mutant anesthetic-resistant receptor knockin or knockout mice models has failed to produce animals resistant to the immobilizing effects of anesthetics. Perhaps the critical receptor target responsible for inhaled anesthetic actions has yet to be discovered. Or perhaps anesthetic effects on cell receptors are mediated through nonspecific anesthetic-protein interactions.

Anatomic sites of action

The inhaled agents cause immobility and amnesia, but these distinct end points are achieved via actions at different CNS sites. In an experimental goat model in which the cerebral circulation was isolated from the rest of the body, selective brain isoflurane administration more than doubled the anesthetic requirement for immobility compared with whole-body isoflurane administration. This finding showed that the spinal cord, and not the brain, is principally responsible for preventing movement during surgery with inhaled anesthetics.[36] Within the spinal cord, immobility is most likely produced by depression of locomotor neuronal networks located in the ventral horn.[37] At subanesthetic concentrations, depression of premotor neurons in the spinal cord reduces proprioception[38] and may underlie the incoordination and ataxia commonly observed during inhaled anesthetic recoveries in horses.

In contrast, amnestic effects of inhaled anesthetics are produced by actions within the brain, most probably within the amygdala and hippocampus.[39] Lesions created within the amygdala of rats can block amnestic actions of sevoflurane.[40] On electroencephalography, hippocampal-dependent θ-rhythm frequency slows in proportion to the amnestic effects observed with subanesthetic concentrations of isoflurane in rats.[41] Furthermore, mutant mice lacking the gene encoding either the α_4 or β_3 subunits of $GABA_A$ receptors are resistant to isoflurane depression of hippocampus-dependent learning and memory,[42,43] and antagonism of α_5 subunit-containing $GABA_A$ receptors restores hippocampal-dependent memory during sevoflurane administration.[44] The mechanisms of inhaled anesthetic action responsible for amnesia are different from those responsible for immobility.

Theory: Willie Sutton hypothesis

Willie Sutton, an infamous bank thief who repeatedly escaped from prisons only to be recaptured each time after committing new heists, was asked by a newspaper reporter why he still kept robbing banks. His (apocryphal) reply was: "Because that's where the money is."[45]

Inhaled anesthetics have a large steady-state volume of distribution[5] and can modulate multiple cell targets to reduce cell excitability throughout the body. Glycine receptors,[46] NMDA receptors,[47] and potassium channels[48] likely contribute to immobility because these anesthetic-sensitive receptors are highly expressed within the spinal cord, the anatomic site responsible for immobility. $GABA_A$ receptors likely contribute to amnesia, because these anesthetic-sensitive receptors are highly expressed within the amygdala and hippocampus, the sites of memory formation.[42] Analogous to Willie Sutton, inhalants are agents of opportunity. Anesthetics cause immobility and amnesia by modulating multiple anesthetic-sensitive receptors at these sites, because that is where the receptors are.

The ability to modulate multiple receptors and multiple control points within a single receptor may explain how anesthetics that differ in potency or action among receptor types usually show apparently additive (rather than predicted synergistic) effects in combination.[49,50] Drugs that act principally through a single receptor should be reversible when an antagonist of that receptor is administered, and the antagonist should cause a dose-dependent increase in the anesthetic median effective dose. Although propofol and isoflurane both modulate $GABA_A$ receptors, only propofol shows dose-dependent reversal by $GABA_A$ receptor antagonists.[51] Thus $GABA_A$

receptors might contribute to immobility from isoflurane, but they do not act alone to cause immobility from isoflurane. The contribution of 1 receptor type to anesthesia can depend on the magnitude of contributions from other anesthetic-sensitive receptors. When either GABA$_A$ or glycine receptors are inhibited within the spinal cord, isoflurane or sevoflurane must inhibit more NMDA receptors in order to produce immobility.[52,53] The sum of inhibition at multiple excitatory targets plus potentiation at multiple inhibitory targets depresses CNS function and is most probably responsible for what we observe as general anesthesia.

Anesthetic End Points and Potency

At a minimum, general anesthesia consists of immobility and amnesia,[54] but may also include muscle relaxation, autonomic quiescence, analgesia, and unconsciousness. Inhaled agents achieve most of these end points, but not at the same anesthetic concentration.

Inhaled anesthetics produce immobility at 1 MAC, which is defined as the mean of the highest end-tidal anesthetic concentration that allows movement and the lowest end-tidal anesthetic concentration that prevents movement in response to a painful stimulus.[55] Essentially, MAC represents an EC$_{50}$ for inhaled agents. MAC is increased by hyperthermia, hypernatremia, and CNS stimulants such as ephedrine. Anesthetic MAC is decreased by hypothermia, hyponatremia, severe hypercapnea or hypoxemia or hypotension, hepatic or renal failure, sepsis, senescence, pregnancy, and by many sedatives and other anesthetics. In contrast to MAC-sparing effects in humans and many animals, opioids have little or no effect on inhaled anesthetic potency in horses at clinically relevant doses,[56,57] although opioids at very high doses may increase MAC.[58]

The median anesthetic concentration (in humans) at which wakefulness occurs, defined by voluntary responsiveness to commands, occurs around 0.4 times MAC and is defined as MAC-awake.[59,60] Amnesia occurs at even lower anesthetic concentrations (about 0.3 times MAC).[61,62] Hence, even although movement may inadvertently occur at a sub-MAC anesthetic plane, horses should not form memories of surgical events if the inhalant concentrations are more than 0.4 to 0.5 times MAC.

Inhalants also cause dose-dependent muscle relaxation, although profound relaxation using a nonbalanced technique requires deep anesthetic planes, at which cardiorespiratory side effects are similarly profound. Although inhalants inhibit nicotinic cholinergic receptors and intracellular calcium release, skeletal muscle relaxation is primarily mediated via spinal actions rather than via direct actions on the muscle itself.[63]

Autonomic responses to surgical stimuli are manifested clinically by hypertension, tachycardia, or tachypnea. This occurs because peri-MAC anesthetic doses that cause depression of ventral horn spinal neurons and that prevent movement do not affect afferent nerve conduction or dorsal horn input.[64,65] As with profound muscle relaxation, deep anesthetic planes with inhalants alone produce autonomic quiescence, but at severe cost to cardiorespiratory function.

To the extent that they interfere with the motivational-affective dimension of pain,[66] inhaled anesthetics prevent horses from experiencing pain at concentrations higher than MAC. In addition, anesthetic concentrations between 0.8 and 1.0 times MAC decrease (but do not ablate) windup and central sensitization and so may help prevent heightened postoperative pain sensitivity; however, higher concentrations of contemporary ether anesthetics offer no further benefit in this regard.[67,68] Inhaled anesthetic concentrations between 0.4 and 0.8 times MAC decrease withdrawal responses to noxious stimuli, but lower concentrations cause hyperalgesia, with a peak effect at

0.1 times MAC.[69,70] This is the result of potent nicotinic cholinergic receptor inhibition by modern inhaled agents.[71] For horses recovering from anesthesia, low end-tidal inhalant concentrations could enhance postoperative pain and could contribute to poor recovery quality.

It is difficult to define at what anesthetic concentration unconsciousness occurs, in part, because unconsciousness itself is difficult to define. Intuitively, it must occur over the wide concentration range between MAC-awake and depths that produce an isoelectric electroencephalogram.[72] However, the extent to which a horse experiences consciousness, the types and number of sensory-neural inputs responsible for consciousness, and the perception of consciousness are all undoubtedly different from that of the human experience, such as defined by Descartes: *Cogito ergo sum* ("I think, therefore I am"). It may not be possible to definitively test for the presence or absence of consciousness when administering drugs that act via the CNS to produce immobility and amnesia.[54] The study of inhaled agents and consciousness thus remains as much the domain of philosophers as it does anesthesiologists.

Anesthetic Side Effects

Respiratory

All agents cause dose-dependent hypoventilation. As a species, horses are more sensitive to the respiratory-depressant effects of volatile anesthetics than are dogs, cats, or humans. Lightly anesthetized horses at concentrations around MAC commonly have arterial CO_2 tensions greater than 65 mm Hg and may require ventilatory support. Isoflurane doses ranging between 1 and 2 times MAC linearly decrease respiratory rate,[73] but sevoflurane and desflurane concentrations higher than 1.5 times MAC may be associated with a high incidence of apnea as a result of greater respiratory depression.[74,75] Tidal volume also decreases with dose, and this response is most steep higher than 1.5 times MAC. Temporal increases in respiratory depression during the first 2 hours of anesthesia parallel reductions in respiratory rate.[76]

Compared with isoflurane, greater respiratory depression from sevoflurane delays anesthetic washout, despite a lower sevoflurane blood:gas partition coefficient.[77] In this manner, sevoflurane pharmacodynamics can adversely modify its own pharmacokinetics.[5]

Cardiovascular

All agents cause dose-dependent hypotension (**Fig. 4**). Although the modern ether-type anesthetics are potent vasodilators, reductions in blood pressure higher than 1 MAC are largely caused by dose-dependent decreases in stroke volume and cardiac output.[73–75] When ventilated to maintain isocapnea, cardiac output is better preserved between 1.0 and 1.5 times MAC with desflurane and sevoflurane than with isoflurane. However, at concentrations higher than 1.5 times MAC, cardiac output is significantly higher with desflurane than with either isoflurane or sevoflurane.[73–75] Desflurane is associated with increased sympathetic tone, particularly after large concentration changes,[78] which might mask some of the hypotension observed with other agents. During the first 2 hours of anesthesia, at least with isoflurane in horses, there are also time-dependent increases in stroke volume, cardiac output, and blood pressure, which may be the result of endogenous β-adrenergic receptor activation.[79]

When anesthesia is induced and maintained using only an inhaled anesthetic, mean blood pressure is often 70 mm Hg or greater at light to moderate anesthetic planes (see **Fig. 4**). However, when combined with sedative hypnotics such as α_2-agonists or acepromazine, hypotension is likely.[80,81] Because induction and maintenance with an inhalant alone are uncommon (and often impractical) and because horses

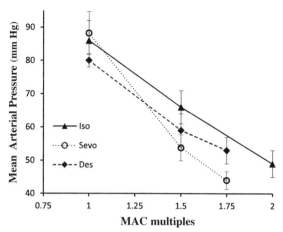

Fig. 4. Direct mean arterial blood pressure as a function of anesthetic dose expressed as multiples of MAC for isoflurane, sevoflurane, and desflurane. (*Data from* Refs.[73–75])

require higher tissue perfusion pressures for adequate blood flow to dependent muscle having high intracompartmental pressure, a positive inotrope is often necessary to support a mean arterial pressure higher than 70 mm Hg under clinical conditions.[82]

CNS
The brain, cerebrospinal fluid, and cerebral blood volume are contained within the rigid calvarium, and because horses have very high intracranial elastance, even a small uncompensated increase in volume of any of these components causes a large increase in intracranial pressure.[83] The difference between mean arterial pressure and intracranial pressure is the cerebral perfusion pressure (the driving pressure for blood flow into the brain). If increased intracranial pressure is not accompanied by similar increases in mean arterial pressure, the cerebral perfusion pressure decreases, possibly putting the patient at risk for cerebral ischemia.

Intracranial pressure in awake horses remains constant irrespective of head position,[84] but cerebral vasodilation during inhalant anesthesia causes large increases in intracranial pressure (sometimes similar in magnitude to values seen in patients with severe head trauma), which is exacerbated by dorsal recumbency, head-down positioning, hypercapnea during spontaneous ventilation, and anesthetic time during controlled ventilation.[18,85–87] In many species, inhaled anesthetics interfere with compensatory vasomotor responses to changes in cerebral perfusion pressure, resulting in either uncontrolled excess or inadequate tissue perfusion. Over a wide range of perfusion pressures, isoflurane-anesthetized horses maintain regional cerebral blood flow relatively constant, albeit at a low flow, which may still place animals at risk for tissue hypoxia.[88] Blood flow to the thoracolumbar spinal cord is particularly low, and further reduction may predispose to postanesthetic myelomalacia in horses.[89]

Visceral organs
Aside from the formation of potentially nephrotoxic metabolites discussed previously (see section on sevoflurane), undesirable effects on visceral organs principally arise from decreased cardiac output and blood flow redistribution to other parts of the animal. Without inotropic support, for example, isoflurane in ponies dose-dependently reduces renal perfusion, to the point that blood flow is less than half of

awake values at 1.5 times MAC. Blood flow to the small intestine and colon is halved by only 1.1 times MAC isoflurane compared with awake measurements, but higher anesthetic concentrations do not further reduce flow.[90] What effect such reductions might have in bowel that is already compromised, as in the equine patient with intestinal colic, remains unknown. Although hepatic arterial flow is unaffected, dose-dependent reductions in intestinal perfusion by modern ether-type anesthetics cause similar reductions in portal venous and total hepatic blood flow.[91] As a result, inhaled anesthetics can decrease hepatic clearance of many drugs, including other anesthetics.

SUMMARY

Inhaled anesthetics provide an effective means to produce immobility, amnesia, and muscle relaxation in horses undergoing surgical and diagnostic procedures. They offer many advantages, including favorable washout kinetics, elimination that is not dependent on hepatic or renal function, and the ability to indirectly monitor real-time effect-site concentrations by measuring alveolar (end-tidal) anesthetic gas concentrations. At the same time, these agents present several potential challenges in horses, including profound cardiovascular and respiratory depression and the requirement of large-volume anesthetic delivery circuits that slow anesthetic uptake and delay changes to anesthetic inspired concentrations and depth.

REFERENCES

1. Henderson A, Cherry WA. Experiments on the effects of ether in the horse. Lancet 1847;49:396–7.
2. Johnston GM, Eastment JK, Wood JL, et al. The confidential enquiry into perioperative equine fatalities (CEPEF): mortality results of Phases 1 and 2. Vet Anaesth Analg 2002;29:159–70.
3. Langbein T, Sonntag H, Trapp D, et al. Volatile anaesthetics and the atmosphere: atmospheric lifetimes and atmospheric effects of halothane, enflurane, isoflurane, desflurane and sevoflurane. Br J Anaesth 1999;82:66–73.
4. Steffey EP, Woliner MJ, Howland D. Accuracy of isoflurane delivery by halothane-specific vaporizers. Am J Vet Res 1983;44:1072–8.
5. Brosnan RJ, Steffey EP, Escobar A. Effects of hypercapnic hyperpnea on recovery from isoflurane or sevoflurane anesthesia in horses. Vet Anaesth Analg 2012;39:335–44.
6. Driessen B, Zarucco L, Steffey EP, et al. Serum fluoride concentrations, biochemical and histopathological changes associated with prolonged sevoflurane anaesthesia in horses. J Vet Med A Physiol Pathol Clin Med 2002;49:337–47.
7. Kharasch ED, Subbarao GN, Cromack KR, et al. Sevoflurane formulation water content influences degradation by Lewis acids in vaporizers. Anesth Analg 2009;108:1796–802.
8. Steffey EP, Mama KR, Brosnan RJ, et al. Effect of administration of propofol and xylazine hydrochloride on recovery of horses after four hours of anesthesia with desflurane. Am J Vet Res 2009;70:956–63.
9. Lockwood G. Theoretical context-sensitive elimination times for inhalation anaesthetics. Br J Anaesth 2010;104:648–55.
10. Fang ZX, Eger EI 2nd, Laster MJ, et al. Carbon monoxide production from degradation of desflurane, enflurane, isoflurane, halothane, and sevoflurane by soda lime and Baralyme. Anesth Analg 1995;80:1187–93.

11. Andrews JJ, Johnston RV Jr. The new Tec6 desflurane vaporizer. Anesth Analg 1993;76:1338–41.

12. Andrews JJ, Johnston RV Jr, Kramer GC. Consequences of misfilling contemporary vaporizers with desflurane. Can J Anaesth 1993;40:71–6.

13. Steffey EP, Howland D Jr. Rate of change of halothane concentration in a large animal circle anesthetic system. Am J Vet Res 1977;38:1993–6.

14. Solano AM, Brosnan RJ, Steffey EP. Rate of change of oxygen concentration for a large animal circle anesthetic system. Am J Vet Res 2005;66:1675–8.

15. Eger EI 2nd. Anesthetic uptake and action. Baltimore (MD): Williams & Wilkins; 1974.

16. Stoelting RK, Longnecker DE. The effect of right-to-left shunt on the rate of increase of arterial anesthetic concentration. Anesthesiology 1972;36:352–6.

17. Saidman LJ, Eger EI 2nd. The influence of ventilation-perfusion abnormalities upon the uptake of inhalation anesthetics. Clin Anesth 1967;1:79–87.

18. Brosnan RJ, Esteller-Vico A, Steffey EP, et al. Effects of head-down positioning on regional central nervous system perfusion in isoflurane-anesthetized horses. Am J Vet Res 2008;69:737–43.

19. Eger EI 2nd, Saidman LJ. Illustrations of inhaled anesthetic uptake, including intertissue diffusion to and from fat. Anesth Analg 2005;100:1020–33.

20. Eger EI 2nd. Age, minimum alveolar anesthetic concentration, and minimum alveolar anesthetic concentration-awake. Anesth Analg 2001;93:947–53.

21. Sonner JM, Antognini JF, Dutton RC, et al. Inhaled anesthetics and immobility: mechanisms, mysteries, and minimum alveolar anesthetic concentration. Anesth Analg 2003;97:718–40.

22. Nunn JF, Sturrock JE, Wills EJ, et al. The effect of inhalational anaesthetics on the swimming velocity of *Tetrahymena pyriformis*. J Cell Sci 1974;15:537–54.

23. Livingston JS. On the anaesthetic effects of chloroform, ether, and amylene, on sensitive plants. Transactions of the Botanical Society Edinburgh 1860;6:323–5.

24. Cullen SC, Gross EG. The anesthetic properties of xenon in animals and human beings, with additional observations on krypton. Science 1951;113:580–2.

25. Brosnan R, Gong D, Cotten J, et al. Chirality in anesthesia II: stereoselective modulation of ion channel function by secondary alcohol enantiomers. Anesth Analg 2006;103:86–91.

26. Won A, Oh I, Brosnan R, et al. Hypothermia decreases ethanol MAC in rats. J Anesth 2006;20:247–50.

27. Brosnan RJ, Eger EI 2nd, Laster MJ, et al. Anesthetic properties of carbon dioxide in the rat. Anesth Analg 2007;105:103–6.

28. Brosnan RJ, Yang L, Milutinovic PS, et al. Ammonia has anesthetic properties. Anesth Analg 2007;104:1430–3.

29. Won A, Oh I, Liao M, et al. The minimum alveolar anesthetic concentration of 2-, 3-, and 4-alcohols and ketones in rats: relevance to anesthetic mechanisms. Anesth Analg 2006;102:1419–26.

30. Overton CE. Studies of narcosis. London: Chapman and Hall; 1991.

31. Miller KW, Pang KY. General anaesthetics can selectively perturb lipid bilayer membranes. Nature 1976;263:253–5.

32. Eger EI 2nd, Saidman LJ, Brandstater B. Temperature dependence of halothane and cyclopropane anesthesia in dogs: correlation with some theories of anesthetic action. Anesthesiology 1965;26:764–70.

33. Pohorille A, Wilson MA, New MH, et al. Concentrations of anesthetics across the water-membrane interface; the Meyer-Overton hypothesis revisited. Toxicol Lett 1998;100–101:421–30.

34. Cantor RS. Breaking the Meyer-Overton rule: predicted effects of varying stiffness and interfacial activity on the intrinsic potency of anesthetics. Biophys J 2001;80: 2284–97.
35. Franks NP, Lieb WR. Do general anaesthetics act by competitive binding to specific receptors? Nature 1984;310:599–601.
36. Antognini JF, Schwartz K. Exaggerated anesthetic requirements in the preferentially anesthetized brain. Anesthesiology 1993;79:1244–9.
37. Jinks SL, Atherley RJ, Dominguez CL, et al. Isoflurane disrupts central pattern generator activity and coordination in the lamprey isolated spinal cord. Anesthesiology 2005;103:567–75.
38. Barter LS, Mark LO, Antognini JF. Proprioceptive function is more sensitive than motor function to desflurane anesthesia. Anesth Analg 2009;108:867–72.
39. Eger EI 2nd, Xing Y, Pearce R, et al. Isoflurane antagonizes the capacity of flurothyl or 1,2-dichlorohexafluorocyclobutane to impair fear conditioning to context and tone. Anesth Analg 2003;96:1010–8.
40. Alkire MT, Nathan SV. Does the amygdala mediate anesthetic-induced amnesia? Basolateral amygdala lesions block sevoflurane-induced amnesia. Anesthesiology 2005;102:754–60.
41. Perouansky M, Rau V, Ford T, et al. Slowing of the hippocampal theta rhythm correlates with anesthetic-induced amnesia. Anesthesiology 2010;113:1299–309.
42. Rau V, Iyer SV, Oh I, et al. Gamma-aminobutyric acid type A receptor alpha 4 subunit knockout mice are resistant to the amnestic effect of isoflurane. Anesth Analg 2009;109:1816–22.
43. Rau V, Oh I, Liao M, et al. Gamma-aminobutyric acid type A receptor beta3 subunit forebrain-specific knockout mice are resistant to the amnestic effect of isoflurane. Anesth Analg 2011;113:500–4.
44. Zurek AA, Bridgwater EM, Orser BA. Inhibition of alpha5 gamma-aminobutyric acid type A receptors restores recognition memory after general anesthesia. Anesth Analg 2012;114:845–55.
45. Sutton W, Linn E. Where the money was. New York: Viking Press; 1976.
46. Zhang Y, Laster MJ, Hara K, et al. Glycine receptors mediate part of the immobility produced by inhaled anesthetics. Anesth Analg 2003;96:97–101.
47. Stabernack C, Sonner JM, Laster M, et al. Spinal N-methyl-d-aspartate receptors may contribute to the immobilizing action of isoflurane. Anesth Analg 2003;96: 102–7.
48. Heurteaux C, Guy N, Laigle C, et al. TREK-1, a K+ channel involved in neuroprotection and general anesthesia. EMBO J 2004;23:2684–95.
49. Eger EI 2nd, Tang M, Liao M, et al. Inhaled anesthetics do not combine to produce synergistic effects regarding minimum alveolar anesthetic concentration in rats. Anesth Analg 2008;107:479–85.
50. Brosnan RJ, Pham TL. Does anesthetic additivity imply a similar molecular mechanism of anesthetic action at N-methyl-D-aspartate receptors? Anesth Analg 2011;112:568–73.
51. Sonner JM, Zhang Y, Stabernack C, et al. GABA(A) receptor blockade antagonizes the immobilizing action of propofol but not ketamine or isoflurane in a dose-related manner. Anesth Analg 2003;96:706–12.
52. Brosnan RJ. GABA(A) receptor antagonism increases NMDA receptor inhibition by isoflurane at a minimum alveolar concentration. Vet Anaesth Analg 2011;38: 231–9.
53. Brosnan RJ, Thiesen R. Increased NMDA receptor inhibition at an increased Sevoflurane MAC. BMC Anesthesiol 2012;12:9.

54. Eger EI 2nd, Sonner JM. Anaesthesia defined (gentlemen, this is no humbug). Best Pract Res Clin Anaesthesiol 2006;20:23–9.

55. Eger EI 2nd, Saidman LJ, Brandstater B. Minimum alveolar anesthetic concentration: a standard of anesthetic potency. Anesthesiology 1965;26:756–63.

56. Pascoe PJ, Steffey EP, Black WD, et al. Evaluation of the effect of alfentanil on the minimum alveolar concentration of halothane in horses. Am J Vet Res 1993;54: 1327–32.

57. Thomasy SM, Steffey EP, Mama KR, et al. The effects of i.v. fentanyl administration on the minimum alveolar concentration of isoflurane in horses. Br J Anaesth 2006;97:232–7.

58. Steffey EP, Eisele JH, Baggot JD. Interactions of morphine and isoflurane in horses. Am J Vet Res 2003;64:166–75.

59. Dwyer R, Bennett HL, Eger EI 2nd, et al. Effects of isoflurane and nitrous oxide in subanesthetic concentrations on memory and responsiveness in volunteers. Anesthesiology 1992;77:888–98.

60. Chortkoff BS, Eger EI 2nd, Crankshaw DP, et al. Concentrations of desflurane and propofol that suppress response to command in humans. Anesth Analg 1995;81: 737–43.

61. Kandel L, Chortkoff BS, Sonner J, et al. Nonanesthetics can suppress learning. Anesth Analg 1996;82:321–6.

62. Sonner JM, Xing Y, Zhang Y, et al. Administration of epinephrine does not increase learning of fear to tone in rats anesthetized with isoflurane or desflurane. Anesth Analg 2005;100:1333–7.

63. Ginz HF, Zorzato F, Iaizzo PA, et al. Effect of three anaesthetic techniques on isometric skeletal muscle strength. Br J Anaesth 2004;92:367–72.

64. Kim J, Yao A, Atherley R, et al. Neurons in the ventral spinal cord are more depressed by isoflurane, halothane, and propofol than are neurons in the dorsal spinal cord. Anesth Analg 2007;105:1020–6.

65. Larrabee MG, Posternak JM. Selective action of anesthetics on synapses and axons in mammalian sympathetic ganglia. J Neurophysiol 1952;15: 91–114.

66. Melzack R, Casey KL. Sensory, motivational, and control determinants of pain: a new conceptual model. In: Kenshalo D, editor. The skin senses. Springfield, Illinois: Thomas; 1967. p. 423–43.

67. O'Connor TC, Abram SE. Inhibition of nociception-induced spinal sensitization by anesthetic agents. Anesthesiology 1995;82:259–66.

68. Mitsuyo T, Dutton RC, Antognini JF, et al. The differential effects of halothane and isoflurane on windup of dorsal horn neurons selected in unanesthetized decerebrated rats. Anesth Analg 2006;103:753–60.

69. Zhang Y, Eger EI 2nd, Dutton RC, et al. Inhaled anesthetics have hyperalgesic effects at 0.1 minimum alveolar anesthetic concentration. Anesth Analg 2000; 91:462–6.

70. Sonner J, Li J, Eger EI 2nd. Desflurane and nitrous oxide, but not nonimmobilizers, affect nociceptive responses. Anesth Analg 1998;86:629–34.

71. Flood P, Sonner JM, Gong D, et al. Isoflurane hyperalgesia is modulated by nicotinic inhibition. Anesthesiology 2002;97:192–8.

72. Alkire MT, Hudetz AG, Tononi G. Consciousness and anesthesia. Science 2008; 322:876–80.

73. Steffey EP, Howland D Jr. Comparison of circulatory and respiratory effects of isoflurane and halothane anesthesia in horses. Am J Vet Res 1980;41: 821–5.

74. Steffey EP, Mama KR, Galey FD, et al. Effects of sevoflurane dose and mode of ventilation on cardiopulmonary function and blood biochemical variables in horses. Am J Vet Res 2005;66:606–14.

75. Steffey EP, Woliner MJ, Puschner B, et al. Effects of desflurane and mode of ventilation on cardiovascular and respiratory functions and clinicopathologic variables in horses. Am J Vet Res 2005;66:669–77.

76. Steffey EP, Hodgson DS, Dunlop CI, et al. Cardiopulmonary function during 5 hours of constant-dose isoflurane in laterally recumbent, spontaneously breathing horses. J Vet Pharmacol Ther 1987;10:290–7.

77. Soares JH, Brosnan RJ, Fukushima FB, et al. Solubility of haloether anesthetics in human and animal blood. Anesthesiology 2012;117:48–55.

78. Weiskopf RB, Moore MA, Eger EI 2nd, et al. Rapid increase in desflurane concentration is associated with greater transient cardiovascular stimulation than with rapid increase in isoflurane concentration in humans. Anesthesiology 1994;80: 1035–45.

79. Dunlop CI, Steffey EP, Miller MF, et al. Temporal effects of halothane and isoflurane in laterally recumbent ventilated male horses. Am J Vet Res 1987;48: 1250–5.

80. Steffey EP, Kelly AB, Farver TB, et al. Cardiovascular and respiratory effects of acetylpromazine and xylazine on halothane-anesthetized horses. J Vet Pharmacol Ther 1985;8:290–302.

81. Steffey EP, Pascoe PJ, Woliner MJ, et al. Effects of xylazine hydrochloride during isoflurane-induced anesthesia in horses. Am J Vet Res 2000;61: 1225–31.

82. Raisis AL. Skeletal muscle blood flow in anaesthetized horses. Part II: effects of anaesthetics and vasoactive agents. Vet Anaesth Analg 2005;32:331–7.

83. Brosnan RJ, LeCouteur RA, Steffey EP, et al. Intracranial elastance in isoflurane-anesthetized horses. Am J Vet Res 2004;65:1042–6.

84. Brosnan RJ, LeCouteur RA, Steffey EP, et al. Direct measurement of intracranial pressure in adult horses. Am J Vet Res 2002;63:1252–6.

85. Brosnan RJ, Steffey EP, LeCouteur RA, et al. Effects of body position on intracranial and cerebral perfusion pressures in isoflurane-anesthetized horses. J Appl Physiol 2002;92:2542–6.

86. Brosnan RJ, Steffey EP, LeCouteur RA, et al. Effects of ventilation and isoflurane end-tidal concentration on intracranial and cerebral perfusion pressures in horses. Am J Vet Res 2003;64:21–5.

87. Brosnan RJ, Steffey EP, LeCouteur RA, et al. Effects of duration of isoflurane anesthesia and mode of ventilation on intracranial and cerebral perfusion pressures in horses. Am J Vet Res 2003;64:1444–8.

88. Brosnan RJ, Steffey EP, Lecouteur RA, et al. Effects of isoflurane anesthesia on cerebrovascular autoregulation in horses. Am J Vet Res 2011;72:18–24.

89. Trim CM. Postanesthetic hemorrhagic myelopathy or myelomalacia. Vet Clin North Am Equine Pract 1997;13:73–7.

90. Manohar M, Gustafson R, Goetz TE, et al. Systemic distribution of blood flow in ponies during 1.45%, 1.96%, and 2.39% end-tidal isoflurane-O2 anesthesia. Am J Vet Res 1987;48:1504–10.

91. Frink EJ Jr, Morgan SE, Coetzee A, et al. The effects of sevoflurane, halothane, enflurane, and isoflurane on hepatic blood flow and oxygenation in chronically instrumented greyhound dogs. Anesthesiology 1992;76:85–90.

92. Laster MJ, Fang Z, Eger EI 2nd. Specific gravities of desflurane, enflurane, halothane, isoflurane, and sevoflurane. Anesth Analg 1994;78:1152–3.

93. Kharasch ED, Powers KM, Artru AA. Comparison of Amsorb, sodalime, and Baralyme degradation of volatile anesthetics and formation of carbon monoxide and compound a in swine in vivo. Anesthesiology 2002;96:173–82.
94. Steffey EP, Howland D Jr, Giri S, et al. Enflurane, halothane, and isoflurane potency in horses. Am J Vet Res 1977;38:1037–9.
95. Johnson CB, Taylor PM. Comparison of the effects of halothane, isoflurane and methoxyflurane on the electroencephalogram of the horse. Br J Anaesth 1998; 81:748–53.

Balanced Anesthesia and Constant-Rate Infusions in Horses

Alexander Valverde, DVM, DVSc

KEYWORDS

- Partial intravenous anesthesia • Total intravenous anesthesia • Alpha-2 agonist
- Opioids • Lidocaine • Ketamine • Benzodiazepine • Guaifenesin

KEY POINTS

- Injectable anesthetics with analgesic properties are useful additions to the muscle-relaxant and depressive effects on the central nervous system of volatile anesthetics in balanced anesthetic techniques.
- Reduced doses of individual drugs are possible in balanced anesthetic techniques because of the synergistic or additive effects.
- Pharmacokinetic data generated in horses for injectable anesthetics allow administration of injectable anesthetics using constant-rate infusions to achieve steady-state plasma concentrations and predictable pharmacodynamic effects during volatile anesthesia.
- The use of balanced techniques for the maintenance of anesthesia should also have positive effects during the recovery period that allow for controlled and safe recoveries in horses.

Balanced anesthesia consists of administering a combination of anesthetic drugs and anesthetic adjuvants to provide the patient with the desired effects of these drugs while minimizing their adverse side effects, such that analgesia, hypnosis, and stable cardiorespiratory function are enhanced.

Balanced anesthesia was first introduced in human anesthesia by incorporating local anesthetic techniques used to provide analgesia with volatile anesthetics used at the time (ether, chloroform, ethyl chloride, nitrous oxide, and ethylene).[1] Soon after, it also included the use of barbiturates and opioids combined with volatile anesthesia, and it was noted how overall balanced anesthesia allowed the use of moderate amounts of several anesthetic drugs rather than a large dose of any of the individual drugs.[1]

The equine literature is recognizing this topic, and several reviews have appeared in the last few years.[2–4] In this article, the concept of balanced anesthesia refers to the combination of volatile anesthesia with at least 1 injectable anesthetic during the

Department of Clinical Studies, Ontario Veterinary College, University of Guelph, 50 Stone Road, Guelph, Ontario N1G 2W1, Canada
E-mail address: valverde@uoguelph.ca

Vet Clin Equine 29 (2013) 89–122
http://dx.doi.org/10.1016/j.cveq.2012.11.004
0749-0739/13/$ – see front matter © 2013 Elsevier Inc. All rights reserved.

maintenance period. The term balanced anesthesia is considered interchangeable with partial intravenous anesthesia (PIVA). The use of exclusively injectable anesthetic drugs (total intravenous anesthesia [TIVA]) or volatile anesthetics to maintain anesthesia is described in articles elsewhere in this issue.

One important concept that should be observed with balanced techniques is that patients may exhibit a lesser degree of central nervous system (CNS) depression resulting from the analgesic and relaxation properties of some of the injectable anesthetics, which facilitates handling of the patient on a lighter plane of anesthesia; however, this may predispose to awareness, although this concept is impossible to determine in veterinary patients. Awareness is the result of inadequate general anesthesia that does not provide unconsciousness and prevention of recall during surgical stimulation.

The incidence of awareness during insufficient anesthesia is estimated at 0.0068% to 0.13% in human patients,[5,6] for whom the use of muscle relaxants for paralysis is more frequent than in veterinary patients, and probably a major contributing factor to inadequate anesthetic depth and inability to recognize signs of a light plane of anesthesia.[7] In human anesthesia, anesthetic techniques that do not involve volatile anesthetic drugs or use low end-tidal anesthetic concentrations rely excessively on the use of intraoperative opioids and muscle relaxants. These techniques are preferentially used in critical patients (American Society of Anesthesiologists physical status >3) and are more likely to result in awareness.[5,6,8] Likewise, patients who have received reduced doses of premedication, induction, and maintenance anesthetics are also more likely to show awareness along with signs of hypertension, tachycardia, or purposeful movement,[9] although these signs are not always associated with awareness during anesthesia.[8]

The use of balanced techniques in critical patients could be falsely associated with a higher risk because these techniques tend to be selected more often for unstable cases to avoid the depressive cardiorespiratory effects that are induced by exclusive or excessive use of volatile anesthesia. Mortality studies in horses have shown an increased risk (4 to 10 times) for emergency cases in comparison with elective cases.[10,11] Use of total volatile anesthesia is also associated with a higher risk of mortality in comparison with TIVA.[12] Because critical cases tend to require longer anesthesia time than elective cases, it is likely that balanced techniques are selected more often than total volatile or intravenous techniques to meet patients' requirements for analgesia, support of cardiorespiratory function, and anesthetic depth, which may lend false bias toward a negative correlation between use of balanced techniques and survival.

In a recent retrospective study, mares with dystocia that received guaifenesin-xylazine-ketamine or α_2-agonist–ketamine before recovery from volatile anesthesia tended to have 25 and 9 times higher odds of death, respectively, than those receiving only an α_2-agonist.[13] The critical intraoperative condition of this population of patients often dictates lighter planes of volatile anesthesia that need to be combined with injectable intravenous anesthetics for adequate maintenance, which could result in a greater level of sedation and ataxia during recovery. These factors are probably major ones in the reported outcome, and should not be misinterpreted as inadequate anesthetic techniques.

PHARMACOKINETIC PRINCIPLES

The effects or actions elicited by a drug are part of the pharmacodynamics, whereas drug concentrations in plasma, blood, or tissues, and the distribution and clearance of the drug, are part of its pharmacokinetic profile. Injectable anesthetic drugs used as part of balanced techniques can be administered as single intermittent doses or as a single bolus followed by a constant-rate infusion (CRI) throughout the maintenance period. A CRI of a specific drug can provide predictable plasma concentrations (steady-state concentrations) and predictable pharmacodynamic actions. Similar to a volatile anesthetic delivered through a precision vaporizer to maintain a constant end-tidal concentration, the delivery of an injectable anesthetic as a CRI can maintain plasma or blood concentrations that reflect those in specific target tissues (ie, brain) to obtain a particular desired effect.

A drug delivered as a CRI achieves a steady-state concentration when the elimination rate does not surpass the administration rate and vice versa, and is achieved when the drug is fully distributed at equilibrium throughout the body, known as the volume of distribution at steady state (V_d^{ss}).[14] The time frame at which steady-state concentrations are achieved corresponds to the equivalent of 5 terminal half-lives or 3 time constants of the specific drug if a bolus dose (loading dose) was not administered before the CRI.[15] The purpose of the bolus dose is to fill the volume of distribution and facilitate the matching of delivery and clearance of the drug, so that steady-state concentrations are achieved promptly.

There are 2 ways to administer a CRI:

- Fixed infusion rate. A fixed infusion rate is easy to implement and assumes that a steady state is achieved based on adequate distribution that matches clearance. However, as compartments (tissues) are saturated and the infusion continues at the same rate, it is possible to exceed clearance and achieve higher than expected plasma concentrations. Therefore, adjustments in the CRI may be necessary over time for this modality.
- Target infusion rate. For this type of infusion, the rate is adjusted according to the specific rate constants that govern the drug's movement between compartments, based on saturation of the tissues, as determined in previous pharmacokinetic studies for the study population. Target infusions are therefore more difficult to establish in clinical situations, because knowledge of specific pharmacokinetic constants is required as well as a target-controlled infusion system consisting of a syringe pump and computer program. For this reason, fixed infusion rates are used more commonly than target-controlled rates in equine anesthesia.

Factors to consider during a CRI of any drug include knowledge of plasma concentrations that are associated with a particular desired effect (ie, analgesia or degree of sedation), the terminal half-life, the volume of distribution at steady state, and the clearance. All these terms are summarized in the following formulas.

$$D = C_p^{ss} \times V_d^{ss}$$ Formula 1

To calculate the loading dose (D) it is necessary to know the desired plasma concentration at steady state (C_p^{ss}) and the volume of distribution (V_d^{ss}) of the drug.

$$CRI = C_p^{ss} \times Cl_\beta$$ Formula 2

To calculate the CRI it is necessary to know the desired plasma concentration and the rate at which the drug is eliminated (clearance, Cl_β), where clearance is:

$$Cl_\beta = \beta \times V_d^{ss}$$ Formula 3

where the elimination constant (β) is derived from the terminal half-life ($t_{1/2}$):

$$t_{1/2} = \frac{0.693}{\beta} \qquad \text{Formula 4}$$

so that:

$$\beta = \frac{0.693}{t_{1/2}} \qquad \text{Formula 5}$$

Using published data for anesthetic drugs of interest to balanced techniques, it is possible to estimate useful loading doses and CRI; however, because pharmacokinetics are often determined under research conditions, without the influence of other drugs or disease, one should be cautious about the possible deviations that may result from altering blood flow to organs responsible for biotransformation and clearance of drugs when other drugs have been administered or when there are alterations in the health status of the patient. For example, the pharmacokinetics of fentanyl differed between conscious and isoflurane-anesthetized horses, with a smaller V_d^{ss} and higher clearance during anesthesia, despite similar terminal half-lives in both conditions,[16] whereas xylazine had a longer terminal half-life and lower clearance in halothane-anesthetized horses than in conscious ponies.[17–19] Similarly, lidocaine showed higher blood concentrations, lower clearance, and smaller V_d^{ss} in healthy sevoflurane-anesthetized than in conscious horses[20] but, by contrast, those same pharmacokinetic parameters were similar between conscious horses and horses with colic under sevoflurane anesthesia.[21]

With regard to concurrent administration of different injectable drugs, individual plasma concentrations may not be affected by concurrent administration (eg, administration of an intravenous bolus of flunixin 2 hours after a loading dose and CRI of lidocaine in conscious healthy horses[22]), or may show different pharmacokinetic parameters (eg, a longer terminal half-life for xylazine despite no change in clearance rate when morphine is administered simultaneously in halothane-anesthetized horses[19]).

CARDIORESPIRATORY FUNCTION DURING BALANCED ANESTHESIA

Balanced anesthesia techniques provide a combination of the cardiorespiratory effects observed during TIVA and volatile anesthesia. Cardiorespiratory function tends to be better with TIVA techniques than with volatile anesthesia.[23,24] Usually blood pressure is higher with TIVA because of the continuous use of α_2-agonists, which increase systemic vascular resistance; cardiac output (the product of heart rate and stroke volume) is similar between both techniques even when α_2-agonists reduce heart rate, but at the same time can preserve stroke volume, whereas volatile anesthetics maintain heart rate but reduce stroke volume.[23–25] The effects on arterial blood gases are also similar between both techniques.[24]

Balanced anesthesia preserves cardiovascular function but has the potential to depress respiratory function to a greater extent than TIVA or volatile anesthesia. Most studies describing balanced anesthesia techniques under research or clinical conditions have used mechanical ventilation; therefore, the effects of balanced techniques on respiratory function have not been well defined. In one study, isoflurane-anesthetized horses administered a dexmedetomidine CRI tended to need more mechanical ventilatory support to prevent prolonged apnea and maintain normocapnia to slight hypercapnia compared with horses on isoflurane alone,[26] but in another study, opposite effects were seen in isoflurane-anesthetized horses receiving a detomidine CRI versus isoflurane alone.[27]

INJECTABLE ANESTHETICS COMMONLY USED FOR BALANCED ANESTHESIA

Infusions developed for standing sedation can be used in the anesthetized horse to enhance CNS depression and anesthetic depth and therefore help decrease volatile anesthetic requirements (minimum alveolar concentration [MAC]). It is also possible to benefit from the sedative and analgesic effects of these injectable anesthetics in the postoperative period during recovery by preventing early uncontrolled attempts and therefore improve the quality of recovery.

Doses of individual anesthetics used for balanced techniques can be similar to those used for standing sedation, but in general are lower than doses used for TIVA. The adjustment in doses is based, among other factors, on the requirements for volatile anesthesia, required duration of anesthesia, expected degree of pain, and preference/experience of the anesthetist with the different drugs included in the balanced technique.

In a recent review on the use of injectable anesthetics and analgesics by practitioner members of the American Association of Equine Practitioners, it was reported that xylazine as a sedative drug followed by ketamine and diazepam was the preferred induction protocol for short-term anesthesia (20 minutes' duration), whereas for long-term anesthesia (>30 minutes' duration) a mixture of guaifenesin, ketamine, and xylazine or isoflurane was used most commonly.[28] In this review of balanced anesthesia all of these drugs are described, in addition to other α_2-agonists, lidocaine, and opioids. Background basic information on drugs and doses used for sedative, PIVA, or TIVA purposes is provided to help better understand the implications of doses, and the resultant pharmacokinetics and pharmacodynamics elicited by those doses and the interactions between drugs.

α_2-Agonists

Most balanced anesthesia techniques include the use of an α_2-agonist (xylazine, romifidine, medetomidine, dexmedetomidine, or detomidine) because of their potent sedative and analgesic effects (**Tables 1–3**). The uses and effects of α_2-agonists have been recently reviewed for equine patients.[29] Possible cardiovascular effects of α_2-agonists include a decrease in heart rate, an initial increase in systemic vascular resistance and blood pressure followed by a decrease, an initial decrease in cardiac output and respiratory rate followed by recovery to baseline, and transient decreases in partial pressure of arterial oxygen, and these effects may vary with respect to their administration to the conscious or the anesthetized patient.[26,27,29–31]

The potent effects of α_2-agonists on heart rate, blood pressure, and cardiac output can be exacerbated in the presence of volatile anesthetics; however, it seems that sevoflurane or isoflurane in combination with α_2-agonists results in less cardiorespiratory depression than halothane in combination with α_2-agonists. The sparing effect (decrease in MAC of the volatile anesthetic) induced by α_2-agonists allows for similar or better cardiovascular function at equipotent doses than the volatile anesthetic alone. For example, in horses anesthetized with end-tidal concentrations of 2.8% to 3.1% sevoflurane and supported with dobutamine, cardiac indices were similar to those in horses receiving a CRI of guaifenesin-ketamine-medetomidine combined with 1.4% to 1.6% end-tidal sevoflurane.[32]

Sedative CRI doses of α_2-agonists used in balanced techniques do not affect cardiac output significantly in horses maintained at values close to 1 MAC. Cardiac

Table 1
Doses of α_2-agonists used in horses for sedation, and partial (PIVA) or total (TIVA) intravenous general anesthesia in clinical and research studies, and doses calculated from available pharmacokinetic data

	Bolus Loading Dose (IV)	CRI Dose Used	CRI Calculated[a]	Other Injectable Anesthetics Included in CRI	Purpose of CRI and Other Drugs Included in Those Protocols
Xylazine	0.25–1.0 mg/kg	0.6–0.72 mg/kg/h (10–12 µg/kg/min)	0.12–1 mg/kg/h (2–16 µg/kg/min)	None	Standing sedation[44,45]
		1.2 mg/kg/h (20 µg/kg/min)	0.12–1 mg/kg/h (2–16 µg/kg/min)	Ketamine	After discontinuation of sevoflurane or isoflurane anesthesia[48,49]
		2.1–4.2 mg/kg/h (35–70 µg/kg/min)	2.4–3.9 mg/kg/h (40–65 µg/kg/min)	Ketamine	TIVA Xylazine, guaifenesin[50]
Romifidine	80 µg/kg	30 µg/kg/h (0.5 µg/kg/min)	18–30 µg/kg/h[b] (0.3–0.5 µg/kg/min)	None or butorphanol	Standing sedation[51]
	80 µg/kg	18 µg/kg/h (0.3 µg/kg/min)	18–30 µg/kg/h[b] (0.3–0.5 µg/kg/min)		PIVA Diazepam, ketamine, isoflurane (1.0–1.6% end-tidal)[52]
	0.1 mg/kg	82.5 µg/kg/h (1.4 µg/kg/h)	18–30 µg/kg/h[b] (0.3–0.5 µg/kg/min)	Ketamine Guaifenesin	TIVA ketamine[24]
Medetomidine	5 µg/kg	3.5–5 µg/kg/h	2.4–6 µg/kg/h	None or morphine	Standing sedation[31,53]
	7 µg/kg or Xylazine 1 mg/kg or Romifidine 50 µg/kg	2.75–5 µg/kg/h	2.4–6 µg/kg/h	None or butorphanol or Lidocaine or Ketamine or Guaifenesin	PIVA Xylazine, romifidine, diazepam, ketamine, isoflurane (0.65%–1.1% end-tidal), sevoflurane (1.5% end-tidal)[32–34,43,56]
Dexmedetomidine	3.5 µg/kg	1–1.75 µg/kg/h	1–2.5 µg/kg/h[b]	None	PIVA Midazolam, ketamine, isoflurane (1.5% end-tidal)[26,58]

Detomidine	15 μg/kg	8.5 μg/kg/h	13–38 μg/kg/h	Butorphanol	Standing sedation[62]
	10–30 μg/kg	5–11 μg/kg/h	13–38 μg/kg/h	None	PIVA
					Diazepam, ketamine acepromazine, guaifenesin, thiamylal, isoflurane (1% end-tidal) or halothane (0.6–1.1% end-tidal)[27,63,64]

Xylazine: Therapeutic plasma concentrations of 340–800 ng/mL (PIVA or standing sedation) or 2150–3440 ng/mL (TIVA); clearance of 6 or 20 mL/kg/min.[17–19,44–47,50]

Medetomidine: Therapeutic plasma concentration of 1.0–1.5 ng/mL; clearance of 40 or 67 mL/kg/min.[42,53]

Detomidine: Therapeutic plasma concentration of 10–30 ng/mL; clearance of 21 mL/kg/min.[59–61,63]

Abbreviations: CRI, constant-rate infusion; IV, intravenous.

a Dose calculated from available pharmacokinetic data (CRI = Therapeutic dose × Clearance).

b Dose recommended based on clinical information.

Table 2
Doses of lidocaine, ketamine, and opioids used in horses for sedation, and partial (PIVA) or total (TIVA) intravenous general anesthesia in clinical and research studies, and doses calculated from available pharmacokinetic data

	Bolus Loading Dose (IV)	CRI Dose Used	CRI Calculated[a]	Other Injectable Anesthetics Included in CRI	Purpose of CRI and Other Drugs Included in Those Protocols
Lidocaine	1.5–5 mg/kg	1.5–6 mg/kg/h (25–100 µg/kg/min)	4.5 mg/kg/h (75 µg/kg/min)	None or medetomidine or ketamine or morphine	PIVA Acepromazine, detomidine, xylazine, romifidine, levomethadone, midazolam, diazepam, ketamine, isoflurane (end-tidal 0.59–1.1%), halothane (1.2% end-tidal)[33,34,43,67,68,71,74]
Ketamine	0.3 mg/kg	3.6 mg/kg/h (60 µg/kg/min)	1.9 mg/kg/h (32 µg/kg/min)	Xylazine	After discontinuation of sevoflurane or isoflurane anesthesia[48,49]
	3 mg/kg	1.0–3.6 mg/kg/h (17–60 µg/kg/min)	1.9 mg/kg/h (32 µg/kg/min)	Lidocaine or medetomidine or morphine or midazolam	PIVA Xylazine, romifidine, morphine, diazepam, midazolam, isoflurane (0.59–1.0% end-tidal), sevoflurane (1.7% end-tidal)[43,71,74,124]
	2–2.2 mg/kg	2–9 mg/kg/h (33–150 µg/kg/min)	1.9 mg/kg/h (32 µg/kg/min)	None or xylazine or romifidine or guaifenesin or midazolam or diazepam	TIVA Xylazine or romifidine, midazolam, guaifenesin, and ketamine[24,25,50,123]

Opioids					
Morphine	0.05 mg/kg	0.03 mg/kg/h (0.5 µg/kg/min)	0.04–0.07 mg/kg/h (0.6–1.2 µg/kg/min)	Medetomidine	Sedation[31]
	0.15 mg/kg	0.1 mg/kg/h (1.7 µg/kg/min)	0.04–0.07 mg/kg/h (0.6–1.2 µg/kg/min)	None	PIVA Romifidine, diazepam, ketamine, halothane[108,110]
Butorphanol	25 µg/kg	25 µg/kg/h	31.5 µg/kg/h	Medetomidine	PIVA Medetomidine, diazepam, ketamine, isoflurane (1.06% end-tidal)[56]

Lidocaine: Therapeutic plasma concentration of 3000 ng/mL; clearance of 25 mL/kg/min.[20,21,66]
Ketamine: Therapeutic plasma concentration of 1000 ng/mL; clearance of 32 mL/kg/min.[86]
Morphine: Therapeutic plasma concentration of 15–30 ng/mL; clearance of 40 mL/kg/min.[105,112–114]
Butorphanol: Therapeutic plasma concentration of 25 ng/mL; clearance of 21 mL/kg/min.[102]
[a] Dose calculated from available pharmacokinetic data (CRI = Therapeutic dose × Clearance).

Table 3
Doses of benzodiazepines and guaifenesin used in horses for partial (PIVA) or total (TIVA) intravenous general anesthesia in clinical and research studies, and doses recommended based on clinical information

	Bolus Loading Dose (IV)	CRI Dose Used	CRI Recommended[a]	Other Injectable Anesthetics Included in CRI	Purpose of CRI and Other Drugs Included in Those Protocols
Diazepam	None	0.11 mg/kg/h (1.8 µg/kg/min)	20 µg/kg/h[b] (0.33 µg/kg/min)	Xylazine and ketamine	TIVA Xylazine, ketamine[123]
Midazolam	40 µg/kg	20 µg/kg/h (0.33 µg/kg/min)	20 µg/kg/h[b] (0.33 µg/kg/min)	Ketamine and medetomidine	PIVA Medetomidine, ketamine, sevoflurane (1.5% end-tidal)[124]
	0.1 mg/kg	0.12 mg/kg/h (2 µg/kg/min)	20 µg/kg/h[b] (0.33 µg/kg/min)	Xylazine and ketamine	TIVA Xylazine, ketamine[126]
Guaifenesin	None	25 mg/kg/h (0.42 mg/kg/min)	25 mg/kg/h (0.42 mg/kg/min)	Medetomidine and ketamine	PIVA Medetomidine, diazepam, ketamine, sevoflurane (1.5% end-tidal)[32]
	2.2 mg/kg	50–100 mg/kg/h (0.8–1.7 mg/kg/min)	25 mg/kg/h (0.42 mg/kg/min)	Romifidine Ketamine	TIVA Romifidine, ketamine[24,123,125,128]

Guaifenesin: Therapeutic plasma concentration of 50,104 ng/mL; estimated clearance of 8.3 mL/kg/min based on an average half-life of 75 minutes and a V_d of 0.9 L/kg.[126–128]

[a] Dose calculated from available pharmacokinetic data (CRI = Therapeutic dose × Clearance).
[b] Dose recommended based on clinical information.

indices of 53 to 55 mL/kg/min in horses under 1.1% end-tidal isoflurane combined with 5 μg/kg/h of medetomidine and 50 μg/kg/min (3 mg/kg/h) of lidocaine,[33] or with 3.5 μg/kg/h of medetomidine alone,[34] were similar to values of 48 to 65 mL/kg/min obtained in horses sedated with a bolus of medetomidine (5 μg/kg) and morphine (50 μg/kg) followed by a CRI of medetomidine-morphine (5–30 μg/kg/h) for laparoscopic surgery.[31]

Use of α_2-agonists during pregnancy has been a concern because of early evidence for increases in intrauterine pressure as a result of increased uterine contractions in mares.[35] However, different studies have demonstrated their safety at different stages of pregnancy.[36–39] The author uses them as part of balanced techniques in pregnant mares undergoing elective or emergency anesthesia.

Horses administered CRIs of α_2-agonists tend to produce vast amounts of urine, owing to hyperglycemia from hypoinsulinemia and a reduced secretion rate of arginine vasopressin.[40–42] Therefore, it is recommended that urine output be monitored and, if possible, to routinely catheterize the bladder and empty it during anesthesia for procedures longer than 1 hour, to prevent the horse from retaining urine and voiding in the recovery stall and/or causing discomfort that affects the quality of recovery.[33]

Although ideally the bolus dose and subsequent CRI should consist of the same α_2-agonist, some anesthetists do not necessarily use the same α_2-agonist for both purposes. A loading dose with xylazine or romifidine has been followed by a CRI of medetomidine in some studies to maintain receptor occupancy,[33,43] on the assumption that clinical effects are maintained by the 2 α_2-agonists because of the interaction of the agonist with the specific receptor, as long as the terminal half-life of the drug used for the loading dose is not exceeded before the start of the CRI with the second α_2-agonist.

Xylazine

Pharmacokinetics Xylazine has a terminal half-life of 75 minutes in conscious ponies after an intravenous dose of 1.1 mg/kg and of 50 minutes in conscious horses after an intravenous dose of 0.6 mg/kg, with a clearance of 19 to 21 mL/kg/min in ponies and horses.[17,18] Anesthesia seems to affect the pharmacokinetics of xylazine, because in halothane-anesthetized horses an intravenous dose of 0.5 mg/kg increased the terminal half-life to 118 minutes and decreased the clearance to 6 mL/kg/min.[19] In the latter study, concurrent administration of intravenous morphine (0.1 or 0.2 mg/kg) increased the half-life of xylazine to approximately 150 minutes, although not statistically significant, and did not affect clearance.[19]

CRI use for sedation Plasma concentrations of 340 to 800 ng/mL have been associated with sustained standing sedation, as assessed by constant degree of head drop, using CRIs of 0.69 to 0.72 mg/kg/h (11–12 μg/kg/min) after an intravenous loading dose of 1 mg/kg,[44,45] and serum concentrations of 300 to 500 ng/mL were measured after a loading dose of 0.25 mg/kg and a CRI of 0.6 mg/kg/h (10 μg/kg/min).[46]

CRI use for PIVA Xylazine (0.5–1 mg/kg, intravenously) decreases the MAC of halothane or isoflurane by approximately 20% to 35% in a dose-dependent and time-dependent fashion.[19,47]

Using the concept of balanced anesthesia, horses were discontinued from 90 minutes of sevoflurane or isoflurane administration and then administered a CRI for 30 minutes of 1.2 mg/kg/h (20 μg/kg/min) of xylazine and 3.6 mg/kg/h (60 μg/kg/min) of ketamine after a bolus dose of 0.15 mg/kg xylazine and 0.3 mg/kg ketamine, to maintain anesthetic depth while the volatile anesthetic was eliminated, before allowing horses to recover, which resulted in better recoveries than in horses receiving sevo-flurane, but not isoflurane, without the CRI.[48,49]

CRI use for TIVA Plasma concentrations of 2150 to 3440 ng/mL were measured during CRIs of 2.1 to 4.2 mg/kg/h (35–70 µg/kg/min) of xylazine combined with ketamine at 5.4 to 7.2 mg/kg/h (90–120 µg/kg/min) administered for approximately 1 hour, after induction with xylazine (0.75 mg/kg), guaifenesin, and ketamine. These concentrations were associated with adequate immobilization and cardiorespiratory function, and with very good to excellent recoveries.[50] Horses stood up 1 hour after stopping the CRI, with plasma concentrations of 1030 ng/mL for the group receiving the highest CRI of xylazine. One group of horses that did not receive xylazine in the CRI, but only the induction dose (0.75 mg/kg) and a CRI of ketamine at (9 mg/kg/h [150 µg/kg/min]), stood up with plasma concentrations of 780 ng/mL within 33 minutes after stopping the CRI.[50]

Defining a CRI for PIVA Because of the wide variation in plasma concentrations between standing sedative techniques (300–780 ng/mL) and TIVA techniques (2150–3440 ng/mL), the anesthetist needs to define the purpose of including xylazine in the CRI, that is, analgesia or anesthesia or marked sedation. For balanced techniques it is likely that desired effects include those associated with sedative doses in order to avoid excessive cardiorespiratory depression that results from combining volatile anesthesia with high doses of α_2-agonists. Therefore, the author usually attempts to calculate CRIs for balanced techniques based on plasma concentrations reported during sedation. For example, using formula 2, to achieve a concentration of 800 ng/mL a CRI of 1.0 mg/kg/h (16 µg/kg/min) is necessary if the clearance of 20 mL/kg/min determined in conscious horses is used,[17,18] but the dose is 0.3 mg/kg/h (5 µg/kg/min) if the clearance of 6 mL/kg/min determined in anesthetized horses is used (see **Table 1**).[19,47] Clinically the author uses doses of 0.5 to 1.0 mg/kg/h (8–16 µg/kg/min) xylazine, the lower end of the dose range, if other drugs such as ketamine (1–2 mg/kg/h [16.7–33.3 µg/kg/min]) are included in the balanced technique.

Romifidine
Pharmacokinetics There is no information on the specific pharmacokinetics of romifidine. Plasma concentrations of approximately 30 ng/mL were measured during steady state of a CRI for standing sedation.[51]

CRI for sedation For standing sedation, administration of 80 µg/kg romifidine resulted in adequate sedation that was further maintained at a steady state with additional single doses for 2 hours, resulting in a calculated CRI of 30 µg/kg/h (0.5 µg/kg/min).[51]

CRI for PIVA A CRI of 18 µg/kg/h (0.3 µg/kg/min) in isoflurane-anesthetized horses induced with 80 µg/kg romifidine and a combination of diazepam (0.1 mg/kg) and ketamine (3 mg/kg) allowed elective surgery with end-tidal concentrations between 1% and 1.6%, whereas a similar group without the CRI required end-tidal concentrations between 1.6% and 2.2% that resulted in lower arterial blood pressures and higher demand for dobutamine administration.[52]

CRI for TIVA Induction with romifidine, 0.1 mg/kg and ketamine, 2.2 mg/kg, followed by CRIs of romifidine (82.5 µg/kg/h [1.38 µg/kg/min]), ketamine (6.6 mg/kg/h [110 µg/kg/min]) and guaifenesin (100 mg/kg/h [1.7 mg/kg/min]) for the first 30 minutes, and then reduced to 50 mg/kg/h (0.84 mg/kg/min) of guaifenesin and unaltered rates of romifidine and ketamine for the next 45 minutes, provided satisfactory results, with better blood pressures and indirect indicators of stroke volume than in horses induced in a similar fashion but maintained on 0.95% end-tidal halothane.[24]

Defining a CRI for PIVA The lack of information on the pharmacokinetics of romifidine makes it difficult to recommend a specific CRI dose for balanced anesthesia. One simple way of choosing a CRI dose clinically is to estimate the duration of action (eg, for sedation) of a predetermined dose and repeat that dose per unit of time while adjusting it for the amount of drug that may still be present in blood and tissues; therefore, it is recommended that the dose be underestimated in subsequent administrations. For example, the effects of a single intravenous bolus of 80 μg/kg on sedation decreased after approximately 40 minutes,[51] and boluses of only 20 μg/kg were necessary to regain the degree of sedation. Because other drugs are likely to be involved during balanced anesthesia, a sedative dose lower than the full one (80–120 μg/kg) is recommended. Doses reported for sedation or PIVA (18–30 μg/kg/h [0.3–0.5 μg/kg/min]) seem to be appropriate for horses on volatile anesthesia (see **Table 1**).

Medetomidine

Pharmacokinetics The pharmacokinetic parameters of medetomidine have been determined in conscious ponies after an intravenous dose of 7 μg/kg and in horses after an intravenous dose of 10 μg/kg.[42,53] Medetomidine has a V_d^{ss} of 2.2 L/kg in ponies and of 1.9 L/kg in horses, as well as one of the shortest terminal half-lives (51 minutes in ponies; 29 minutes in horses) and highest clearances (67 mL/kg/min in ponies; 40 mL/kg/min in horses) among α_2-agonists, which facilitates its administration as part of a CRI.[42,53]

CRI for sedation Medetomidine has been recommended at an intravenous loading dose of 5 μg/kg and CRI of 3.5 μg/kg/h to provide standing sedation in ponies.[42] It has also been administered at a CRI of 5 μg/kg/h after the same loading dose for standing laparoscopic surgery.[31]

CRI for PIVA A CRI of 3.5 μg/kg/h reduced isoflurane end-tidal concentrations by 20% when compared with horses not receiving it during surgery,[54] and by 28% in research ponies under desflurane anesthesia.[55]

Several studies using balanced techniques with medetomidine have used induction protocols with medetomidine, romifidine, or xylazine, diazepam and ketamine, followed by CRIs with medetomidine alone, medetomidine with lidocaine, medetomidine with lidocaine and ketamine, or medetomidine with ketamine and guaifenesin. The doses of medetomidine in these studies range between 1.25 and 5 μg/kg/h.[32–34,43,53]

One study induced horses with medetomidine (7 μg/kg), diazepam (0.02 mg/kg), and ketamine (2.2 mg/kg) followed by a CRI of medetomidine (3.5 μg/kg/h) and 1.05% end-tidal isoflurane for elective surgeries of less than 2 hours, and compared them with horses with added butorphanol (loading dose of 25 μg/kg and CRI of 25 μg/kg/h). Cardiorespiratory function, requirements for inotropic support with dobutamine, the number of rescue doses with ketamine, recovery scores, and time to standing (51–55 minutes) were similar in both groups, but time to extubation was significantly longer in the horses that had received butorphanol (26 vs 20 minutes).[56] Of note, isoflurane requirements in the group receiving butorphanol were not affected (1.06%).[56]

In another study, horses received intravenous doses of 1 mg/kg xylazine, 0.02 mg/kg diazepam, and 2 mg/kg ketamine, and were maintained for approximately 2 hours with a CRI of medetomidine (5 μg/kg/h) with lidocaine (2 mg/kg intravenous loading dose followed by a CRI of 50 µg/kg/min [3 mg/kg/h]) or a CRI of lidocaine alone (same dose), and 1.1% end-tidal isoflurane for arthroscopic surgery.[33] Horses receiving medetomidine and lidocaine had better arterial blood pressures but similar cardiac output and heart rate to those receiving lidocaine alone. Recovery times to standing were longer (54 vs 22 minutes) but of better quality in the group that had received both medetomidine and lidocaine.[33]

During elective surgeries, it was easier to maintain a surgical plane of anesthesia and use lower end-tidal isoflurane concentrations in a group of horses that received a CRI of medetomidine (3.5 µg/kg/h) than in those receiving a CRI of lidocaine (2 mg/kg intravenous loading dose followed by 50 µg/kg/min [3 mg/kg/h]), after induction with intravenous xylazine (1 mg/kg) or medetomidine (7 µg/kg) combined with diazepam (0.02 mg/kg) and ketamine (2.2 mg/kg).[34] Cardiac output and heart rate were higher in the lidocaine group.[34] Recoveries were longer, but of better quality, in the medetomidine group (59 vs 39 minutes).[34]

Adding a CRI of medetomidine of 3.6 µg/kg/h for the first 50 minutes and then reduced to 2.75 µg/kg/h to CRIs of ketamine (33 µg/kg/min [2 mg/kg/h]) and lidocaine (33 µg/kg/min [2 mg/kg/h] at a loading dose of 1.5 mg/kg for the first 50 minutes and then reduced to 25 µg/kg/min [1.5 mg/kg/h]) for both drugs, to horses undergoing elective surgery during isoflurane anesthesia, after induction with romifidine (50 µg/kg), levomethadone (50 µg/kg), diazepam (0.1 mg/kg), and ketamine (3 mg/kg), reduced the median end-tidal isoflurane concentration an additional 35% in comparison with horses without the medetomidine (1% vs 0.65%).[43] It also resulted in lower doses of dobutamine needed to support blood pressure, but there was no difference in recovery scores between the 2 groups.[43]

More complex techniques have also included triple drips. Horses administered 5 µg/kg medetomidine, 0.04 mg/kg diazepam, and 2.5 mg/kg ketamine intravenously for induction were then maintained with a CRI of guaifenesin at 25 mg/kg/h (0.42 mg/kg/min), ketamine at 1 mg/kg/h (16.7 µg/kg/min), medetomidine at 1.25 µg/kg/h, and 1.5% sevoflurane during right carotid translocation surgery.[32] In this study, 50% less end-tidal concentration (1.5% vs 3%) was required than in horses induced in a similar fashion but maintained on sevoflurane alone, which contributed to better mean arterial blood pressures (>70 mm Hg) without inotropic support and cardiac outputs that were at least 70% of conscious values.[32] Time to recovery after approximately 4 hours of infusion was less than 1 hour and was similar to that for horses maintained on sevoflurane alone, but the benefit lay in there being fewer attempts to standing compared with the balanced technique (1.5 vs 3).[32]

Defining a CRI for PIVA Medetomidine plasma concentrations of 1.0 to 1.5 ng/mL at steady state are recommended in ponies for standing sedation[53] and, based on the clearance values (40 or 67 mL/kg/min), these concentrations can be achieved with an intravenous bolus of 2 to 3 µg/kg using formula 1, with an average V_d^{ss} of 2 L/kg, followed by a CRI of 2.4 to 6 µg/kg/h using the product of the desired plasma concentration and the clearance as stated in formula 2 (see **Table 1**). Similar rates have been used in anesthetized horses with good success, using the assumption that pharmacokinetic data remain unchanged; however, as already mentioned, variations between conscious and anesthetized states have been detected for other α_2-agonists (eg, xylazine).[19,47]

Dexmedetomidine

Pharmacokinetics The terminal half-life of a single intravenous dose of 3.5 µg/kg dexmedetomidine is shorter (20 vs 29 minutes) in mature ponies (4–5 years) than in older ponies (19–23 years), because of higher clearance. These half-lives are significantly shorter than for medetomidine (51 minutes)[30,53] and allow rapid adjustments in the anesthetic depth to meet patient requirements; however, it also means that on discontinuation of the CRI the patient may arouse more rapidly than for other α_2-agonists, although studies in dogs have shown that duration of sedation was longer after 20 μg/kg dexmedetomidine than after 40 μg/kg medetomidine, despite lower plasma concentrations and a shorter terminal half-life of dexmedetomidine (47 vs 58 minutes).[57]

CRI for sedation Based on similar sedative effects, an intravenous dose of 3.5 μg/kg dexmedetomidine is equipotent to 5 to 10 μg/kg medetomidine.[30] Therefore, balanced anesthesia protocols with dexmedetomidine use a lower dose than for medetomidine but are expected to cause the same degree of CNS depression. The author uses 50% of the dose used for CRIs of medetomidine, resulting in doses of 1.75 to 2.5 μg/kg/h.

CRI for PIVA In research ponies dexmedetomidine CRIs of 1 and 1.75 μg/kg/h after intravenous induction with dexmedetomidine at 3.5 μg/kg, midazolam at 0.06 mg/kg, and ketamine at 2.2 mg/kg, and maintenance with 1.5% end-tidal isoflurane resulted in slight decreases in cardiac output and heart rate, and no change in blood pressure with respect to baseline.[58] In the clinical setting during surgery, using the same anesthetic protocol and a dexmedetomidine CRI of 1.75 μg/kg/h, heart rate and arterial oxygen tensions were lower than in horses not receiving the CRI, but cardiac output, oxygen delivery, and arterial blood pressure were similar in both groups at similar end-tidal isoflurane requirements.[26] In the latter study, dexmedetomidine (0.875 μg/kg) was administered intravenously to both groups of horses before the recovery period, but horses that had received the CRI during surgery made fewer attempts at standing and had better recoveries despite similar times.[26]

Defining CRI for PIVA Based on the sedative and PIVA CRI doses, a dose of 1 to 2.5 μg/kg/h is recommended.

Detomidine
Pharmacokinetics The terminal half-life of detomidine after intravenous administration of 30 μg/kg to conscious horses is 26 minutes with a clearance of 12 mL/kg/min and a V_d of 0.47 L/kg,[59] whereas doses of 10 μg/kg and 20 μg/kg intravenously in conscious horses resulted in median terminal half-lives of 40 and 54 minutes, clearances of 33 and 21 mL/kg/min, and V_d^{ss} of 1.6 and 1.2 L/kg, respectively.[60] Differences between the 2 studies may be due to measurements in plasma[59] as opposed to serum.[60]

CRI for sedation Sustained standing sedation of approximately 60 minutes, as assessed by head drop and an increase in mechanical nociceptive thresholds to pressure applied to the scapular spine or elbow, was achieved after a single intravenous dose of 30 μg/kg that resulted in plasma concentrations of 10 to 30 ng/mL.[61]

A dose-dependent increase in duodenal distension and colorectal distension thresholds was demonstrated in conscious horses after intravenous administration of 10 to 20 μg/kg, which was more obvious with the higher dose and correspondingly higher serum concentrations.[60] Serum concentrations of 17.4 ng/mL were associated with this visceral analgesia, whereas one-tenth (1.73 ng/mL) of these serum concentrations were associated with sedation.[60] Using the pharmacokinetic data obtained from this study, to achieve serum concentrations of 17.4 ng/mL with a clearance of 21 mL/kg/min a CRI of 22 μg/kg/h would be required (formula 2).

A lower CRI dose of detomidine (8.54 μg/kg/h) after a loading dose of 15 μg/kg and 0.03 mg/kg butorphanol resulted in adequate standing sedation and analgesia during experimental abdominal insufflation with CO_2.[62]

CRI for PIVA In halothane-anesthetized horses an average infusion rate of 11 μg/kg/h achieved plasma detomidine concentrations at a steady state of 25.2 ng/mL, which reduced the halothane requirement (MAC) in horses by 33%.[63]

In horses undergoing elective surgery after intravenous induction with detomidine (10 μg/kg), midazolam (0.06 mg/kg), and ketamine (2.2 mg/kg), and maintained with isoflurane and a CRI of detomidine (5 μg/kg/h), lower heart rates and oxygen delivery as well as higher systemic vascular resistance were recorded in comparison with a group of horses without the CRI, but there were no differences in blood pressure, cardiac index, isoflurane requirements, or quality of recovery between the 2 groups.[27] Fifty percent of horses in the placebo group required dobutamine administration to maintain blood pressure above 70 mm Hg, which may have altered the other cardiovascular parameters in this group. All horses in this study received an intravenous bolus of 2.5 μg/kg detomidine before recovery, which may have masked differences between both groups in the quality of recovery.[27] The anesthetist was blinded to the CRI, and no differences were found in isoflurane requirements during surgery (approximately 1% end-tidal for both groups)[37] despite the reported MAC-sparing effect of detomidine for halothane-anesthetized horses of 33%[63] and 23%[64] with a CRI of 11 μg/kg/h.

Defining a CRI for PIVA A CRI dose of 13 to 38 μg/kg/h would be necessary to maintain plasma concentrations associated with sustained sedation and effective analgesia (10–30 ng/mL) based on the mid-value for clearances reported for detomidine (21 mL/kg/min) (formula 2) and seem appropriate to obtain a significant MAC reduction, because lower doses were not associated with a MAC-sparing effect (see **Table 1**).

Lidocaine

Benefits of lidocaine include analgesia, minimal cardiovascular effects in the horse, and anti-inflammatory actions. The analgesic and anti-inflammatory effects of intravenous lidocaine have been recently summarized in a review on equine pain management[65] and include blockade of Na^+ channels, muscarinic antagonism through acetylcholine release in the cerebrospinal fluid, inhibition of glycine receptors, reduction in the production of excitatory amino acids, inhibition of N-methyl-D-aspartate (NMDA) and neurokinin receptors, reduction in the production of thromboxane A_2, promotion of the release of endogenous opioids, and promotion of the release of adenosine triphosphate to attenuate the response to endothelial and vascular cytokines.

These diverse effects justify the common use of intravenous lidocaine in anesthetic protocols with or without the use of volatile anesthetics, α_2-agonists, and ketamine.[33,66–74] The interactions of lidocaine with α_2-agonists have already been mentioned in the sections on the use of α_2-agonists, and the interactions of lidocaine with ketamine are discussed in the section on ketamine.

Pharmacokinetics

The terminal half-life and clearance of lidocaine after intravenous administration of a bolus loading dose of 1.3 mg/kg and a CRI of 50 μg/kg/min (3 mg/kg/h), delivered for 105 minutes to conscious horses, are 79 minutes and 29 mL/kg/min, respectively; and 54 minutes and 15 mL/kg/min, respectively, in horses anesthetized with sevoflurane vaporizer settings between 2.88% and 3.88%.[20] Using the same bolus dose and CRI in horses undergoing abdominal emergency surgery under sevoflurane anesthesia, but administered the rate for 60 to 90 minutes, a terminal half-life and clearance of 65 minutes and 25 mL/kg/min, respectively, were determined.[21] Similarly, in conscious horses administered the same bolus dose followed by 6 hours of the same CRI, the clearance ranged between 29 and 36 mL/kg/min with plasma concentrations between 1370 and 1780 ng/mL.[22]

Some of the initial studies on the pharmacokinetics of lidocaine were aimed at establishing its use as a prokinetic and anti-inflammatory drug in horses with ileus or enteritis, using a dose that achieved plasma concentrations of 1000 to 2000 ng/mL. An intravenous dose of 1.3 mg/kg and a CRI of 50 μg/kg/min (3 mg/kg/h) were recommended from pilot studies.[75] The V_d^{ss} of lidocaine in conscious and anesthetized horses are 0.79 and 0.4 L/kg, respectively,[20] and to achieve those desired plasma concentrations a loading dose of 0.79 to 1.58 mg/kg in the conscious horse and of 0.4 to 0.8 mg/kg in the anesthetized horse is necessary, according to formula 1. These doses are in contrast to those reported in other studies that administered a higher intravenous loading dose (2–5 mg/kg) and CRI of 50 to 100 μg/kg/minutes (3–6 mg/kg/h) for TIVA techniques or to achieve higher MAC reductions through analgesic and/or sedative effects.[33,34,66–70,73]

CRI for sedation
The administration of lidocaine results in negligible sedation. However, horses may show signs of visual dysfunction, tremors, and ataxia at plasma concentrations of 1850 to 4530 ng/mL.[76] Furthermore, the degree of ataxia induced by xylazine was enhanced by lidocaine administration of a bolus of 1.3 mg/kg and a CRI of 25 or 50 μg/kg/min (1.5 or 3 mg/kg/h).[77]

In horses the analgesic effects have been demonstrated using pain models; using thermal stimulation applied to the horse's withers, a somatic analgesic effect was demonstrated with an intravenous dose of 2 mg/kg followed by a CRI of 50 μg/kg/min (3 mg/kg/h) that resulted in plasma concentrations of 916 to 951 ng/mL; however, using a model of colorectal and duodenal distension, no visceral analgesic effect was obtained.[69] During transcutaneous electrical stimulation of the palmar nerve, lidocaine at an intravenous dose of 1.3 mg/kg and a CRI of 25 or 50 μg/kg/min (1.5 or 3 mg/kg/h) enhanced the analgesic effects of an intravenous loading dose of 0.55 mg/kg and a CRI of 1.1 mg/kg/h (18.3 μg/kg/min) of xylazine.[77]

CRI for PIVA
Lidocaine administered as a low infusion rate with an intravenous bolus dose of 2.5 mg/kg and a CRI of 50 μg/kg/min (3 mg/kg/h) or as a high infusion rate with an intravenous bolus of 5 mg/kg and a CRI of 100 μg/kg/min (6 mg/kg/h) decreased the MAC of halothane in a linear fashion up to a serum concentration of 7000 ng/mL, with the greatest influence at concentrations greater than 5000 ng/mL, which decreased MAC by 50% to 70%, whereas concentrations of 2100 to 3500 ng/mL decreased MAC by 30% to 50%, and concentrations of less than 2000 ng/mL provided a maximum MAC reduction of 20%.[66]

An intravenous bolus of 1.3 mg/kg followed by a CRI of 50 μg/kg/min (3 mg/kg/h) decreased the MAC of sevoflurane by 27% at plasma concentrations of approximately 2000 ng/mL.[78] Clinically this MAC-sparing effect of lidocaine has also been shown for isoflurane-anesthetized horses that received a bolus dose of 2.5 mg/kg and a CRI of 50 μg/kg/min (3 mg/kg/h), whereby a 25% reduction was correlated with lidocaine plasma concentrations of 2140 to 4230 ng/mL.[67]

Ponies undergoing castration using 1.2% end-tidal halothane anesthesia and administered a lidocaine intravenous bolus of 5 mg/kg followed by a CRI of 100 μg/kg/min (6 mg/kg/h) after induction achieved serum concentrations of 1500 to 3000 ng/mL, which resulted in no electroencephalographic median frequency activity or total amplitude during surgery, both previously observed in horses that did not receive lidocaine during castration, suggesting that lidocaine both prevented a cortical response through antinociceptive effects and caused CNS depression (sedative effect).[68,79]

Defining a CRI for PIVA

Using values included in the pharmacokinetic data provided here, to achieve plasma concentrations of 3000 ng/mL that provide an approximate 30% reduction in MAC, and assuming a clearance of 25 mL/kg/min, a CRI of 75 μg/kg/min (4.5 mg/kg/h) would be required according to formula 2 (see **Table 2**).

Recommendations during anesthesia for discontinuing the CRI at least 30 minutes before the start of the recovery period have been made in view of a negative interaction between volatile anesthetics and the effects of lidocaine on tremors and ataxia, which results in low quality of recovery.[70] Because of the reported terminal half-life (54–79 minutes),[20,21] interrupting the infusion 30 minutes before the start of recovery and the additional time the horse requires for the first movement in recovery allow for plasma concentrations to decrease to levels below those associated with side effects. For example, plasma concentrations were only 300 to 325 ng/mL 60 minutes after stopping a CRI of 50 μg/kg/min (3 mg/kg/h) in horses anesthetized with isoflurane or sevoflurane.[20,70]

The rate of administration of the intravenous bolus loading dose varies between studies: 20 minutes,[69] 15 minutes,[20,21,34,70,78] 10 minutes,[33,67,71,74] 5 minutes,[66,77] 3 minutes,[76] and 1 minute.[73] The rate of administration seems more relevant in conscious horses because of the effects of lidocaine on muscle tone (ataxia) and the occurrence of visual dysfunction from CNS effects,[70,73] but is less relevant in the anesthetized horse because these symptoms are blunted and not observed. The horse is also less sensitive to adverse cardiovascular effects elicited by lidocaine in other species.[73]

Because of the depressive effects of α_2-agonists on intestinal motility, which may predispose to ileus,[80,81] concurrent administration with lidocaine may prove useful in high-risk patients, such as colics, owing to the prokinetic effects of lidocaine in this subpopulation.[72,75,82]

Ketamine

Ketamine can be used at anesthetic or subanesthetic doses to derive benefit from its analgesic effects. Analgesia results from noncompetitive binding and allosteric modifications to the phencyclidine site of NMDA excitatory glutamate receptors involved in nociceptive transmission, and from decreasing activity of brain structures that respond to noxious stimuli.[83,84] At subanesthetic doses, its analgesic efficacy is preserved and does not cause any of the side effects that have been associated with doses that produce dissociative anesthesia, such as tremors, tonic spasticity, or convulsive seizures.

Anesthetic doses usually preserve adequate cardiovascular function including blood pressure, heart rate, and cardiac output.[49,50,85,86]

Pharmacokinetics

The terminal half-life of ketamine in halothane-anesthetized horses after intravenous administration of 2.2 mg/kg combined with 1.1 mg/kg xylazine was determined to be 66 minutes with a clearance of 31 mL/kg/min,[87] whereas the terminal half-life was 42 minutes in horses administered only ketamine and xylazine, with a clearance of 27 mL/kg/min.[88] In horses maintained on a CRI of ketamine for 1 hour at 40 μg/kg/min (2.4 mg/kg/h) since 5 minutes after induction with intravenous detomidine (20 μg/kg) and ketamine (2.2 mg/kg) and maintenance with halothane for castration, a terminal half-life of 46 minutes, a clearance of 32 mL/kg/min, and a V_d^{ss} of 1.4 L/kg were determined.[86]

Use of long-term CRI of ketamine at 6.7 and 13.3 μg/kg/min (0.4 mg/kg/h and 0.8 mg/kg/h) of ketamine for 6 hours each, in ascending or descending order, to conscious horses yielded a combined terminal half-life for both infusions of only 4.7 minutes, with maximum plasma concentrations of 67 ng/mL during the low CRI and 137 ng/mL during the high CRI[89]; however, no loading dose was used in this study. By contrast, administration in conscious horses of an intravenous loading dose of 0.8 mg/kg administered over 10 minutes, followed by 0.6 mg/kg over the next 10 minutes, then 0.5 mg/kg over the next 10 minutes, and 0.4 mg/kg over the last 10 minutes before starting a CRI of 25 μg/kg/min (1.5 mg/kg/h) to complete 6 hours of ketamine administration, resulted in a terminal half-life of 67 minutes with a clearance of 53 mL/kg/min after achieving initial plasma concentrations of approximately 400 ng/mL during the loading phase and of 235 ng/mL during the CRI.[90]

The use of the S-ketamine enantiomer has been recommended for CRI in horses over the racemic mixture of ketamine, because the S-enantiomer is eliminated faster than the mixture and may also result in better recoveries.[3,91]

CRI for sedation

Sedative effects of low doses of ketamine have not been demonstrated in horses; however, analgesia and manipulations may be facilitated by its combination with α2-agonists and opioids.[89,90,92]

Horses administered a cumulative dose of 2.3 mg/kg over 40 minutes (CRI of 57 μg/kg/min [3.4 mg/kg/h]) showed weight shifting between the forelimbs during the infusion, but these signs disappeared subsequently when the CRI was decreased to 25 μg/kg/min (1.5 mg/kg/h).[90]

Plasma concentrations of at least 60 to 160 ng/mL have been associated with sub-anesthetic analgesic effects of ketamine in people,[93,94] but equivalent analgesic concentrations have not yet been determined in horses.

CRI for PIVA

Plasma concentrations higher than 1200 ng/mL are associated with anesthetic effects in horses,[88] and significant reductions in the MAC of halothane are achieved at plasma concentrations of 1000 ng/mL and reach a maximum 37% reduction at 10,800 ng/mL.[95]

Horses castrated under halothane and a CRI of ketamine for 1 hour at 40 μg/kg/min (2.4 mg/kg/h) since 5 minutes after an induction intravenous dose of 2.2 mg/kg had plasma concentrations of 1300 to 2040 ng/mL at the end of the CRI, which declined rapidly once the infusion was interrupted 15 minutes before the end of surgery, so that recovery to standing was uneventful and was achieved within 42 minutes of discontinuing halothane.[86]

The effects of ketamine and lidocaine on MAC have recently been determined in horses induced with intravenous doses of 1.1 mg/kg xylazine and 3 mg/kg ketamine in a crossover study; one group received the CRI of ketamine and lidocaine and a second group received a placebo. The CRI was started within 20 minutes of induction and included 50 μg/kg/min (3 mg/kg/h) ketamine combined with 50 μg/kg/min

(3 mg/kg/h) lidocaine (intravenous loading dose of 2 mg/kg).[74] MAC determinations were started 1 hour after induction, and values were 49% lower (1.25% vs 0.64%) in the group that received the combined ketamine and lidocaine CRI.[74] Clinically a combined CRI of ketamine and lidocaine also resulted in 38% reduction in isoflurane requirements when compared with a group of horses on placebo (0.97% vs 1.57%) undergoing surgery for approximately 80 minutes. Horses receiving the ketamine and lidocaine CRI had better planes of anesthesia with fewer events that indicated light planes, such as need for rescue analgesia or supplemental intravenous thiopental to control nystagmus or movement, and also required less inotropic support than horses on isoflurane alone.[71] In the latter study, anesthesia was induced with intravenous romifidine (80 μg/kg), diazepam (0.1 mg/kg), and ketamine (3 mg/kg), followed by the combined CRI of ketamine and lidocaine at rate of 60 μg/kg/min [3.6 mg/kg/h]) ketamine and 40 μg/kg/min [2.4 mg/kg/h] lidocaine (intravenous loading dose of 1.5 mg/kg) for the first 50 minutes, then reduced to 50 μg/kg/min (3 mg/kg/h) ketamine and 33 μg/kg/min (2 mg/kg/h) lidocaine before discontinuing the rates 15 minutes from the end of surgery.[71]

In a similar study, horses underwent elective surgery during isoflurane anesthesia with a median end-tidal isoflurane concentration of 1%, after induction with romifidine (50 μg/kg), levomethadone (50 μg/kg), diazepam (0.1 mg/kg), and ketamine (3 mg/kg), followed by CRIs of ketamine (33 μg/kg/min [2 mg/kg/h]) and lidocaine (33 μg/kg/min [2 mg/kg/h]; loading dose of 1.5 mg/kg) for the first 50 minutes, with CRI then being reduced to of 25 μg/kg/min (1.5 mg/kg/h) for both drugs.[43]

CRI for TIVA

Horses maintained on TIVA with a combination of ketamine at doses of 90 to 150 μg/kg/min (5.4–9 mg/kg/h) and xylazine at 2.1 to 4.2 mg/kg/h (35–70 μg/kg/min) had plasma concentrations of 2180 to 5020 ng/mL during the infusion and concentrations of 360 to 1050 ng/mL at the time of standing during recovery, whereby the highest values corresponded to the highest CRI of ketamine.[50]

Defining a CRI for PIVA

To achieve a plasma concentration of 1000 ng/mL, a CRI of 32 μg/kg/min (1.9 mg/kg/h) is necessary using a clearance of 32 mL/kg/min,[86] but if the first-order constants of transfer and elimination generated in one study[87] are used as described in the study that determined the effect of ketamine on MAC,[95] then a CRI of 116 μg/kg/min (7 mg/kg/h) is necessary for the first 8 minutes, subsequently reduced to 111 μg/kg/min (6.7 mg/kg/h) to achieve that same target concentration of 1000 ng/mL (see **Table 2**). This type of discrepancy is common when reviewing pharmacokinetic studies and, as mentioned earlier, they are partly due to the presence of other drugs and differences between aiming target plasma concentrations and delivering a fixed CRI.

The effect of ketamine on the CNS (excitement) and the likelihood of muscle rigidity are of concern during recovery of horses; therefore, administration of excessive doses close to the recovery period should be avoided. The studies described here on the use of CRI in conscious horses[89–91] demonstrate that low doses (6.7–25 μg/kg/min [0.4–1.5 mg/kg/h]) are well tolerated. Furthermore, the use of ketamine combined with α_2-agonists during the transition from inhalational anesthesia to consciousness does not affect the quality of recovery when clinical doses are used. In one study, 3.3 intravenous boluses consisting each of 66 mg ketamine and 33 mg xylazine (total of 218 mg ketamine) were administered to horses during a period of 29 minutes after discontinuation of isoflurane administration, with no adverse effects on recovery.

This dose corresponds to 0.45 mg/kg for the mean weight of the horses (478 kg) or approximately 16 μg/kg/min.[33]

In another study, administration of 60 μg/kg/min (3.6 mg/kg/h) ketamine in combination with xylazine (1.2 mg/kg/h [20 μg/kg/min]), after intravenous loading doses of 0.15 mg/kg xylazine and 0.3 mg/kg ketamine, was used to maintain anesthesia in horses for an additional 30 minutes after discontinuation of sevoflurane or isoflurane anesthesia, and had no impact on recovery in isoflurane-anesthetized horses and improved recoveries in sevoflurane-anesthetized horses when compared with placebo groups.[48,49]

Information on the effects of ketamine on recovery without the use of α_2-agonists can be inferred from the following 2 studies. In one study, horses administered a combined CRI of ketamine (50 μg/kg/min [3 mg/kg/h]) and lidocaine (50 μg/kg/min [3 mg/kg/h]) until isoflurane anesthesia was interrupted at an end-tidal concentration of 0.62% had similar recovery scores and times to standing to horses that received a placebo CRI and started recovery with 1.32% end-tidal isoflurane.[74] Likewise, in a study with horses maintained on TIVA after induction with xylazine, guaifenesin, and ketamine, ketamine doses of 90 to 150 μg/kg/min (5.4–9 mg/kg/h) were combined in different ratios with xylazine at 2.1 to 4.2 mg/kg/h (35–70 μg/kg/min), and there was also one group of horses that only received a CRI of ketamine at 150 μg/kg/min (9 mg/kg/h). The horses that received ketamine alone had the shortest time to standing during recovery (33 minutes) and recovery scores of 4.3 out of 5, whereas inclusion of xylazine with ketamine in the TIVA prolonged the time to standing during recovery (46–69 minutes) but improved recoveries (4.4–5 out of 5).[50]

Opioids

Morphine and butorphanol are the opioids most commonly used in balanced techniques although overall, opioids are used less frequently than the other groups of drugs mentioned previously. The analgesic actions of opioids in horses have been recently reviewed[96]; opioid receptors present in laminae I and II of the dorsal horn of the spinal cord are responsible for analgesia through inhibition of the release of substance P from C nociceptive fibers and, to a lesser extent, A-δ fibers.[97]

In horses, excitatory effects of opioids on the CNS may predominate over their analgesic effect, especially in horses that are pain-free, have received higher than required doses of the opioid, or are inadequately sedated before administration of the opioid. Excitatory manifestations include increased locomotor activity (pacing, pawing), muzzle tremors, muscle twitching, head jerks, and raised tail in conscious horses,[96,98–102] and inconsistent changes in inhalational requirements (MAC), including increased MAC in anesthetized horses that are only administered inhalational anesthetics.[103–106]

Because the adverse effects of opioids seem to be more related to overdosing,[96] it is likely that their use in balanced techniques would become more popular in the future, either as a single bolus injection, single intermittent doses, or single bolus followed by a CRI. Therefore, their use in such modes of administration is presented herein.

Morphine
Pharmacokinetics An intravenous dose of 0.1 mg/kg morphine administered to conscious horses had a terminal half-life of 88 minutes using venous samples,[107] whereas intravenous doses of 0.25 mg/kg and 2 mg/kg administered to isoflurane-anesthetized horses had terminal half-lives of 40 and 60 minutes, respectively, and V_d^{ss} of 1.2 and 1.9 L/kg, respectively, using arterial samples.[105] The clearance of morphine in anesthetized horses is approximately 40 mL/kg/min.[105]

Concurrent administration of intravenous xylazine (0.5 mg/kg) and morphine (0.1 or 0.2 mg/kg) in halothane-anesthetized horses increased the terminal half-life and decreased the clearance of morphine, when compared with the available data for morphine alone in isoflurane-anesthetized horses.[19,105] Xylazine and an intravenous dose of 0.1 mg/kg morphine resulted in a half-life of 95 minutes and a clearance of 13 mL/kg/min, whereas xylazine and an intravenous dose of 0.2 mg/kg morphine had a half-life of 105 minutes and a clearance of 12 mL/kg/min.[19]

CRI for sedation Intravenous morphine loading doses of 0.05 to 0.15 mg/kg followed by CRIs of 0.03 to 0.1 mg/kg/h (0.5–1.7 μg/kg/min) have been shown to be safe and effective for analgesia in clinical conditions.[31,74,108] Based on pharmacokinetic studies, behavioral locomotor changes are not elicited with morphine plasma concentrations that result from 0.1 mg/kg intravenously, while analgesia is still achieved.[107]

CRI for PIVA Intravenous administration of morphine (0.25 or 2 mg/kg) to isoflurane-anesthetized horses increased, decreased, or did not change MAC in different animals. Mean MAC values decreased by as much as 20% and increased by as much as 28% with the lower dose, and ranged between a decrease of 19% and an increase of 56% with the higher dose.[105] The addition of a CRI of morphine (0.1 mg/kg/h [1.7 μg/kg/min]) after a loading dose of 0.15 mg/kg only improved an additional 4% (from 49% to 53%) the isoflurane MAC reduction elicited by a combined CRI of ketamine (50 μg/kg/min [3 mg/kg/h]) and lidocaine (50 μg/kg/min [3 mg/kg/h]) in horses,[74] probably because a near maximum decrease in MAC was already reached.

Epidural administration of 0.1 mg/kg morphine consistently decreased halothane requirements by 14% in ponies,[109] indicating that at this dose the central excitatory effects are not present, thus emphasizing the point that the use of lower doses of morphine provides more consistent analgesic effects and less frequency of excitatory effects, as well as minimal cardiorespiratory effects.

Horses undergoing elective surgery under halothane anesthesia and administered a CRI of morphine (0.1 mg/kg/h [1.7 μg/kg/min]) after induction with romifidine (0.1 mg/kg), morphine (0.15 mg/kg), ketamine (2.2 mg/kg), and diazepam (0.05 mg/kg) tended to receive fewer and lower doses of additional anesthetic drugs and had better recoveries (fewer attempts to sternal and standing and shorter time to standing) than horses treated in a similar fashion that did not receive morphine.[108,110] Similarly, single intravenous injection of 0.1 to 0.17 mg/kg morphine to horses anesthetized for soft-tissue and orthopedic procedures with romifidine, ketamine, diazepam, and halothane did not increase the risk of side effects in the intraoperative or postoperative period when compared with horses that did not receive it.[111]

Defining a CRI for PIVA Morphine plasma concentrations of 14.7 to 16 ng/mL in humans[112,113] and 30 ng/mL in dogs[114] have been determined as minimum effective analgesic concentrations; however, such data are not available in horses. Using formula 2, to achieve plasma concentrations of 15 to 30 ng/mL, a CRI of 36 to 72 μg/kg/h (0.6–1.2 μg/kg/min) is necessary using a clearance of 40 mL/kg/min, as reported for horses anesthetized with isoflurane alone,[105] and a loading dose of 0.02 to 0.04 mg/kg (20–40 μg/kg) using an average V_d^{ss} of 1.5 L/kg (formula 1) (see **Table 2**). Using a clearance of 12 mL/kg/min, as reported for horses anesthetized with halothane that had also received xylazine at the time of morphine administration,[19] the calculated CRI necessary to achieve plasma concentrations of 15 to 30 ng/mL is 11 to 22 μg/kg/h (0.18–0.36 μg/kg/min).

In conscious horses, ideal analgesic conditions with minimal cardiorespiratory effects or behavioral alterations were achieved by administration of a loading dose of 0.05 mg/kg (50 µg/kg) of morphine followed by a CRI of 0.03 mg/kg/h (0.5 µg/kg/min) in combination with 5 µg/kg/h of medetomidine for 3 hours in horses undergoing standing laparoscopy.[31]

Butorphanol

Pharmacokinetics The terminal half-life of a single intravenous dose of butorphanol (0.1–0.13 mg/kg) administered to conscious horses is 44 minutes, with a clearance of 21 mL/kg/min and a V_d^{ss} of 1 L/kg.[102]

CRI for sedation Lower doses of butorphanol appear to be preferable (loading dose of 17.8 µg/kg, CRI of 23.7 µg/kg/h) to a single injection at a higher dose (0.1–0.13 mg/kg [100–130 µg/kg]) in obtaining fewer adverse behavioral and gastrointestinal effects.[102]

For standing sedation, the addition of a bolus (18 µg/kg) and CRI (25 µg/kg/h) of butorphanol to horses sedated with xylazine (1 mg/kg) or romifidine (80 µg/kg) increased the degree of ataxia and incidents of horses falling down in the xylazine group, and did not affect the requirements of additional doses of xylazine in both groups in maintaining steady sedation.[45,51]

CRI for PIVA Similar to the effects of morphine, administration of single intravenous doses of 22, 44, or 50 µg/kg butorphanol to halothane-anesthetized horses or ponies resulted in individual MAC values that were higher, lower, or unchanged, and did not produce an overall significant change in MAC.[103,104] The effects of a CRI of butorphanol on the MAC of volatile anesthetics have not been determined in horses.

Defining a CRI for PIVA Plasma concentrations of 25 ng/mL obtained in one study after a dose 0.1 to 0.13 mg/kg[102] were associated with analgesia against superficial and visceral stimuli from other study,[99] and a loading dose of 17.8 µg/kg and a CRI of 23.7 µg/kg/h were recommended.[102] However, using formulas 1 and 2, with a clearance and V_d^{ss} of 21 mL/kg/min and 1 L/kg, respectively, the calculated loading dose to achieve that target plasma concentration should be 25 µg/kg and the CRI should be 31.5 µg/kg/h (see **Table 2**).

The analgesic and sedative effects of butorphanol in horses or ponies are sometimes difficult to separate. Castration of ponies completed in less than 10 minutes under injectable anesthesia, which included addition of intravenous butorphanol (0.1 mg/kg) as part of the anesthetic induction protocol with acepromazine, detomidine, diazepam, and ketamine, resulted in longer recoveries but similar pain scores in the postoperative period, compared with ponies administered the same anesthetic protocol without butorphanol.[115] In another study, butorphanol (0.05 mg/kg [50 µg/kg], intravenously) administered as part of the premedication of ponies castrated in less than 15 minutes under injectable anesthesia with romifidine and ketamine seemed superior to morphine (0.1 mg/kg, intravenously) or placebo, based on a surgical plane that was easier to maintain; however, there were no differences in the quality or time to recovery between the groups.[116]

Fentanyl

Pharmacokinetics Administration of intravenous fentanyl (2 mg) to adult conscious horses (464–585 kg) resulted in a terminal half-life of 130 minutes, a clearance of 6 mL/kg/min, and a V_d^{ss} of 0.7 L/kg.[117] Administration of 2.8 µg/kg fentanyl followed by a CRI of 2.4 µg/kg/h to conscious horses resulted in a terminal half-life of 49 minutes, a clearance of 16 mL/kg/min, and a V_d^{ss} of 0.8 L/kg.[46] Differences in the data from these studies were attributed to the use of liquid chromatography/mass spectrometry (capable of separating fentanyl from its metabolites) in one study[46] versus radioimmunoassay in the other study.[117]

CRI for PIVA Fentanyl decreased the MAC of isoflurane in horses by 18% (from 1.51% to 1.37%) at plasma concentrations of 13.3 ng/mL, but had no effect on MAC at plasma concentrations of 0.7 ng/mL or 8.4 ng/mL,[106] despite the fact that concentrations of 1 to 2 ng/mL are analgesic in other species.[118,119] Administration of a single intravenous dose of fentanyl of approximately 4 μg/kg can maintain serum fentanyl concentrations of at least 1 ng/mL for up to 2 to 3 hours,[117] but the effects of a CRI of fentanyl have not been determined in horses.

Defining a CRI for PIVA Using a nociceptive somatic (thermal threshold) and visceral (colorectal and duodenal distension) model, fentanyl administration did not provide significant analgesic effects despite serum concentrations of 2.5 ng/mL at steady state, and increasing the dose resulted in behavioral adverse effects.[46] If concentrations of at least 1 ng/mL are in fact analgesic in horses, based on formulas 1 and 2 and using the pharmacokinetic data generated by one of the studies[117] would indicate that a CRI of 0.36 μg/kg/h after a loading dose of 0.7 μg/kg is necessary, but if the data generated by the other study[46] are used, then a loading dose of 0.8 μg/kg and a CRI of 0.96 μg/kg/h would be necessary.

Benzodiazepines

Benzodiazepines potentiate γ-aminobutyric acid (GABA) responses at the $GABA_A$ receptor site, located on the postsynaptic and presynaptic membrane, by allosterically modulating GABA binding. This process results in enhanced chloride influx at the GABA receptor and hyperpolarization of the cell, which makes the cell refractory to stimulation. Benzodiazepines are used in adult horses mostly for their effects on muscle relaxation, and are included in induction protocols with ketamine to counteract the effects of ketamine on increasing muscle tone. Benzodiazepines have the potential for reducing the doses of other induction drugs, but are rarely used in sedative standing procedures in adult horses owing to the potential for ataxia. In foals, benzodiazepines induce reliable sedation and, despite the risk of ataxia, are used frequently to facilitate handling because size/weight is less of an issue and foals can be kept recumbent manually.

Benzodiazepines include diazepam, midazolam, and zolazepam. Zolazepam is available in combination with tiletamine.

Diazepam
Pharmacokinetics Although the pharmacokinetics of diazepam are known in horses and foals, and reported here, there is no specific information on desired plasma concentrations associated with their use in balanced anesthetic techniques.

Administration of approximately 0.18 mg/kg intravenous diazepam to 3 conscious adult horses resulted in terminal half-life values of 6.9, 9.7, and 21.6 hours, clearances of 7, 7.5, and 10 mL/kg/min, and V_d^{ss} of 1.6, 2.9, and 2.4 L/kg, respectively, for the 3 horses.[85] In adult horses suffering from colic and administered intravenous doses of 0.05 to 0.08 mg/kg as part of the premedication, a terminal half-life of 7.5 to 13.2 (mean of 10.2) hours, a clearance of 1.9 to 3.4 (mean of 3) mL/kg/min, and V_d^{ss} of 2 to 2.3 (mean of 2.1) L/kg were determined.[120]

In foals administered 0.25 mg/kg intravenous diazepam at ages 4, 21, 42, and 84 days, terminal half-lives of 4, 3.5, 5, and 3.5 hours, clearances of 5, 8.6, 7.3, and 8.4 mL/kg/min, and V_d^{ss} of 1.6, 2.7, 3, and 2.6 L/kg, respectively, were determined for the 4 age groups.[121]

CRI for sedation Diazepam at intravenous doses of 0.05 to 0.4 mg/kg had minimum effects on cardiopulmonary parameters in conscious horses, although signs of relaxation occur with all doses, and significant ataxia and recumbency is reported with doses of 0.2 mg/kg or higher.[84]

CRI for PIVA The effects of diazepam on inhalation anesthetic requirements have been determined in ponies. The MAC value for halothane was 29% lower than control values at the time of determination, after intravenous administration of a single dose 0.044 mg/kg diazepam.[122] The effect of a CRI of diazepam on MAC for volatile anesthetics has not been determined in horses.

CRI for TIVA Diazepam has been included in one protocol for TIVA that also included ketamine and xylazine administered as a CRI after induction with xylazine (1.1 mg/kg) and ketamine (2.2 mg/kg). The CRI was administered, without a loading dose, at a rate of 0.11 mg/kg/h (1.8 μg/kg/min) diazepam, 1.1 mg/kg/h (18.3 μg/kg/min) xylazine, and 2.2 mg/kg/h (36.7 μg/kg/h) ketamine, and administered for up to 1 hour or until the horse assumed spontaneous lateral recumbency.[123] The degree of anesthesia was considered less adequate, in regard of muscle relaxation and duration of anesthesia and analgesia, than for a CRI of guaifenesin (18 mg/kg/min [110 mg/kg/h]) with the same doses of xylazine and ketamine.[123]

Defining a CRI for PIVA Because of the prolonged terminal half-life of diazepam and the lack of information on target concentrations that are desired, a conservative approach is recommended, using a CRI dose lower than described for the TIVA technique, until this information becomes available. In addition, the muscle relaxation obtained from volatile anesthetics should preclude the use of drugs with those same properties. A dose of 20 μg/kg/h (0.33 μg/kg/min) seems appropriate, based on a study using this dose for midazolam with a PIVA technique[124] and the similarities between both benzodiazepines (see **Table 3**).

Midazolam
Pharmacokinetics There is no information on the pharmacokinetics of midazolam in horses.

CRI for PIVA In horses undergoing carotid translocation surgery under sevoflurane anesthesia with midazolam as a CRI of 20 μg/kg/h (0.33 μg/kg/min) combined with 1 mg/kg/h (16.7 μg/kg/min) ketamine and 1.25 μg/kg/h medetomidine, an end-tidal sevoflurane of 1.7% was necessary for this type of surgery,[124] which is very similar that of a previous study by the same group in which 1.5% sevoflurane was required when guaifenesin (25 mg/kg/h [0.42 mg/kg/min]) was used instead of midazolam, with the same rates for the other drugs.[32] In addition, the recovery characteristics after 4 hours of infusion were similar between the 2 studies.[32,123] The investigators selected the dose of midazolam based on a previous report that determined similar muscle-relaxant effects of 0.1 mg/kg diazepam with 100 mg/kg guaifenesin[125] and the use of similar doses between diazepam and midazolam in equine patients.

CRI for TIVA Midazolam has been used for TIVA combinations in horses undergoing elective surgery, at a CRI of 0.12 mg/kg/h (2 μg/kg/min) in horses anesthetized with xylazine (1 mg/kg), midazolam (0.1 mg/kg), and ketamine (2.2 mg/kg) that also received a CRI of xylazine 1 mg/kg/h (16 μg/kg/min) and ketamine 2 mg/kg/h (33 μg/kg/min). All horses had near excellent recoveries after approximately 1 hour of anesthesia.[126]

Defining a CRI for PIVA Clinically, doses of midazolam are similar to doses of diazepam; however, based on the information available for midazolam, it seems that midazolam at 0.1 mg/kg compares better with guaifenesin than with diazepam in terms of muscle relaxation.[123,125] However, it is difficult to confirm this information based on the differences in design and objectives of the different studies. As is the case for diazepam, it seems prudent to use a dose lower than described for the TIVA technique until this information becomes available, and to consider if it is really necessary to use a drug with muscle-relaxant properties in the presence of volatile anesthetics. A dose of 20 μg/kg/h (0.33 μg/kg/min) as used in PIVA techniques seems appropriate (see **Table 3**).

Guaifenesin (Glyceryl Guaiacolate)

Guaifenesin has mostly been used for TIVA techniques because of its excellent muscle-relaxant properties through central actions. It is usually combined in triple drips that involve the use of ketamine and an α_2-agonist.

The cardiorespiratory effects of guaifenesin include a decrease in blood pressure and partial pressure of arterial oxygen, and no changes in other variables including heart rate, respiratory rate, arterial pH, partial pressure of arterial carbon dioxide, and cardiac output.[126]

Pharmacokinetics

Plasma concentrations of 238,000 ng/mL have been associated in ponies with recumbency and complete muscle relaxation that does not include the diaphragm, and was achieved with a dose of 109 mg/kg.[127] In horses, plasma concentrations of 313,000 ng/mL were measured during lateral recumbency induced by a dose of 134 mg/kg, whereas concentrations of 277,000 ng/mL were measured when xylazine (1.1 mg/kg) preceded a dose of 88 mg/kg guaifenesin to induce lateral recumbency.[126] Half-lives for both groups of horses were approximately 77 minutes, and there were no differences in the half-lives of geldings versus mares or time to standing, although geldings required a higher dose (163 mg/kg) than mares (111 mg/kg) when no premedication was used.[126] In ponies, stallions also required higher doses than mares (130 vs 108 mg/kg) and were associated with longer half-lives (84 vs 60 minutes) and longer times to standing (82 vs 54 minutes).[126] The apparent volume of distribution (V_d) is approximately 0.9 L/kg in ponies.[127]

For a TIVA technique that included romifidine and ketamine with guaifenesin at doses of 50 to 100 mg/kg/h (0.84–1.7 mg/kg/min), plasma concentrations of 230,000 ng/mL were maintained during the infusion.[24] In another study, plasma concentrations were 120,000 ng/mL 20 minutes after administration of 75 mg/kg and had decreased to 67,000 ng/mL 2 hours after administration, at the time of standing,[50] whereas in ponies, standing occurred at concentrations of 154,000 ng/mL at 54 to 82 minutes.[127]

Plasma concentrations of approximately 30% of corresponding plasma concentrations in mares were measured in neonates at the time of delivery, indicating significant crossing of the placental barrier.[126]

CRI for PIVA

As already mentioned, one study used a triple drip (guaifenesin, medetomidine, and ketamine) in a balanced technique with sevoflurane, using a guaifenesin dose of 25 mg/kg/h (0.42 mg/kg/min).[32] In this study, end-tidal sevoflurane was decreased 50% in comparison with horses maintained on sevoflurane alone.[32]

CRI for TIVA

Higher doses of guaifenesin are used for TIVA techniques, usually between 100 and 137.5 mg/kg/h (1.7–2.3 mg/kg/min).[24,123,128] A CRI of guaifenesin (110 mg/kg/h [1.8 mg/kg/min]), with 1.1 mg/kg/h (18.3 μg/kg/min) of xylazine and 2.2 mg/kg/h

(36.7 µg/kg/h) of ketamine, administered for approximately 1 hour following induction with 1.1 mg/kg xylazine and 2.2 mg/kg ketamine, resulted in an excellent degree of anesthesia with regard to muscle relaxation and duration of anesthesia and analgesia, and only a mild decrease in blood pressure was noted with respect to a TIVA that included diazepam instead of guaifenesin.[123]

Similarly, in ponies induction with a mixture of guaifenesin (55 mg/kg), xylazine (0.55 mg/kg), and ketamine (1.1 mg/kg), followed by a CRI of guaifenesin at 137.5 mg/kg/h (2.3 mg/kg/min), xylazine at 1.4 mg/kg/h (23 µg/kg/min), and ketamine 2.8 mg/kg/h (46 µg/kg/min), decreased mean arterial blood pressure throughout the infusion, decreased cardiac output only in the first 5 minutes, and had no significant effects on heart rate.[128]

Defining a CRI for PIVA

Although the use of guaifenesin in combination with other injectable anesthetics may result in significant MAC reduction, its value still needs to be proved in PIVA techniques that already include a muscle relaxant in the volatile anesthetics. For this reason the author recommends the use of lower doses (25 mg/kg/h [0.42 mg/kg/min]) if the use is strictly necessary (see **Table 3**). Using formulas 2–4, a dose of 25 mg/kg/h should result in plasma concentrations of 50,104 ng/mL, assuming an average half-life of 75 minutes for the different studies mentioned here and a V_d of 0.9 L/kg.

SUMMARY AND CLINICAL RELEVANCE

The benefits obtained from a balanced anesthetic technique are the result of the individual effects elicited by each drug included in the combination. The use of more than I drug in the maintenance of general anesthesia has the theoretical advantage of allowing lower individual doses and, in some instances, additive or synergistic effects between the drugs. Main effects that are desired include unconsciousness with muscle relaxation, analgesia, and stable cardiorespiratory function during the maintenance period. During the recovery phase, it is ideal that these drugs have minimum interference and, if possible, still provide analgesia and calm recoveries.

Understanding the pharmacokinetics of drugs used for balanced techniques helps in administering the best doses to obtain those desired effects. Understanding the pharmacodynamics of each drug allows one to choose the ideal combination for each patient.

REFERENCES

1. Lundy JS. Useful anesthetic agents and methods. J Am Med Assoc 1931;97(1): 25–31.
2. Muir WW, Yamashita K. Balanced anesthesia in horses. Proceedings of the Annual Convention of the AAEP 2000;46:98–9.
3. Bettschart-Wolfensberger R, Larenza MP. Balanced anesthesia in the equine. Clin Tech Equine Pract 2007;6(2):104–10.
4. Ratajczak K, Szmigielska M, Henklewski R, et al. Znieczulenie zrównoważone u koni. Med Weter 2011;67(9):604–8 [in Polish].
5. Sebel PS, Bowdle TA, Ghoneim MM, et al. The incidence of awareness during anesthesia: a multicenter United States study. Anesth Analg 2004;99(3):833–9.
6. Pollard RJ, Coyle JP, Gilbert RL, et al. Intraoperative awareness in a regional medical system: a review of 3 years' data. Anesthesiology 2007;106(2):269–74.
7. Manzier J. Awareness, muscle relaxants and balanced anaesthesia. Can Anaesth Soc J 1979;26(5):386–93.

8. Domino KB, Posner KL, Caplan RA, et al. Awareness during anesthesia: a closed claims analysis. Anesthesiology 1999;90(4):1053–61.

9. Ghoneim MM, Block RI, Haffarnan M, et al. Awareness during anesthesia: risk factors, causes and sequelae: a review of reported cases in the literature. Anesth Analg 2009;108(2):527–35.

10. Mee AM, Cripps PJ, Jones RS. A retrospective study of mortality associated with general anaesthesia in horses: elective procedures. Vet Rec 1998;142(11): 275–6.

11. Mee AM, Cripps PJ, Jones RS. A retrospective study of mortality associated with general anaesthesia in horses: emergency procedures. Vet Rec 1998;142(12): 307–9.

12. Johnston GM, Eastment JK, Wood JL, et al. The confidential enquiry into perioperative equine fatalities (CEPEF): mortality results of Phases 1 and 2. Vet Anaesth Analg 2002;29(4):159–70.

13. Rioja E, Cernicchiaro N, Costa MC, et al. Perioperative risk factors for mortality and length of hospitalization in mares with dystocia undergoing general anesthesia: a retrospective study. Can Vet J 2012;53(5):502–10.

14. Roberts F, Freshwater-Turner D. Pharmacokinetics and anaesthesia. Cont Educ Anaesth Crit Care Pain 2007;7(1):25–9.

15. Hill SA. Pharmacokinetics of drug infusions. Cont Educ Anaesth Crit Care Pain 2004;4(3):76–80.

16. Thomasy SM, Mama KR, Whitley K, et al. Influence of general anaesthesia on the pharmacokinetics of intravenous fentanyl and its primary metabolite in horses. Equine Vet J 2007;39(1):54–8.

17. Garcia-Villar R, Toutain PL, Alvinerie M, et al. The pharmacokinetics of xylazine hydrochloride: an interspecific study. J Vet Pharmacol Ther 1981; 4(2):87–92.

18. Dyer DC, Hsu WH, Lloyd WE. Pharmacokinetics of xylazine in ponies: influence of yohimbine. Arch Int Pharmacodyn Ther 1987;289(1):5–10.

19. Bennett RC, Steffey EP, Kollias-Baker C, et al. Influence of morphine sulfate on the halothane sparing effect of xylazine hydrochloride in horses. Am J Vet Res 2004;65(4):519–26.

20. Feary DJ, Mama KR, Wagner AE, et al. Influence of general anesthesia on pharmacokinetics of intravenous lidocaine infusion in horses. Am J Vet Res 2005; 66(4):574–80.

21. Feary DJ, Mama KR, Thomasy S, et al. Influence of gastrointestinal tract disease on pharmacokinetics of lidocaine after intravenous infusion in anesthetized horses. Am J Vet Res 2006;67(2):317–22.

22. Waxman SJ, KuKanich GB, Milligan M, et al. Pharmacokinetics of concurrently administered intravenous lidocaine and flunixin in healthy horses. J Vet Pharmacol Ther 2012;35(4):413–6.

23. Luna SP, Taylor PM, Wheeler MJ. Cardiovascular, endocrine and metabolic changes in ponies undergoing intravenous or inhalation anesthesia. J Vet Pharmacol Ther 1996;19(4):251–8.

24. McMurphy RM, Young LE, Marlin DJ, et al. Comparison of the cardiopulmonary effects of anesthesia maintained by continuous infusion of romifidine, guaifenesin, and ketamine with anesthesia maintained by inhalation of halothane in horses. Am J Vet Res 2002;63(12):1655–61.

25. Hubbell JA, Aarnes TK, Lerche P, et al. Evaluation of a midazolam-ketamine-xylazine infusion for total intravenous anesthesia in horses. Am J Vet Res 2012;73(4):470–5.

26. Gozalo-Marcilla M, Schauvliege S, Segaert S, et al. Influence of a constant rate infusion of dexmedetomidine on cardiopulmonary function and recovery quality in isoflurane anaesthetized horses. Vet Anaesth Analg 2012;39(1):49–58.

27. Schauvliege S, Gozalo-Marcilla M, Verryken K, et al. Effects of a constant rate infusion of detomidine on cardiovascular function, isoflurane requirements and recovery quality in horses. Vet Anaesth Analg 2011;38(6):544–54.

28. Hubbell JA, Saville WJ, Bednarski RM. The use of sedatives, analgesic and anaesthetic drugs in the horse: an electronic survey of members of the American Association of Equine Practitioners (AAEP). Equine Vet J 2010;42(6):487–93.

29. Valverde A. Alpha-2 agonists for pain therapy in horses. Vet Clin North Am Equine Pract 2010;26(3):515–32.

30. Bettschart-Wolfensberger R, Freeman SL, Bowen IM, et al. Cardiopulmonary effects and pharmacokinetics of i.v. dexmedetomidine in ponies. Equine Vet J 2005;37(1):60–4.

31. Solano AM, Valverde A, Desrochers A, et al. Behavioural and cardiorespiratory effects of a constant rate infusion of medetomidine and morphine for sedation during standing laparoscopy in horses. Equine Vet J 2009;41(2):153–9.

32. Yamashita K, Satoh M, Umikawa A, et al. Combination of continuous intravenous infusion using a mixture of guaifenesin-ketamine-medetomidine and sevoflurane anesthesia in horses. J Vet Med Sci 2000;62(3):229–35.

33. Valverde A, Rickey E, Sinclair M, et al. Comparison of cardiovascular function and quality of recovery in isoflurane-anaesthetised horses administered a constant rate infusion of lidocaine or lidocaine and medetomidine during elective surgery. Equine Vet J 2010;42(3):192–9.

34. Ringer SK, Kalchofner K, Boller J, et al. A clinical comparison of two anaesthetic protocols using lidocaine or medetomidine in horses. Vet Anaesth Analg 2007;34(4):257–68.

35. Schatzmann U, Jozzfck H, Stauffer JL, et al. Effects of alpha 2-agonists on intra-uterine pressure and sedation in horses: comparison between detomidine, romifidine and xylazine. Zentralbl Veterinarmed A 1994;41(7):523–9.

36. Katila T, Oijala M. The effect of detomidine (Domosedan) on the maintenance of equine pregnancy and foetal development: ten cases. Equine Vet J 1988;20(5):323–6.

37. Jedruch J, Gajewski Z, Kuussaari J. The effect of detomidine hydrochloride on the electrical activity of uterus in pregnant mares. Acta Vet Scand 1989;30(3):307–11.

38. Luukkanen L, Katila T, Koskinen E. Some effects of multiple administration of detomidine during the last trimester of equine pregnancy. Equine Vet J 1997;29(5):400–2.

39. Araujo RR, Ginther OJ. Vascular perfusion of reproductive organs in pony mares and heifers during sedation with detomidine or xylazine. Am J Vet Res 2009;70(1):141–8.

40. Tranquilli WJ, Thurmon JC, Neff-Davis CA, et al. Hyperglycemia and hypoinsu-linemia during xylazine-ketamine anesthesia in Thoroughbred horses. Am J Vet Res 1984;45(1):11–4.

41. Alexander SL, Irvine CH. The effect of the alpha-2-adrenergic agonist, clonidine, on secretion patterns and rates of adrenocorticotropic hormone and its secreta-gogues in the horse. J Neuroendocrinol 2000;12(9):874–80.

42. Grimsrud KN, Mama KR, Steffey EP, et al. Pharmacokinetics and pharmacody-namics of intravenous medetomidine in the horse. Vet Anaesth Analg 2012;39(1):38–48.

43. Kempchen S, Kuhn M, Spadavecchia C, et al. Medetomidine continuous rate intravenous infusion in horses in which surgical anaesthesia is maintained with isoflurane and intravenous infusions of lidocaine and ketamine. Vet Anaesth Analg 2012;39(3):245–55.

44. Kollias-Baker CA, Court MH, Willimas LL. Influence of yohimbine and tolazoline on the cardiovascular, respiratory, and sedative effects of xylazine in the horse. J Vet Pharmacol Ther 1993;16(3):350–8.

45. Ringer SK, Portier KG, Fourel I, et al. Development of a xylazine constant rate infusion with or without butorphanol for standing sedation of horses. Vet Anaesth Analg 2012;39(1):1–11.

46. Sanchez LC, Robertson SA, Maxwell LK, et al. Effect of fentanyl on visceral and somatic nociception in conscious horses. J Vet Intern Med 2007;21(5):1067–75.

47. Steffey EP, Pascoe PJ, Woliner MJ, et al. Effects of xylazine hydrochloride during isoflurane-induced anesthesia in horses. Am J Vet Res 2000;61(10):1225–31.

48. Wagner AE, Mama KR, Steffey EP, et al. A comparison of equine recovery characteristics after isoflurane or isoflurane followed by a xylazine-ketamine infusion. Vet Anaesth Analg 2008;35(2):154–60.

49. Wagner AE, Mama KR, Steffey EP, et al. Evaluation of infusions of xylazine with ketamine or propofol to modulate recovery following sevoflurane anesthesia in horses. Am J Vet Res 2012;73(3):346–52.

50. Mama KR, Wagner AE, Steffey EP, et al. Evaluation of xylazine and ketamine for total intravenous anesthesia in horses. Am J Vet Res 2005;66(6):1002–7.

51. Ringer SK, Portier KG, Fourel I, et al. Development of a romifidine constant rate infusion with or without butorphanol for standing sedation of horses. Vet Anaesth Analg 2012;39(1):12–20.

52. Kuhn M, Köhler L, Fenner A, et al. Isofluran-Reduktion und Beeinflussung kardiovaskulärer und pulmonaler Parameter durch kontinuierliche Romifidin-Infusion während der Narkose bei Pferden—Eine klinische Studie. Pferdeheilkunde 2004;20(6):511–6 [in German].

53. Bettschart-Wolfensberger R, Clarke KW, Vainio O, et al. Pharmacokinetics of medetomidine in ponies and elaboration of a medetomidine infusion regime which provides a constant level of sedation. Res Vet Sci 1999;67(1):41–6.

54. Neges K, Bettschart-Wolfensberger R, Müller J, et al. The isoflurane sparing effect of a medetomidine constant rate infusion in horses. Vet Anaesth Analg 2003;30(2):93–4.

55. Bettschart-Wolfensberger R, Jäggin-Schmucker N, Lendl C, et al. Minimal alveolar concentration of desflurane in combination with an infusion of medetomidine for the anaesthesia of ponies. Vet Rec 2001;148(9):264–7.

56. Bettschart-Wolfensberger R, Dicht S, Vullo C, et al. A clinical study on the effect in horses during medetomidine-isoflurane anaesthesia, of butorphanol constant rate infusion on isoflurane requirements, on cardiopulmonary function and on recovery characteristics. Vet Anaesth Analg 2011;38(3):186–94.

57. Kuusela E, Raekallio M, Anttila M, et al. Clinical effects and pharmacokinetics of medetomidine and its enantiomers in dogs. J Vet Pharmacol Ther 2000;23(1):15–20.

58. Gozalo-Marcilla M, Schauvliege S, Duchateau L, et al. Cardiopulmonary effects of two constant rate infusions of dexmedetomidine in isoflurane anesthetized ponies. Vet Anaesth Analg 2010;37(4):311–21.

59. Grimsrud KN, Mama KR, Thomasy SM, et al. Pharmacokinetics of detomidine and its metabolites following intravenous and intramuscular administration in horses. Equine Vet J 2009;41(4):361–5.

60. Elfenbein JR, Sanchez LC, Robertson SA, et al. Effect of detomidine on visceral and somatic nociception and duodenal motility in conscious adult horses. Vet Anaesth Analg 2009;36(2):162–72.
61. Mama KR, Grimsrud K, Snell T, et al. Plasma concentrations, behavioural and physiological effects following intravenous and intramuscular detomidine in horses. Equine Vet J 2009;41(8):772–7.
62. Cruz AM, Kerr CL, Bouré LP, et al. Cardiovascular effects of insufflation of the abdomen with carbon dioxide in standing horses sedated with detomidine. Am J Vet Res 2004;65(3):357–62.
63. Dunlop CI, Daunt DA, Chapman PL, et al. The anesthetic potency of 3 steady-state plasma levels of detomidine in halothane anesthetized horses. In: Proceedings of the 4th International Congress of Veterinary Anaesthesia. Utrecht (The Netherlands): 1991. p. 7.
64. Wagner AE, Dunlop CI, Heath RB, et al. Hemodynamic function during neurectomy in halothane anesthetized horses with or without constant dose detomidine infusion. Vet Surg 1992;21(3):248–55.
65. Doherty TJ, Seddighi MR. Local anesthetics as pain therapy in horses. Vet Clin North Am Equine Pract 2010;26(3):533–49.
66. Doherty T, Frazier D. Effect of lidocaine on halothane minimum alveolar concentration in ponies. Equine Vet J 1998;30(4):300–3.
67. Dzikiti TB, Hellebrekers LJ, van Dijk P. Effects of intravenous lidocaine on isoflurane concentration, physiological parameters, metabolic parameters and stress-related hormones in horses undergoing surgery. J Vet Med A Physiol Pathol Clin Med 2003;50(4):190–5.
68. Murrell JC, White KL, Johnson CB, et al. Investigation of the EEG effects of intravenous lidocaine during halothane anaesthesia in ponies. Vet Anaesth Analg 2005;32(4):212–21.
69. Robertson SA, Sanchez LC, Merritt AM, et al. Effect of systemic lidocaine on visceral and somatic nociception in conscious horses. Equine Vet J 2005;37(3):122–7.
70. Valverde A, Gunkel C, Doherty TJ, et al. Effect of a constant rate infusion of lidocaine on the quality of recovery from sevoflurane or isoflurane general anaesthesia in horses. Equine Vet J 2005;37(6):559–64.
71. Enderle AK, Levionnois OL, Kuhn M, et al. Clinical evaluation of ketamine and lidocaine intravenous infusions to reduce isoflurane requirements in horses under general anaesthesia. Vet Anaesth Analg 2008;35(4):297–305.
72. Cook VL, Blikslager AT. Use of systemically administered lidocaine in horses with gastrointestinal tract disease. J Am Vet Med Assoc 2008;232(8):1144–8.
73. Sinclair M, Valverde A. Use of intravenous lidocaine with short-term anaesthesia with xylazine, diazepam/ketamine for castration in horses under field conditions. Equine Vet J 2009;41(2):149–52.
74. Villalba M, Santiago I, Gomez de Segura IA. Effects of constant rate infusion of lidocaine and ketamine, with or without morphine, on isoflurane MAC in horses. Equine Vet J 2011;43(6):721–6.
75. Malone E, Ensink J, Turner T, et al. Intravenous continuous infusion of lidocaine for treatment of equine ileus. Vet Surg 2006;35(1):60–6.
76. Meyer G, Lin HC, Hanson RR, et al. Effects of intravenous lidocaine overdose on cardiac electrical activity and blood pressure in the horse. Equine Vet J 2001;33(5):434–7.
77. Fernandes de Souza JF, Raposo-Monteiro E, Campagnol D, et al. Evaluation of nociception, sedation, and cardiorespiratory effects of a constant rate infusion

of xylazine alone or in combination with lidocaine in horses. J Equine Vet Sci 2012;32(6):339–45.

78. Rezende ML, Wagner AE, Khursheed R, et al. Effects of intravenous administration of lidocaine on the minimum alveolar concentration of sevoflurane in horses. Am J Vet Res 2011;72(4):446–51.

79. Murrell JC, Johnson CB, White KL, et al. Changes in the EEG during castration in horses and ponies anaesthetized with halothane. Vet Anaesth Analg 2003;30(3): 138–46.

80. Merritt AM, Burrow JA, Hartless CS. Effect of xylazine, detomidine, and a combination of xylazine and butorphanol on equine duodenal motility. Am J Vet Res 1998;59(5):619–23.

81. Sutton DG, Preston T, Christley RM, et al. The effects of xylazine, detomidine, acepromazine and butorphanol on equine solid phase gastric emptying rate. Equine Vet J 2002;34(5):486–92.

82. Torfs S, Delesalle C, Dewulf J, et al. Risk factors for equine postoperative ileus and effectiveness of prophylactic lidocaine. J Vet Intern Med 2009;23(3):606–11.

83. Himmelseher S, Durieux ME. Ketamine for perioperative pain management. Anesthesiology 2005;102(1):211–20.

84. Muir WW. NMDA receptor antagonists and pain: ketamine. Vet Clin North Am Equine Pract 2010;26(3):565–78.

85. Muir WW, Sams RA, Huffman RH, et al. Pharmacodynamic and pharmacokinetic properties of diazepam in horses. Am J Vet Res 1982;43(10):1756–62.

86. Flaherty D, Nolan A, Reid J, et al. The pharmacokinetics of ketamine after a continuous infusion under halothane anesthesia in horses. J Vet Anaesth 1998;25(1):31–6.

87. Waterman AE, Robertson SA, Lane JG. Pharmacokinetics of intravenously administered ketamine in the horse. Res Vet Sci 1987;42(2):162–6.

88. Kaka JS, Klavano PA, Hayton WL. Pharmacokinetics of ketamine in the horse. Am J Vet Res 1979;40(7):978–81.

89. Fielding CL, Brumbaugh GW, Matthews NS, et al. Pharmacokinetics and clinical effects of a subanesthetic continuous rate infusion of ketamine in awake horses. Am J Vet Res 2006;67(9):1484–90.

90. Lankveld DP, Driessen B, Soma LR, et al. Pharmacodynamic effects and pharmacokinetic profile of a long-term continuous rate infusion of racemic ketamine in healthy conscious horses. J Vet Pharmacol Ther 2006;29(6):477–88.

91. Larenza MP, Peterbauer C, Landoni MF, et al. Stereoselective pharmacokinetics of ketamine and norketamine after constant rate infusion of a subanesthetic dose of racemic ketamine or S-ketamine in Shetland ponies. Am J Vet Res 2009;70(7):831–9.

92. Wagner AE, Mama KR, Contino EK, et al. Evaluation of sedation and analgesia in standing horses after administration of xylazine, butorphanol, and subanesthetic doses of ketamine. J Am Vet Med Assoc 2011;238(12):1629–33.

93. Clements JA, Nimmo WS, Grant IS. Bioavailability, pharmacokinetics, and analgesic activity of ketamine in humans. J Pharm Sci 1982;71(5):539–42.

94. Strigo IA, Duncan GH, Bushnell MC, et al. The effects of racemic ketamine on painful stimulation of skin and viscera in human subjects. Pain 2005;113(3): 255–64.

95. Muir WW 3rd, Sams R. Effects of ketamine infusion on halothane minimal alveolar concentration in horses. Am J Vet Res 1992;53(10):1802–6.

96. Clutton RE. Opioid analgesia in horses. Vet Clin North Am Equine Pract 2010; 26(3):493–514.

97. Yaksh TL. Multiple opiate receptor systems in brain and spinal cord. Part I. Eur J Anaesthesiol 1984;1(2):171–99.
98. Muir WW, Skarda RT, Sheehan WC. Hemodynamic and respiratory effects of xylazine-morphine sulfate in horses. Am J Vet Res 1979;40(10):1417–20.
99. Kalpravidh M, Lumb WV, Wright M, et al. Analgesic effects of butorphanol in horses: dose-response studies. Am J Vet Res 1984;45(2):211–6.
100. Clarke KW, Paton BS. Combined use of a detomidine with opiates in the horse. Equine Vet J 1988;20(5):331–4.
101. Nolan AM, Besley W, Reid J, et al. The effects of butorphanol on locomotor activity in ponies: a preliminary study. J Vet Pharmacol Ther 1994; 17(4):323–6.
102. Sellon DC, Monroe VL, Roberts MC, et al. Pharmacokinetics and adverse effects of butorphanol administered by single intravenous injection or continuous intravenous infusion in horses. Am J Vet Res 2001;62(2):183–9.
103. Matthews NS, Lindsay SL. Effect of low-dose butorphanol on halothane minimum alveolar concentration in ponies. Equine Vet J 1990;22(5):325–7.
104. Doherty TJ, Geiser DR, Rohrbach BW. Effect of acepromazine and butorphanol on halothane minimum alveolar concentration in ponies. Equine Vet J 1997; 29(5):374–6.
105. Steffey EP, Eisele JH, Baggot JD. Interactions of morphine and isoflurane in horses. Am J Vet Res 2003;64(2):166–75.
106. Thomasy SM, Steffey EP, Mama KR, et al. The effects of i.v. fentanyl administration on the minimum alveolar concentration of isoflurane in horses. Br J Anaesth 2006;97(2):232–7.
107. Combie JD, Nugent TE, Tobin T. Pharmacokinetics and protein binding of morphine in horses. Am J Vet Res 1983;44(5):870–4.
108. Clark L, Clutton RE, Blissitt KJ, et al. Effects of peri-operative morphine administration during halothane anaesthesia in horses. Vet Anaesth Analg 2005; 32(1):10–5.
109. Doherty TJ, Geiser DR, Rohrbach BW. Effect of high volume epidural morphine, ketamine and butorphanol on halothane minimum alveolar concentration in ponies. Equine Vet J 1997;29(5):370–3.
110. Clark L, Clutton RE, Blissitt KJ, et al. The effects of morphine on the recovery of horses from halothane anaesthesia. Vet Anaesth Analg 2008;35(1):22–9.
111. Mircica E, Clutton RE, Kyles KW, et al. Problems associated with perioperative morphine in horses: a retrospective case analysis. Vet Anaesth Analg 2003; 30(3):147–55.
112. Dahlström B, Tamsen A, Paalzow L, et al. Patient-controlled analgesic therapy, Part IV: pharmacokinetic and analgesic plasma concentrations of morphine. Clin Pharmacokinet 1982;7(3):266–79.
113. Gourlay G, Willis R, Lamberty JA. A double-blind comparison of the efficacy of methadone and morphine in postoperative pain control. Anesthesiology 1986; 64(3):322–7.
114. Lucas AN, Firth AV, Anderson GA, et al. Comparison of the effects of morphine administered by constant-rate intravenous infusion or intermittent intramuscular injection in dogs. J Am Vet Med Assoc 2001;218(6):884–91.
115. Love EJ, Taylor PM, Clark C, et al. Analgesic effect of butorphanol in ponies following castration. Equine Vet J 2009;41(6):552–6.
116. Corletto F, Raisis AA, Brearley JC. Comparison of morphine and butorphanol as pre-anesthetic agents in combination with romifidine for field castration in ponies. Vet Anaesth Analg 2005;32(1):16–22.

117. Maxwell LK, Thomasy SM, Slovis N, et al. Pharmacokinetics of fentanyl following intravenous and transdermal administration in horses. Equine Vet J 2003;35(5): 484–90.
118. Shibutani K, Inchiosa MA Jr, Sawada K, et al. Pharmacokinetic mass of fentanyl for postoperative analgesia in lean and obese patients. Br J Anaesth 2005; 95(3):377–83.
119. Robertson SA, Taylor PM, Sear JW, et al. Relationship between plasma concentrations and analgesia after intravenous fentanyl and disposition after other routes of administration in cats. J Vet Pharmacol Ther 2005;28(1):87–93.
120. Shini S, Klaus AM, Hapke HJ. Elimination of diazepam after intravenous injection in the horse. Dtsch Tierarztl Wochenschr 1997;104(1):22–5.
121. Norman WM, Court MH, Greenblatt DJ. Age-related changes in the pharmacokinetic disposition of diazepam in foals. Am J Vet Res 1997;58(8):878–80.
122. Matthews NS, Dollar NS, Shawley RV. Halothane-sparing effect of benzodiazepines in ponies. Cornell Vet 1990;80(3):259–65.
123. Baetge CL, Matthews NS, Carroll GL. Comparison of 3 total intravenous anesthetic infusion combinations in adult horses. Intern J Appl Res Vet Med 2007; 5(1):1–8.
124. Kushiro T, Yamashita K, Umar MA, et al. Anesthetic and cardiovascular effects of balanced anesthesia using constant rate infusion of midazolam-ketamine-medetomidine with inhalation of oxygen-sevoflurane (MKM-OS anesthesia) in horses. J Vet Med Sci 2005;67(4):379–84.
125. Brock N, Hildebrand SV. A comparison of xylazine-diazepam-ketamine and xylazine-guaifenesin-ketamine in equine anesthesia. Vet Surg 1990;19(6): 468–74.
126. Hubbell JA, Muir WW, Sams RA. Guaifenesin: cardiopulmonary effects and plasma concentrations in horses. Am J Vet Res 1980;41(11):1751–5.
127. Davis LE, Wolff WA. Pharmacokinetics and metabolism of glyceryl guaiacolate in ponies. Am J Vet Res 1970;31(3):469–73.
128. Greene SA, Thurmon JC, Tranquilli WJ, et al. Cardiopulmonary effects of continuous intravenous infusion of guaifenesin, ketamine, and xylazine in ponies. Am J Vet Res 1986;47(11):2364–7.

Total Intravenous Anesthesia in Horses

Phillip Lerche, BVSc, PhD

KEYWORDS

- Alpha-2 adrenoceptor agonist • Ketamine • Guaifenesin • Midazolam • Horse
- Total intravenous anesthesia (TIVA)

KEY POINTS

- Total intravenous anesthesia (TIVA) is useful for procedures less than 60 minutes in duration to avoid accumulation of drugs leading to poorer recoveries.
- TIVA protocols use multiple drugs infused at the same time to provide unconsciousness, muscle relaxation, and analgesia.
- Cardiorespiratory depression tends to be minimal during TIVA using clinically useful doses.
- Recovery from TIVA is generally smooth and predictable.

INTRODUCTION

The sole use of intravenous (IV) drugs to induce and maintain anesthesia in the horse (total intravenous anesthesia [TIVA]) is the most common means used to anesthetize equids.[1]

TIVA has several benefits compared with inhalational anesthesia:

- Ease of use
- Reduced cost, because expensive anesthetic equipment is not required
- Useful to provide anesthesia distant from an oxygen source (field anesthesia)
- No requirement for scavenging, or risk of operator exposure to, anesthetic inhalant gases
- Better cardiovascular function (higher cardiac index and arterial blood pressure)
- Lesser stress response
- Recovery is generally smoother and more predictable

TIVA also has disadvantages:

- Cumulative effects of IV drugs leading to weaker or poor-quality recoveries for anesthetic episodes lasting longer than 1 hour

Department of Veterinary Clinical Sciences, The Ohio State University, 601 Vernon Tharp Street, Columbus, OH 43210, USA
E-mail address: lerche.1@osu.edu

Vet Clin Equine 29 (2013) 123–129
http://dx.doi.org/10.1016/j.cveq.2012.11.008
0749-0739/13/$ – see front matter © 2013 Published by Elsevier Inc.

- Control of anesthetic depth is easier with inhalant anesthesia
- Oxygen supplementation is harder to provide under field anesthesia conditions
- Relies on liver metabolism for clearance
- Availability of IV drugs may be limited

THE IDEAL INJECTABLE ANESTHETIC DRUG

An ideal drug for TIVA in the horse would:

- Provide muscle relaxation, analgesia, and unconsciousness
- Be water soluble
- Not accumulate, being rapidly metabolized to inactive metabolites
- Be nontoxic to tissues
- Be free of side effects
- Allow a smooth recovery
- Be readily available
- Be economical to use.

However, the ideal injectable anesthetic drug does not exist. The equine anesthetist therefore makes use of combinations of drugs, with an understanding of their pharmacology, to achieve these goals.

TECHNIQUES FOR TIVA IN HORSES

Pharmacokinetic and pharmacodynamic information on many of the drugs discussed in this article are discussed in the article on balanced anesthesia and constant rate infusions. At the time of writing, several of the drugs discussed in this article are unavailable in some parts of the United States because of manufacturing and distribution issues.

INDUCTION OF ANESTHESIA

Regardless of the technique selected for maintenance of anesthesia, induction typically follows the same pattern. It is essential that all personnel involved understand how to use any equipment that may be used (swing doors, ropes, tables, hoists) as well as how to handle the horse as it transitions from the standing position to recumbency. The person controlling the horse's head during this time has an essential job, and should be familiar with the anesthetic induction process.

Adequate sedation of the horse before induction is paramount, and is usually achieved with an alpha-2 adrenoceptor agonist, several of which are available (**Table 1**).[2–4] Signs of appropriate sedation are related to the muscle-relaxing and sedative effects of this drug class. Muscle relaxation, which may be less noticeable with romifidine, leads to ataxia, a wide-based stance, knuckling at the carpal joints, lowering of the head, and drooping of the lip, whereas sedation leads to a decreased

Table 1	
Alpha-2 agonists used for preanesthetic medication in horses	
Drug	**Dose**
Xylazine	0.4–1.1 mg/kg, IV
Detomidine	0.005–0.03 mg/kg, IV
Romifidine	0.06–0.1 mg/kg, IV

level of responsiveness to external stimuli. Alpha-2 agonist drugs also provide analgesia.[5]

Sedation can be enhanced by combining an alpha-2 agonist with the opioid analgesic butorphanol (0.04 mg/kg IV). Butorphanol and the alpha-2 agonists are water soluble and can be combined in 1 syringe for ease of administration.

Anesthesia in horses is typically induced with ketamine, a dissociative anesthetic agent with analgesic properties attributed to its action as an N-methyl-D-aspartate (NMDA) receptor antagonist. A benzodiazepine (midazolam, diazepam) can be added to ketamine to provide additional muscle relaxation, because muscle rigidity may be seen following induction of anesthesia with ketamine. As an alternative, the muscle relaxant guaifenesin can be delivered to good effect before ketamine is administered (**Table 2**).

The length of surgical time following anesthesia with a single dose of ketamine is up to 15 minutes, allowing short procedures to be completed without need for additional drug administration in most horses. Recovery from an alpha-2 adrenoceptor agonist plus ketamine induction is typically smooth, and occurs within 20 to 25 minutes.

Tiletamine and zolazepam (Telazol, Fort Dodge) are longer-lasting dissociative and benzodiazepine drugs that produce similar effects to ketamine combined with a benzodiazepine. Recovery is usually similar to that seen after ketamine, although sometimes less coordinated.[6]

SHORT-TERM TIVA (20 TO 30 MINUTES)

Following a single-dose injectable protocol, it is possible that a procedure may last longer than anticipated, or that the useful anesthetic duration is shorter than expected (the horse returns to consciousness more rapidly than expected). Anesthesia can be extended by administering one-third to one-half of the original doses of alpha-2 and ketamine. This dose can be repeated as needed, but multiple redosing usually leads to longer recovery times.[7]

LONG-TERM TIVA (UP TO 60 MINUTES)

For procedures lasting up to an hour in which TIVA is used, the equine anesthetist usually administers an infusion of combined drugs (coinfusion) to maintain anesthesia. This technique is advantageous because it decreases the peaks and troughs of high and low plasma concentrations of the drugs being infused. By providing a constant plasma concentration once steady state has been reached, toxicity (peaks) and inadequate anesthetic depth (troughs) are avoided.

KETAMINE-BASED PROTOCOLS

Combinations of an alpha-2 agonist, ketamine, and guaifenesin have been in general use for TIVA in horses for more than 25 years. The first combination reported,

Table 2		
Drugs that provide muscle relaxation used with ketamine (2.2 mg/kg IV) for anesthetic induction		
Drug	**IV Dose (mg/kg)**	**Note**
Diazepam	0.04–0.1 mg/kg, IV	Combined in the same syringe as ketamine
Midazolam	0.04–0.1 mg/kg, IV	
Guaifenesin	35–50 mg/kg, IV	Ketamine is given as soon as the horse shows signs of marked ataxia (frequent knuckling at the carpus joints)

guaifenesin, ketamine, and xylazine (GKX) is frequently referred to as triple drip.[8] It is essential that guaifenesin is infused intravenously, and it is recommended that an indwelling intravenous catheter be used because guaifenesin can cause tissue irritation and sloughing if inadvertent extravascular administration occurs. It is important to recognize that the infusion rates that are required to maintain anesthesia may vary with individual horses and with different procedures. Frequent monitoring of patient status (discussed later) and adjustment of infusion rate accordingly is essential.

Availability of other alpha-2 agonists for use in horses has led to other protocols being used, and the term triple drip is sometimes applied to all of these protocols. Triple drip using detomidine may be abbreviated as GKD (guaifenesin, ketamine, and detomidine)[9] and, likewise, when romifidine is part of the protocol, the abbreviation is GKR (**Table 3**).[10]

Guaifenesin formulated at concentrations greater than 10% in water or 5% dextrose solutions may cause hemolysis (leading to hemoglobinuria) and the delayed complication of venous thrombosis. Stabilized 15% guaifenesin solutions are available in some countries and are less likely to cause these problems, although thrombosis may still occur.[11] The availability of commercially prepared guaifenesin in the United States has been limited. Practitioners must therefore either prepare solutions themselves or contract with a pharmacy willing to compound it. A TIVA infusion using midazolam in place of guaifenesin has been evaluated (MKX).[12] Moderate to marked ataxia after standing was a common finding in this study, most likely attributable to midazolam concentrations. The authors recommend using a reduced concentration of midazolam (see **Table 3**). Protocols using xylazine and ketamine alone at various doses to maintain anesthesia in horses for up to one hour has been described (Mama 2005).[13] However these horses may need oxygen

Table 3 Protocols for TIVA infusions			
TIVA	Preparation	Final Concentrations	Infusion Rate (mL/kg/h)
GKX	Add 250mg xylazine and 500–1000 mg ketamine to 500 mL of 5% guaifenesin[a]	G: 50 mg/mL K: 1–2 mg/mL X: 0.5 mg/mL	1.5
GKD	Add 10 mg detomidine and 500–1000 mg of ketamine to 500 mL of 5% guaifenesin[a]	G: 50 mg/mL K: 1–2 mg/mL D: 20 μg/mL	1.2–1.6
GKR	Add 40 mg romifidine and 3.3 g ketamine to 500 mL of 5% guaifenesin[a,b]	G: 50 mg/mL K: 6.6 mg/mL R: 80 μg/mL	1
MKX	Add 25 mg midazolam,[c] 650 mg ketamine and 325 mg xylazine to 500 mL of 0.5% saline[d]	M: 0.05 mg/mL K: 1.3 mg/mL X: 0.65 mg/mL	1.6

Abbreviation: MKX, midazolam, ketamine, and xylazine.

[a] When using 500mL of 10% guaifenesin as the basis, drugs added should be doubled, leading to final concentrations that are doubled, and infusion rate will be halved.

[b] The concentration of romifidine is slightly lower than the original report (80 mg/mL versus 82.5 mg/mL). A higher concentration of guaifenesin was administered for the first 30 minutes in the original report.

[c] Diazepam can NOT be substituted for midazolam because diazepam is not water soluble and may result in the formation of a precipitate.

[d] The final concentrations have been modified from the original report; see text for details.

supplementation. The use of ketamine alone does not provide satisfactory anesthesia and is not recommended.

PROPOFOL

Propofol is a rapidly acting, non-barbiturate, anesthetic agent that is rapidly redistributed and cleared from the plasma by hepatic metabolism. Propofol has also demonstrated extrahepatic clearance that likely occurs in pulmonary and renal tissues. This pharmacokinetic profile makes it a potentially useful drug for maintaining anesthesia as it is rapidly redistributed and cleared so that rapid changes in depth of anesthesia via titration are easily achieved, particularly in species other than horses. Additionally, these same properties allow for a rapid recovery following a single dose or continuous infusion of propofol, and recoveries are typically very smooth.[14] However, in clinical use with horse, TIVA with propofol has variable kinetics and its quality of anesthesia may not be as reliable.[15] Loss of response to noxious stimuli (surgery) may not occur and increasing the dose may result in involuntary muscle movements (myclonus or dystonia).

Propofol is unlikely to replace ketamine for adult or large horses for field anesthesia as large volumes (up to 200ml) are required and induction, even with the use of alpha-2 agonists, often results in dangerous excitement of horses.[16] Additionally hypoventilation can be seen following propofol induction, which, while usually transient, can be problematic if it persists and an oxygen source is not present. It is recommended that oxygen supplementation be available when using propofol in horses.

OTHER DRUGS

Several other anesthetic drugs have been investigated as components of TIVA in horses, including medetomidine, tiletamine, and climazolam. For further reading and review of all the methods that have been used to provide TIVA in horses, the reader is directed elsewhere.[1]

MONITORING DURING TIVA

Given that most TIVA procedures occur in the field, it is usually not possible to monitor patients as invasively as in the clinic setting. At a minimum, depth of anesthesia, heart rate, and respiratory rate should be monitored closely.

Signs of central nervous system activity (eye position and palpebral reflexes) are often difficult to interpret. Horses' eye signs can remain active during TIVA, particularly with protocols using ketamine, and it is common to see tear production and spontaneous blinking.

Signs that the anesthetic plane is getting lighter usually include an increase in respiratory rate and depth, and increasing activity of the eyeball (eg, slow nystagmus progressing to rapid nystagmus) and palpebral reflex (eg, slight response progressing to spontaneous blinking). Physical movement of limbs and stretching or tensing of the neck also indicate a plane of anesthesia that is too light to allow the procedure to continue without potential injury to the horse or personnel. The plane of anesthesia is typically deepened by either increasing the infusion rate or giving additional boluses of ketamine. In addition, TIVA can be augmented with local anesthetic techniques, such as intratesticular lidocaine for castrations.

Anesthesia that is too deep can have any of the following signs: rapid shallow breathing that progresses to apnea or a pattern of Cheyne-Stokes breathing (deeper and sometimes faster breathing followed by a gradual decrease until a temporary apnea occurs, and then cycles again), pulses that are difficult to palpate, and dull eye signs (absent palpebral reflex, centrally positioned globe, absent corneal reflex). Anesthetic plane can be decreased by slowing or stopping the infusion until the appropriate depth has been achieved.

Portable physiologic parameter monitors are available and can be used to supplement physical signs when monitoring horses anesthetized with TIVA. Pulse oximetry can be used to determine pulse rate and the need for oxygen supplementation. Portable electrocardiogram and indirect blood pressure monitors can also be used, particularly in field situations involving critically ill horses.

RECOVERY

Recovery from TIVA relies on redistribution of the drugs away from the central nervous system and metabolism. As plasma concentrations decrease, the level of consciousness of the patient increases until the horse makes a successful attempt to stand.

Recovery from TIVA lasting less than 60 minutes is generally smooth and predictable. Longer durations of infusions lead to accumulation of drugs, longer times to recovery, and a less predictable course of achieving the standing position (additional information can be found in the article on recovery elsewhere in this issue).

PARTIAL INTRAVENOUS ANESTHESIA

Any of the intravenous infusion combinations can also be given during inhalant anesthesia. This technique, which is designed to allow reduction in dose of both injectables and inhalant, thus minimizes the side effects of both, and is referred to as balanced anesthesia, or partial intravenous anesthesia (PIVA).

Anesthetic infusions can be administered at up to one-tenth to one-quarter of the standard TIVA doses, which decreases the likelihood of decreased metabolism and drug accumulation during an inhalant anesthetic lasting several hours. It is essential that patients, as well as the rate of intravenous drug administration, be monitored closely to ensure that the depth of anesthesia does not become excessive. It is also possible that some drug effects are additive, as opposed to being minimized (eg, respiratory depression from ketamine and inhalant anesthetic).

The concentration of inhalant required to maintain an adequate depth of anesthesia can also be decreased by concurrent infusion of other drugs, such as lidocaine, opioids, alpha-2 agonists, and subanesthetic doses of ketamine (see the article on balanced anesthesia and constant rate infusions).

SUMMARY

TIVA is the mainstay of field anesthesia in horses, because cardiorespiratory depression is mild at clinically useful doses, and recovery is smooth in most horses. Drug components are selected to provide unconsciousness, muscle relaxation, and analgesia, and TIVA may induce a lesser stress response than inhalant anesthesia. With an attentive, careful anesthetist, TIVA provides predictable and safe anesthesia for procedures lasting up to 60 minutes.

REFERENCES

1. Muir WW, Hubbell JA. Equine anesthesia. 2nd edition. St Louis (MO): Saunders Elsevier; 2009. p. 260–76.
2. Muir WW, Skarda RT, Milne DW. Evaluation of xylazine and ketamine hydrochloride for anesthesia in horses. Am J Vet Res 1977;38:195–201.

3. Clarke KW, Taylor PM, Watkins SB. Detomidine/ketamine anaesthesia in the horse. Acta Vet Scand Suppl 1986;82:167–79.
4. Kerr CL, McDonnell WN, Young SS. A comparison of romifidine and xylazine when used with diazepam/ketamine for short-duration anesthesia in the horse. Can Vet J 1996;37:601–9.
5. Valverde A. Alpha-2 agonists as pain therapy in horses. Vet Clin North Am Equine Pract 2010;26(3):515–32.
6. Hubbell JA, Bednarski RM, Muir WW. Xylazine and tiletamine-zolazepam anesthesia in horses. Am J Vet Res 1989;50:737–42.
7. McCarty JE, Trim CM, Ferguson D. Prolongation of anesthesia with xylazine, ketamine and guaifenesin in horses: 64 cases (1986-1989). J Am Vet Med Assoc 1990;197:1646–50.
8. Muir WW, Skarda RT, Sheehan W. Evaluation of xylazine, guaifenesin, and ketamine hydrochloride for restraint in horses. Am J Vet Res 1978;39:1274–8.
9. Taylor PM, et al. Total intravenous anaesthesia in ponies using detomidine, ketamine and guaifenesin: pharmacokinetics, cardiopulmonary and endocrine effects. Res Vet Sci 1995;59:17–23.
10. McMurphy RM, et al. Comparison of the cardiopulmonary effects of anesthesia maintained by continuous infusion of romifidine, guaifenesin and ketamine, with anesthesia maintained by inhalation of halothane in horses. Am J Vet Res 2002;63:1655–61.
11. Hall LW, Clarke KW, Trim CM. Veterinary anaesthesia. 10th edition. London: Saunders; 2001. p. 174–5.
12. Hubbell JA, et al. Evaluation of a midazolam-ketamine-xylazine infusion for total intravenous anesthesia in horses. Am J Vet Res 2012;73:470–5.
13. Mama KR, Wagner AE, Steffey EP, et al. Evaluation of xylazine and ketamine for total intravenous anesthesia in horses. Am J Vet Res 2005;66(6):1002–7.
14. Nolan AM, Hall LW. Total intravenous anesthesia in the horse with propofol. Equine Vet J 1985;17:394–8.
15. Boscan P, Rezende ML, Grimsrud K, et al. Pharmacokinetic profile in relation to anaesthesia characteristics after a 5% micellar microemulsion of propofol in the horse. Br J Anaesth 2010;104(3):330–7.
16. Mama KR, Steffey EP, Pascoe PJ. Evaluation of propofol for general anesthesia in premedicated horses. Am J Vet Res 1996;57(4):512–6.

Neuromuscular Blocking Agents and Monitoring in the Equine Patient

Manuel Martin-Flores, DVM, DACVA

KEYWORDS

- Equine • Neuromuscular block • Acceleromyography • Cisatracurium • Vecuronium
- Rocuronium

KEY POINTS

- Neuromuscular blocking agents (NMBA) interrupt transmission at the neuromuscular junction, resulting in paralysis of skeletal musculature.
- NMBA do not contribute to sedation/hypnosis, hence the appropriate level of anesthesia needs to be assessed.
- Neuromuscular blockers may allow for smaller doses of general anesthetics to be administered, because immobility provided solely by general anesthetics may require large doses.
- Residual neuromuscular block is a potential complication every time neuromuscular blocking agents are used, and needs to be addressed before general anesthesia is interrupted.

INTRODUCTION

Neuromuscular blocking agents (NMBA), commonly called muscle relaxants or paralytic agents, compose a unique group of drugs used during general anesthesia: in contrast to most other agents administered during general anesthesia, NMBA do not participate in the provision of sedation, hypnosis, or analgesia, nor do they cross the blood-brain barrier or placenta in significant concentrations. NMBA are largely hydrophilic compounds with limited distribution. The only (intended) effect attributable to these drugs is the relaxation of skeletal muscle, which is achieved by interfering with normal neuromuscular transmission; neurotransmitter released from motor neurons are unable to stimulate skeletal muscle to produce contraction. This specific action results in a patient incapable of producing motor activity, even in response to noxious stimulation. As a consequence, the anesthetist needs to consider that some common

No conflicts of interest declared.

Department of Clinical Sciences, College of Veterinary Medicine, Cornell University, Box 32, Ithaca, NY 14853, USA

E-mail address: mm459@cornell.edu

Vet Clin Equine 29 (2013) 131–154

http://dx.doi.org/10.1016/j.cveq.2012.11.010

0749-0739/13/$ – see front matter © 2013 Elsevier Inc. All rights reserved.

signs used for the assessment of anesthetic depth will be completely abolished; attention must be focused on the maintenance of a suitable depth of hypnosis. Indeed, the inclusion of NMBA when people are anesthetized has resulted in a higher incidence of awareness under anesthesia.[1] For obvious reasons, spontaneous ventilation cannot occur, or at least not efficiently, in the presence of complete or partial neuromuscular block. The administration of NMBA without the means for providing mechanical ventilation (both in terms of equipment and skills) is contraindicated.

The introduction of NMBA into clinical anesthesia occurred only little more than half a century ago, and changed the practice of general anesthesia.[2] This change in anesthetic practice was not without complications: Beecher and Todd[3] documented in 1954 that the inclusion of NMBA in the anesthetic protocol increased mortality. It is not clear whether this was the result of NMBA use, poor use of mechanical ventilation, or reversal from relaxation and/or monitoring. As already mentioned, the use of these agents was also associated with an increase in the incidence of awareness under anesthesia.[1] It should be noted, however, that general volatile anesthetics produce immobility mainly through effects on the spinal cord. Movement in response to noxious stimuli may reflect insufficient analgesia, not insufficient hypnosis. Because awareness occurs as a result of insufficient hypnosis, an argument can be made that awareness under anesthesia occurs not because movement in response to noxious stimulation is blunted by NMBA, but simply because hypnotic agents are not administered in sufficient quantities.

The main purpose for including a NMBA in the anesthetic protocol is to enhance muscle relaxation without the necessity of administering large doses of general anesthetics. Both injectable and inhalational anesthetics may produce sufficient muscle relaxation for most surgical procedures in horses; however, the doses required to abolish muscular responses are considerably higher than those needed to produce hypnosis.[4–6] (More details on end points of inhalational anesthesia, and their relationship to the concentration administered, are discussed in the article written by Brosnan on inhalational anesthetics elsewhere in this issue.) The addition of an NMBA to the anesthetic protocol allows the anesthetist to administer a general anesthetic at doses only sufficient to provide hypnosis. When an analgesic drug is also included, this technique is referred to as balanced anesthesia, whereby all 3 major components of general anesthesia (hypnosis, analgesia, and muscle relaxation) are provided by the combination of different agents, rather than by the administration of a large dose of 1 agent. Because most general anesthetics produce a dose-dependent depression of cardiovascular functions, the reduction in the doses of general anesthetics administered typically results in improved and more stable hemodynamics.

In some cases, administration of NMBA may be actually necessary for some procedures to be completed. Ophthalmologic surgery may require the eye to be immobile, relaxed, and in a central position, which is easily achieved by paralyzing the patient. Fractures or luxations may be easier to be reduced in the absence of muscular tone. Muscle relaxation can aid in the institution of positive-pressure ventilation, and also can prevent substantial increases in intrathoracic pressure that may result from unsynchronized mechanical ventilation over spontaneous breathing from the patient. Profound muscle relaxation may also prevent accidents provoked by a horse's reflex response to noxious stimulation. Equipment damage from horses moving under anesthesia has occurred, implying not only a substantial loss in economic terms but also potential injury to the patient or the staff in the operating room. Anesthesiologists may also administer NMBA in very unstable and critically ill horses during colic surgery to reduce the amount of inhalational agents being used, without the risk of patient movement during surgery, at least until progress has been made in terms of hemodynamic stability. Several of these advantages have been recognized in horses receiving muscle relaxants as part of their anesthetic protocol.[7]

Regardless of whether the NMBA is administered because of necessity for a specific surgical procedure, or simply because the anesthesiologist chooses to include it as part of the anesthetic protocol, one thing is clear: monitoring the depth and duration of muscle relaxation is vital for ensuring that an adequate level of relaxation is achieved, assessing when subsequent doses are needed, and evaluating the extent of recovery of neuromuscular transmission before the patient is extubated and recovery from anesthesia can begin. Residual neuromuscular block is a serious potential complication after an NMBA has been administered, and should be prevented or addressed every time these drugs are used.

ANATOMY AND PHYSIOLOGY OF THE NEUROMUSCULAR JUNCTION

Because NMBA exert their actions by acting as either agonists (depolarizing NMBA) or antagonists (nondepolarazing NMBA) in the neuromuscular junction (NMJ), basic knowledge of the physiology of this synapse is vital for the understanding of neuromuscular block. The NMJ is a well-known and described synapse, and is the site of communication between the nervous and musculoskeletal systems. In general, neuromuscular transmission follows a relatively simple process. When an action potential arrives at the distal end of the motor nerve cell, conformational changes in voltage-gated Ca^{2+} channels allow an influx of Ca^{2+}, increasing its intracellular concentration. Vesicles containing acetylcholine (ACh), which is synthesized and stored by the nerve cell, are mobilized toward the cell membrane. The neurotransmitter contained in the vesicles is released into the cleft that separates the nerve cell and the muscle cell. Once in the synaptic cleft, ACh interacts with nicotinic acetylcholine receptors (nAChR) in the motor endplate. These receptors undergo a conformational change in response to the interaction with ACh, allowing an influx of Na^+; depolarization of the muscle cell follows. The action potential propagates along the muscle cell as more Na^+ channels open, triggering contraction of the skeletal muscle. The effects of ACh in the neuromuscular cleft are almost immediately terminated; the interaction between ACh and the nAChR is very brief, and once ACh disengages from the receptor it is hydrolyzed by the acetylcholinesterase enzyme.[8–10]

Anatomy of the NMJ

Motor neurons are single myelinated cells that reach muscle cells without any other synapses since their emergence at the spinal cord. Myelin is lost as the motor neuron reaches muscular tissue, and branching allows one motor neuron to reach several muscle cells; these muscle cells will constitute a motor unit. Schwann cells cover the branches of the motor neuron at the synapse (**Fig. 1**).

Vesicles containing ACh are localized in the motor neuron, close to the junctional membrane, in a region called the active zone. When Ca^{2+} concentration in the cell increases, as the action potential reaches the distal end of the neuron, vesicles are mobilized toward the membrane, fuse with the membrane, and rupture into the junctional cleft, releasing neurotransmitter by exocytosis. This process occurs very quickly, taking no more than 200 microseconds. The ACh released into the cleft will interact with nAChRs on the postsynaptic membrane. The amount of neurotransmitter released is much larger than the one needed to stimulate the receptors; in other words, ACh is released in excess. Stimulation of the nAChRs produces a depolarization of the endplate, which is also larger than the stimulating threshold. This "greater than required" signal and response happens even when only a fraction of the available

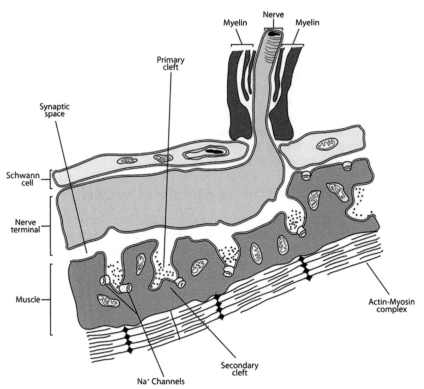

Fig. 1. The adult neuromuscular junction (NMJ). The motor neuron, muscle fiber, and Schwan cells are shown. Vesicles containing acetylcholine (ACh) cluster in proximity to the synaptic membrane in the nerve cell; this area is called the active zone. Folding in the muscle membrane increases the surface area, and nicotinic acetylcholine receptors (nAChR) can be found in the primary and secondary clefts. (*From* Shear TD, Martyn JA. Physiology and biology of neuromuscular transmission in health and disease. J Crit Care 2009;24:7; with permission.)

ACh is being released, and not all of the nAChRs are being stimulated. This mechanism provides the neuromuscular transmission with a great safety margin and a large reserve.[11] (The clinical implications of this safety margin are discussed later.) The amount of quanta released by the motor neuron depends, in part, on the concentration of extracellular Ca^{2+}. In the absence of Ca^{2+}, no ACh is released even after the nerve is stimulated. By the same principle, an increase in the extracellular Ca^{2+} results in the release of a larger amount of neurotransmitter. This concept is vital for the understanding of a physiologic phenomenon called posttetanic facilitation (PTF) and a monitoring technique named posttetanic count (PTC), and is discussed in more detail in the section on monitoring.

Two different pools of vesicles containing ACh can be identified in the motor nerve cell: a pool of readily available vesicles and a reserve pool. Readily available vesicles are found in the active zone, in close proximity to the junctional membrane, and these will release neurotransmitter in response to the arrival of an action potential.

Separated by the junctional cleft, the muscle membrane is also specialized tissue. The muscle cell presents folds, also called clefts; both primary and secondary clefts exist. As a result, the surface of the endplate is quite large. These folds are the site of residence of the nAChRs. In each cleft, close to 5 million nAChRs might be present. Deeper in the folds, Na^+ channels can be found. The region of the muscle cell that is immediately adjacent to the junctional area is called the perijunctional zone. The density of Na^+ channels increases in this area while nAChRs are still present. As a result, the response to activation of nAChRs is efficient, and the propagation of depolarization through the muscle cell is facilitated.[8–10]

Nicotinic acetylcholine receptors
The nAChR is a ligand-gated ion channel consisting of 5 subunit proteins. The nAChR is arranged so that a central pore can change its permeability to ions, depending on whether the receptor interacts with an agonist or not. The nAChR is embedded in the lipid bilayer and is thicker than the membrane, so that it protrudes to both the intracellular and extracellular spaces. These receptors can contain different combinations of subunits, establishing in this way several subpopulations of nAChRs. Some types are found presynaptically and some are found postsynaptically. Presynaptic and postsynaptic receptors mediate different actions pertinent to the use and monitoring of muscle relaxants (more details are given later).

Fetal nAChRs, as well as immature and extrajunctional receptors, present the following subunits: two $\alpha 1$ subunits, and one $\beta 1$, one δ, and one γ subunit ($\alpha 1\beta 1\delta\gamma$). These receptors are present in muscles during decreased levels of activity, as may occur in fetal muscles, or, for example, in individuals following prolonged immobilization, motor neuron injury, or burns. The fetal receptor presents a smaller pore, but a longer time of channel opening, in comparison with the adult form of the nAChR.[8]

Following innervation or return to muscle activity, the γ subunit is replaced by an ε subunit ($\alpha 1\beta 1\delta\varepsilon$); this is the adult or mature receptor, which will not undergo further changes. The nAChRs have 2 binding sites for interaction with agonists (eg, ACh). Sensitivity to neurotransmitter stimulation differs between the fetal and adult forms of the receptor; the fetal receptor is more sensitive to the stimulating effects of an agonist, such as ACh or succinylcholine (SCh), and channel opening is also increased. Fetal receptors also display a resistance to nondepolarizing neuromuscular blockers in comparison with the adult receptor. The same is true for patients with severe burns or denervations, who are more susceptible to the effects of agonists and depolarizing agents (SCh) and are resistant to the effects of nondepolarizing agents, which may indicate a decreased affinity of these receptors to nondepolarizing NMBA (eg, atracurium or vecuronium).[8]

Synaptic cleft and the acetylcholinesterase enzyme
As mentioned previously, the interaction between ACh and the nAChRs is short lived; almost immediately ACh detaches from the receptor into the synaptic cleft. The enzyme acetylcholinesterase is abundant in the synaptic cleft, and rapidly destroys any ACh that did not interact with a receptor or has detached from the receptor. Close to 50% of the ACh secreted is hydrolyzed before it even reaches a nAChR. The acetylcholinesterase enzyme is released by the postsynaptic muscle cell. After no more than 1 millisecond of its secretion, ACh is hydrolyzed into acetate and choline; choline is taken up by the presynaptic neuron and is used for the synthesis of new ACh.

Free ACh in the synaptic cleft may also interact with a presynaptic cholinergic receptor. Little is known about the presynaptic cholinergic receptors, but evidence shows that interaction between muscle relaxants and the presynaptic receptors may be responsible for some of the effects observed after the administration of a nondepolarizing agent. It is possible that depolarizing agents, such as SCh, do not interact with these receptors, explaining in part the differences seen during neuromuscular monitoring when depolarizing and nondepolarizing agents are used. This phenomenon is discussed in further detail in the following paragraphs. For more details on anatomy and physiology of the NMJ, the readers should consult relevant literature by Martyn and colleagues, Shear and Martyn, and Fagerlund and Eriksson.[8–10]

DEPOLARIZING NEUROMUSCULAR BLOCKING AGENTS: SUCCINYLCHOLINE

Neuromuscular blocking drugs can be classified into depolarizing or nondepolarizing agents, according to their mechanism of action. Succinylcholine (SCh) was introduced to clinical anesthesia in 1952, and despite well-known side effects it remains in clinical use as the sole depolarizing neuromuscular blocker. Its rapid onset and brief duration of action has kept SCh available all these years, despite its known drawbacks.

SCh closely resembles ACh, and on interaction with the nAChR it causes depolarization: SCh is an agonist for the nAChR. Prolonged interaction between an agonist (including ACh) and the receptor results in a lack of response to the agonist; this does not occur with ACh because such an interaction is very brief (<1 millisecond). The interaction between SCh and the receptor is much longer because SCh is not hydrolyzed by the acetylcholinesterase enzyme. Because of its agonistic effects, SCh initially produces muscle contractions: Fasciculations are seen on injection of SCh, which reflect a desynchronized depolarization of the muscle membrane.[12] Muscle fasciculations are followed by a refractory period during which relaxation ensues.

The muscle-relaxant effects of SCh are terminated when the drug diffuses out of the NMJ and becomes metabolized by plasma cholinesterase (pseudocholinesterase, or butyrylcholinesterase). This process takes longer than the hydrolysis of ACh that occurs via the acetylcholinesterase enzyme. During this period SCh is available to repeatedly interact with the receptor, perpetuating the period of no response and providing muscular relaxation.

Depolarizing neuromuscular block as caused by SCh is a characteristic one. On administration of SCh, single-twitch tension is decreased. However, the response to high-frequency stimulation, for example, during tetanic stimulation or train-of-four (TOF) stimulation, does not decrease. Fade during TOF monitoring is not observed. This characteristic type of block is named phase 1 block, and it is not reversed by the administration of antagonists such as edrophonium or neostigmine. In fact, administration of such agents may prolong phase 1 blockade, presumably by depressing the effects of plasma cholinesterase.[13]

After larger or repeated doses of SCh are administered, phase 2 blockade ensues. Phase 2 blockade is characterized by a decrease in single-twitch height, as well as the development of a fade in the response to tetanic or TOF stimuli. Phase 2 blockade can be shortened or antagonized by administering edrophonium or neostigmine. More details of phase 1 and 2 blockade are discussed in the section on monitoring.

SCh has a long list of side effects. Cardiac dysrhythmias have been observed after SCh administration to horses. SCh, 0.3 mg/kg (alone or followed by an infusion) caused mild and transient increases in heart rate and blood pressure when given to halothane-anesthetized horses.[14] Muscle fasciculations secondary to SCh administration can cause pain that may extend to the postoperative period. Muscular fasciculations can also result in increases in serum K^+ levels. Increases in serum K^+ concentrations of more than 100% were observed after administration of SCh to horses.[14] Although it is described that SCh can produce increases in intraocular pressure, such increases were transient (<5 minutes) and insignificant when evaluated in horses under halothane anesthesia.[15] Increases in intra-abdominal and intracranial pressure have also been reported in humans after the administration of SCh.

In a different study in ponies, 0.1 mg/kg SCh caused severe increases in heart rate of greater than 100% over preinjection values. An increase of almost 200% was seen in an individual receiving an infusion of the relaxant. These increases in heart rate were accompanied by increases in blood pressure and temperature as well as the development of metabolic acidosis and hypercapnia, despite mechanical ventilation. Muscle fasciculations lasted as long as 5 minutes in some ponies after SCh was administered.[16] The reason for such severe effects in some individuals is not clear, but a distinction between "reactors" and "nonreactors" was made in this study. Many of these side effects resemble signs of malignant hyperthermia (MH), and it should be noted that SCh administration is a known trigger of MH.

Prolonged relaxation after SCh can also result when the activity of plasma cholinesterase is decreased. Decreased plasma cholinesterase activity can occur in horses exposed to organophosphates; indeed, exposure to organophosphates prolongs the duration of action of this relaxant in horses.[17]

The reason SCh has remained a popular agent in clinical anesthesia is attributable to its ultrashort onset and brief duration. In contrast to SCh, nondepolarizing NMBA (see later discussion) have a prolonged onset of action, that is, the time between injection and the development of complete blockade requires a few minutes. Typically at least 3 to 5 minutes are required before significant neuromuscular blocking effects are reached. SCh, on the other hand, can produce profound paralysis, suitable for tracheal intubation, in only 1 minute, with a short duration of action (<10 minutes).[18] Such a profile proves to be advantageous during rapid sequence induction, a technique used under certain circumstances when human subjects are anesthetized. There is no necessity for paralysis when horses are intubated, and because of its short duration and long list of side effects, SCh has little value in equine anesthesia. Sadly a different indication has been proposed for the use of this paralyzing agent in horses: SCh has historically been used to immobilize horses without the use of hypnotic agents. Immobilizing a conscious animal by the administration of an NMBA is simply an inhumane practice, even when performed only minutes before the individual may be euthanized. As stated by Jones and Knottenbelt[19] in their 2001 letter to the editor regarding agents suitable for euthanasia,

> It is our firmly held view that the use of muscle relaxant drugs, such as SCh, is wholly contraindicated on humane grounds. In our opinion, it is totally unacceptable for any animal under any circumstances to be paralyzed while still conscious, even for a minimal period.

The author agrees with and supports this statement.

NONDEPOLARIZING NEUROMUSCULAR BLOCKING AGENTS

Nondepolarizing NMBA are the agents in current use for providing profound relaxation in horses. As the classification indicates, these agents do not produce depolarization of the muscle fibers. Nondepolarizing agents act as antagonists to the postsynaptic nAChR; they bind to the receptor and prevent the interaction between the nAChR and its natural agonist, ACh. Relaxation ensues because contraction simply cannot be evoked by ACh. The nature of this antagonism is competitive, therefore the concentration of the NMBA and ACh at the NMJ will dictate the effects. Nondepolarizing agents need to bind to either one or both α subunits at the ACh-binding site of the nAChR to block the action of ACh.

Nondepolarizing NMBA also exert their actions at presynaptic receptors in the NMJ. The interaction between these agents and the presynaptic receptor appears to be responsible for the development of fade seen during high-frequency nerve stimulation (eg, TOF or tetanus). Through positive and negative feedback, presynaptic receptors mediate the release of ACh according to the concentration of the neurotransmitter in the NMJ. Fade in contractile force during repetitive stimulation may be produced by a decreased release of ACh from the motor neuron caused by the interaction of the NMBA and the presynaptic receptor. Decreases in ACh release also enhance the competitive actions of NMBA at postsynaptic receptors.[12,20]

It was previously pointed out that the NMJ has a wide safety margin, and this has clinical implications. When an NMBA is administered at a low dose, several nAChR might be blocked without the development of clinical signs of relaxation. This situation is possible because activation of only a fraction of the receptors, with the neurotransmitter ACh, is necessary to produce muscle contractions. At least 70% of the nAChR must be blocked before signs of neuromuscular block are evident. Once such a high fraction of receptors has been blocked, relatively small increments of NMBA administration will produce noticeable effects. At this point the safety margin has been overcome, and no more drug is "wasted" in receptors that do not actively participate in the generation of muscle contraction. This phenomenon is the basis for a technique also used to shorten onset time, called priming. Priming was commonly used during intubation of humans, especially with older, slower-acting agents. The priming principle consists in administering only a fraction of the NMBA a few minutes before the balance of the dose is given. The reasoning is that the first fraction of the dose administered will occupy receptors without causing evident signs of blockade. Once the rest of the dose is injected, the drug will bind largely to "active" receptors. The time from injection of the second part of the dose to development of complete paralysis is shorter than if the full dose is administered once.

The second implication of the safety margin presented by the NMJ is that subsequent doses of NMBA will produce an increasingly larger effect. This notion follows the same principle as for the priming technique, and the clinical consequence is that when the effects of an NMBA begin to spontaneously recover, only a fraction of the original dose is needed to reestablish complete blockade. For example, if 0.1 mg/kg of atracurium is given to paralyze a horse, only a fraction of that dose (eg, 0.03–0.05 mg/kg) will be required to produce complete blockade when the effects of the first dose start to dissipate. During a dose-response study in horses, an initial dose of 0.13 mg/kg rocuronium produced an initial 40% depression of the single twitch. Once single-twitch depression was no longer seen, a further dose of only 0.04 mg/kg resulted in a further 80% reduction of the twitch (M. Martin-Flores, personal communication, 2012). In other words, although the second dose was substantially smaller, the subsequent decrease in twitch height was larger.

Historically, nondepolarizing NMBA have been clinically classified into long-acting, intermediate-acting, and short-acting agents. As shorter-acting anesthetic and analgesic agents that allow for quick recovery from anesthesia have been incorporated into clinical practice, long-lasting NMBA have been progressively abandoned. Short-acting nondepolarizing NMBA are also not easy to find. Mivacurium is often classified as a short-acting NMBA. However, this classification might not apply to all species; whereas mivacurium might be a short-acting agent when used in people, its duration of action is certainly not short in dogs.[21] Furthermore, the drug is not currently available in the United States, and literature regarding its use in equine anesthesia is not available. As a result, such a classification is impractical for the equine anesthetist. All modern nondepolarizing NMBA in use can be classified as intermediate-acting drugs. In addition, all NMBA present an onset time that is longer than that of SCh. These agents, therefore, are slower than SCh in producing relaxation; up to 3 to 5 minutes might be required before the full effect is established. To reduce onset time, larger doses can be administered. When dose-finding studies of muscle relaxants are performed, the doses that produce 50% and 95% twitch depression (ED_{50} and ED_{95}, respectively) are usually documented. The ED_{50} is a robust indicator of potency while the ED_{95} is a clinically useful dose; 95% depression of single twitch is typically considered sufficient for intubation and surgical procedures to be performed.[22] Multiples of the ED_{95} are commonly administered to accelerate onset, with the disadvantage that duration of action is also prolonged.

From a chemical viewpoint, NMBA can be divided into benzylisoquinolinium compounds and aminosteroid compounds. This classification is in fact more practical, as agents in each family share common characteristics.

Benzylisoquinolines

Atracurium

Benzylisoquinolinium compounds in current clinical use include atracurium and cisatracurium. Atracurium is a mixture of 10 different isomers of variable potency. Advantages of atracurium include its rapid and predictable metabolism, which is largely independent of hepatic and renal functions. Atracurium is hydrolyzed by nonspecific enzymes involving tissue esterases, which are different from plasma cholinesterase or ACh. Atracurium also undergoes Hoffman elimination, which is a nonenzymatic degradation dependent on pH and temperature. In contrast to SCh, abnormal plasma cholinesterase activity does not affect the elimination of atracurium.[23] Atracurium has been extensively used in horses, and a sizable body of literature is available. In addition, atracurium is probably the most cost-effective muscle relaxant currently available on the market.

When administered in large doses, atracurium has the ability of releasing histamine, which may result in adverse effects such as vasodilation, followed by hypotension and tachycardia. Bronchoconstriction is also a possible complication. Such complications can be prevented by slow administration of the drug or avoidance of large doses. Although histamine release has been commonly observed in people receiving atracurium, it should be noted that large doses are used frequently. During induction of anesthesia, and to accelerate the onset of the muscle relaxants, doses in excess of those needed to produce surgical relaxation are used (ie, twice the ED_{95} or more). Such rapid onset is rarely needed during equine anesthesia. Hence, a dose just sufficient to cause relaxation can be used, and the potential for histamine release minimized.

The effects of atracurium on anesthetized horses have been studied by Hildebrand and colleagues.[24–26] When used in halothane-anesthetized ponies, atracurium, 0.11 mg/kg, produced surgical relaxation (>95% reduction in single-twitch height). Twitch height returned to 10% of baseline after approximately 25 minutes. Further increments of one-half of the dose prolonged paralysis by a slightly longer period. The neuromuscular blocking effects were reversed with edrophonium, 0.5 mg/kg, at the end of the procedure. In adult horses, a lower dose (0.07 mg/kg) produced close to 100% twitch depression during halothane anesthesia, with a duration of less than 15 minutes (for return to 10% height of the single twitch). Surgical relaxation was maintained in horses with an infusion of 0.17 mg/kg/h. In these experiments, force of contraction in response to nerve stimulation was measured.

In horses anesthetized with isoflurane, and in which neuromuscular function was monitored with acceleromyography, atracurium, 0.15 mg/kg, failed to produce complete paralysis; at least one response to TOF stimulation could be detected.[27] At this dose, onset of action of atracurium required at least 6 minutes. Although spontaneous recovery from atracurium-induced paralysis is typically predictable and quick, in 1 of 9 horses the duration of paralysis doubled the average of the other 8 individuals evaluated, without an apparent cause.[27] The reasons for the disagreement in potency between these studies could be attributed to the technique of monitoring and/or the anesthetic technique used. Cardiovascular changes were not noted in these studies. Since its introduction to equine anesthesia, atracurium has been extensively used at doses ranging between 0.07 and 0.2 mg/kg without any major complications being reported.

Cisatracurium

Cisatracurium is one of the 10 isomers that constitute atracurium. Cisatracurium is more potent than atracurium, a smaller dose being necessary to achieve the same effects. Cisatracurium was synthesized in an attempt to decrease the undesirable side effects of atracurium, namely histamine release. The potential for histamine release with cisatracurium is less than with its parent compound, atracurium. Significant histamine release was seen in people only after 8-fold ED_{95} of cisatracurium was tested.[23]

When used in humans, the ED_{95} for cisatracurium is approximately 0.05 mg/kg, well below the ED_{95} of atracurium, which ranges between 0.2 and 0.25 mg/kg. To date, no reports on cisatracurium use in horses are available. The author's team has begun trials with cisatracurium, and pilot data indicate that doses of approximately 0.04 to 0.05 mg/kg may produce close to complete neuromuscular block in horses under isoflurane anesthesia (Martin-Flores, unpublished data). The electromyographic response to approximately 0.04 mg/kg of cisatracurium administered to a horse is shown in **Fig. 2**.

Aminosteroids

Pancuronium, vecuronium, and rocuronium are examples of aminosteroid NMBA that have been used in horses. Although literature exists for pancuronium, its clinical use has been mostly abandoned because of its long duration of action. Only vecuronium and rocuronium are commonly used for muscle relaxation during clinical anesthesia of horses.

Aminosteroid compounds differ from benzylisoquinolines in that their clearance depends on organ function; either hepatic and/or renal functions will determine excretion and, in part, duration of action. Therefore, the possibility for prolonged duration or paralysis caused by hepatic or renal insufficiency, or reduced blow flow to those organs, is increased when these agents are used. However, aminosteroid compounds are not known for releasing histamine, even at large doses. In fact, an advantage of aminosteroids is their cardiovascular stability.

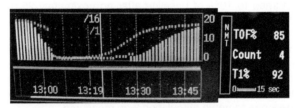

Fig. 2. Electromyographic trace in a horse anesthetized with isoflurane after the administration of cisatracurium, approximately 0.04 mg/kg intravenously. Green dots represent T1 and white vertical bars represent the train-of-four (TOF) ratio. Close to complete paralysis was achieved (T1 depression ~95%), and complete spontaneous recovery occurred after approximately 45 minutes. The panel on the right shows the value for the TOF ratio (85%) and the first twitch of the train (T1; 92%) during recovery from cisatracurium-induced block.

Vecuronium

Vecuronium was introduced to clinical anesthesia almost at the same time as atracurium, and it has been its aminosteroid equivalent ever since. Like atracurium, administration of clinical useful doses of vecuronium in people provides relaxation of intermediate duration (30–45 minutes), without cardiovascular changes. Vecuronium offers a good alternative to atracurium when hemodynamic changes are to be minimized. Vecuronium has also gained popularity as a muscle relaxant in dogs. The use of vecuronium in horses, however, has been limited, and the literature in equine anesthesia is scarce.

The limited experience with vecuronium has revealed some unexpected complications, previously not reported with atracurium. Horses with an apparent resistance to the neuromuscular blocking effects of vecuronium have been encountered; reports reflect that after the administration of 0.05 to 0.1 mg/kg of vecuronium, no decrease in neuromuscular function was observed (**Fig. 3**).[28–30] It was also noted that some individuals in which vecuronium produced no muscle-relaxant effects did become paralyzed after atracurium was administered. The cause if this lack of sensitivity of some horses to vecuronium is not known.

The use of vecuronium to facilitate mechanical ventilation in horses has been reported.[31] In this study, vecuronium, 0.1 mg/kg was given to horses under halothane anesthesia. The duration of action of vecuronium was reported to be only approximately 12 minutes; however, no objective method for monitoring the depth of neuromuscular block was used.

Recently a dose-finding study for vecuronium in isoflurane-anesthetized horses was undertaken.[32] Two main conclusions are noteworthy from this investigation. First, the potency of vecuronium in horses appears to be somewhat less than in other species. Whereas humans, dogs, and cats may be completely paralyzed with 0.05 mg/kg, horses receiving as much as 0.1 mg/kg only reached submaximal block ($\sim$75% twitch depression). In addition, whereas 0.025 mg/kg will produce substantial block in dogs, no effects at all were detected with this dose in the horses evaluated. Hence, higher doses than used in other species would be needed for complete paralysis. Second, even when only partial block was achieved with 0.1 mg/kg, duration of partial relaxation was much longer than expected. One horse recovered spontaneously 2 hours after vecuronium administration, whereas other individuals required pharmacologic antagonism 2 hours or more after vecuronium administration. Furthermore, in those individuals requiring pharmacologic antagonism, large doses of edrophonium were required before reversal was complete. Although doses of edrophonium ranging between 0.1 and 0.5 mg/kg are typically used, one horse required as much as 1.1 mg/kg of edrophonium before recovery from general anesthesia could begin. The author's service abandoned the use of vecuronium in horses after these data were collected. An acceleromyographic trace of prolonged partial block in a horse after 0.1 mg/kg of vecuronium is shown in **Fig. 4**.

Rocuronium

Rocuronium is also an aminosteroid compound that was introduced to the market to satisfy some demand for a nondepolarizing agent with a short onset of action; indeed, the lag between administration and complete paralysis is shorter for rocuronium than for vecuronium. Onset time after vecuronium was administered ranged between 2 and 5.5 minutes, depending on the dose.[32] A dose of rocuronium producing approximately 90% twitch depression in horses had an onset time of only about 2.5 minutes (range 1.5–3.5 minutes). This interval was shortened when the dose was increased (1.5 [0.75–2.5] minutes).[33] Although a higher dose of vecuronium (sufficient to produce

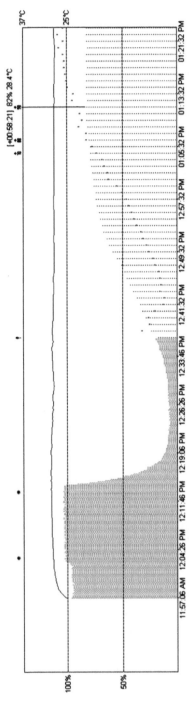

Fig. 3. Resistance to vecuronium in a horse. Vecuronium administration (*first asterisk* on top) produced no depression on the acceleromyographic single-twitch response. Atracurium (*second asterisk*) produced neuromuscular block. The pattern of stimulation was switched to TOF to assess recovery and exclude residual curarization. Return of the TOF ratio to 70%, 80%, and 90% is indicated on top of the trace.

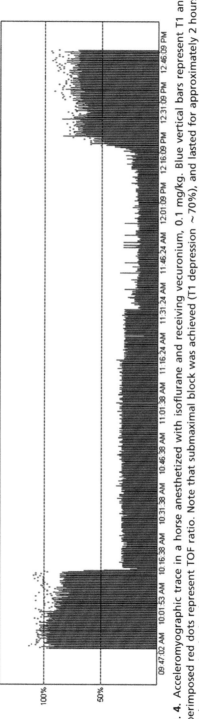

Fig. 4. Acceleromyographic trace in a horse anesthetized with isoflurane and receiving vecuronium, 0.1 mg/kg. Blue vertical bars represent T1 and superimposed red dots represent TOF ratio. Note that submaximal block was achieved (T1 depression ~70%), and lasted for approximately 2 hours. This horse received edrophonium, 1.1 mg/kg (given in increments) until recovery from block was considered adequate before general anesthesia could be discontinued.

complete block) could result in a shorter onset time, such an investigation was not pursued because of the preliminary results found with lower doses.[32]

Although a formal dose-finding study for rocuronium has not yet been reported, doses ranging between 0.2 and 0.6 mg/kg have been used extensively in horses under inhalational anesthesia; doses of 0.2 mg/kg provided approximately 90% twitch depression, and 0.4 and 0.6 mg/kg produced full blockade.[33] Rocuronium-induced block lasted less than 20 minutes with the lower dose, and as much as 1 hour after the highest dose. However, no reports of resistance, excessively prolonged paralysis, or cardiovascular instability have been reported to date. Rocuronium has therefore gained popularity and has become the natural alternative for atracurium. Rocuronium, however, shows certain variability regarding its duration of action. For example, a dose of 0.2 mg/kg had complete recovery times between approximately 5 and 30 minutes. Rocuronium, 0.3 mg/kg, was given to horses undergoing ophthalmologic surgery.[34] The interval between administration and the return to 25% twitch height ranged between 7.7 and 56 minutes. Complete recovery required about 20 to 85 minutes (average of ~35 minutes). However, 2 things should be pointed out. First, whereas longer than expected duration could delay recovery from anesthesia and increase the time under general anesthesia, shorter than expected duration is not a problem during clinical anesthesia, as long as the depth of neuromuscular block is monitored. Incremental doses can be used if neuromuscular block needs to be prolonged. With the use of low doses, prolonged duration of action with rocuronium is an infrequent phenomenon. Second, an agent-specific reversal agent for rocuronium is now available in Europe, and should soon be available in the United States. More details regarding reversal of a nondepolarizing block are discussed later.

MONITORING NEUROMUSCULAR BLOCKADE

Much like any other parameter that can be monitored during general anesthesia, neuromuscular function can also be evaluated, and it is now possible to do so in an objective (and user-friendly) manner. Unfortunately, neuromuscular monitoring has not gained widespread acceptance in operating rooms, regardless of whether humans or animals are being anesthetized, despite the large body of evidence showing the benefits of using these monitors. In brief, neuromuscular monitoring reduces the incidence of complications associated with residual neuromuscular block, allows for tighter titration of NMBA being administered, and provides the anesthetist with necessary information to decide whether reversal with an antagonist can be attempted.

There are several techniques to monitor neuromuscular block, all of which follow the same criterion: because neuromuscular blockers inhibit the transmission between motor nerve cells and muscle fibers, a motor neuron is stimulated and the muscular response is evaluated. The difference in monitoring techniques depends on how the evoked response to nerve stimulation is assessed. The simplest way to monitor depth and recovery of neuromuscular block is through visual or tactile assessment of the response to stimulation with a peripheral nerve stimulator (PNS). This qualitative method does not provide any measurements, but it is certainly useful if its limitations are understood.

A PNS stimulator can be used over the peroneal nerve in the hind limb, the radial nerve in the thoracic limb, or the facial nerve. A close agreement between the pelvic and thoracic limbs for monitoring sites was found, whereas more variable results were obtained when monitoring was performed at the face. Details regarding the placement of electrodes in either location can be found in a study by Mosing and colleagues.[35] Most commonly the peroneal or radial nerve is used. Stimulation at the peroneal nerve produces an extension of the hoof. Stimulation of the radial nerve produces extension of the carpus. Choice of stimulating site usually depends on the surgical procedure and the access to a limb in the operating room.

During nerve stimulation, several patterns of stimulation can be used. The simplest mode is called single twitch. Single twitch is the delivery of a single impulse, which is repeated either every second or every 10 seconds (frequencies of 1 Hz or 0.1 Hz, respectively). Single twitch is commonly used during dose-response studies; depression of the single twitch reflects the magnitude of block. Its clinical utility, however, is limited. To accurately use single twitch as a method for monitoring, twitch height in the absence of relaxation must be established. That is, the height of a single twitch is measured before the NMBA is given. Subsequent reductions in single-twitch measurements are then compared with baseline. Hence, it is evident that single twitch lacks any utility if the response is evaluated only visually, because no measurements can be obtained.

The most commonly used pattern of stimulation during clinical anesthesia is the TOF. TOF was described in 1971 by Ali and colleagues,[36] who stated that repeated stimulation at 2 Hz (ie, every 0.5 seconds) resulted in the progressive loss of contractile force during nondepolarizing neuromuscular block. These trains of stimulation are typically repeated every 10 to 15 seconds. TOF stimulation therefore offers a great advantage; each train behaves as its own control. A baseline value, obtained in the absence of blockade, is not needed. In turn, each time a TOF is delivered, the height of the fourth component of the train (T4) can be compared with that of the first component (T1). By dividing these values, the TOF ratio is obtained (T4/T1). Logically, in the absence of blockade both components should produce equal measurements, and a TOF ratio of 1.0 (or 100%) is recorded. Normal TOF ratios in horses and in the absence of paralysis typically exceed 0.9. Lower values indicate the development of fade and the presence of neuromuscular block, even if partial. When the evaluation is performed only visually, a TOF ratio cannot be measured; however, it is possible to detect fades of 0.5 or less. Values greater than 0.5 are commonly missed, meaning that shallow residual block may go undetected.

Other patterns of stimulation include double burst stimulation (DBS), tetanus, and posttetanic count (PTC). In brief, DBS comprises the administration of 2 brief tetanic impulses separated by a short interval, and was introduced in 1989 with the purpose of increasing the efficacy of detecting residual block when the responses were evaluated subjectively.[37] Because only 2 (and not 4) evoked contractions are seen, and because the contractions last longer, it may be easier to detect residual block with DBS with more efficiency than with TOF. However, such a difference is minimal, and shallow degrees of residual block cannot be detected subjectively with either pattern of stimulation.

Tetanus is infrequently used, and it consists of the delivery of high-frequency stimulation (50 or 100 Hz) lasting typically for 5 seconds (which is painful), resulting in a sustained response. It does not offer clinical advantages over TOF and because of the pain it may provoke, its use during light planes of anesthesia can result in patient movement. In the presence of residual block, fade develops during the duration of the tetanic response. PTC is a method that can be used to assess very deep (or intense) neuromuscular block. Once an NMBA has been administered and no response to TOF stimulation can be elicited, further increments in the depth of blockade cannot be monitored by this method. The PTC offers a possibility for assessing the depth of blockade, even when no responses to TOF can be seen. During PTC, a tetanic stimulus is followed (after a 3-second pause) by several single twitches at 1 Hz.[38] Neurotransmitter release is influenced by the amount of intracellular Ca^{2+}. During a tetanic stimulation, large amounts of Ca^{2+} enter the cell at a higher rate than they leave (in fact, a tetanic stimulus is the summation of several high-frequency stimuli; Ca^{2+} enters the cell with each stimulus). The tetanic stimulation results in the movement of stored ACh to the active zone and the release of a larger than normal amount of ACh during the subsequent single-twitch stimulation (posttetanic facilitation). This large amount of ACh temporarily reverses neuromuscular block and produces noticeable twitches, which otherwise would not have been observed. The number of twitches during PTC is inversely related to the interval before recovery from block occurs.

Because TOF is the most commonly used pattern of stimulation and the most useful during clinical equine anesthesia, the rest of this section discusses this pattern rather than the others. **Fig. 5** shows a representation of single twitch, TOF, and tetanus in a horse during nondepolarizing block.

Visual inspection of evoked muscle contractions provides information useful to the management of neuromuscular block and its reversal. Put simply, if no responses can be elicited during TOF stimulation, relaxation is profound, and pharmacologic reversal with anticholinesterase inhibitors should not be attempted. Surgical relaxation is present when 0 to 2 responses can be elicited during TOF stimulation with a PNS. When all 4 responses are present, the anesthetist can evaluate whether a fade is seen. If a fade can be seen during recovery from nondepolarizing block, residual block

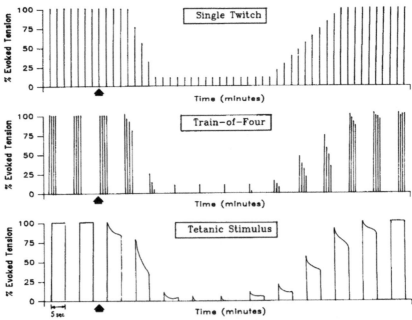

Fig. 5. Mechanomyographic (ie, force measurements) representation of hoof twitch in a horse before, during, and after nondepolarizing neuromuscular blockade. Before administration of neuromuscular blocking agents (*arrow*), single-twitch height and TOF ratio are set to 100%. Similarly, no fade can be seen in response to 5-second tetanic (50 Hz) stimulation. During nondepolarizing block, height of single twitch decreases, and fade appears during TOF and tetanic stimulation. The return of fade to 100% during TOF is the most commonly used technique to assess recovery from nondepolarizing block. (*From* Hildebrand S. Neuromuscular blocking agents in equine anesthesia. Vet Clin North Am Equine Pract 1990;6(3):598; with permission.)

is present and recovery is still incomplete. If no fade is seen, it is uncertain whether residual block is present; this is the first limitation when using subjective neuromuscular monitoring with a PNS. Although in theory lack of fade during TOF stimulation should represent complete recovery from neuromuscular block, visual or tactile inspection of a TOF is not reliable enough to detect low levels of fade. It was first demonstrated in people than when TOF ratio is 0.4 to 0.5 or higher, a fade cannot be visually detected.[39] When this was studied in horses under general anesthesia and recovering from atracurium-induced neuromuscular block, similar results were obtained: even the most experienced anesthesiologists cannot visually detect a fade greater than 0.5.[27] In other words, if one was to decide whether neuromuscular block has been completely reversed based on a visual inspection of TOF stimulation, a horse could be considered reversed when the TOF is only 0.5. Hence, the use of PNS with subjective evaluation of the evoked responses produces useful but limited information. It is a safer approach to use a PNS to judge whether an antagonist should be administered (eg, >2 responses to TOF stimulation present) or whether antagonism should be delayed (eg, no responses present).

Objective monitoring producing actual measurements of evoked responses is obviously preferred. Several techniques are available. Measurement of force constitutes the gold standard and is called mechanomyography (MMG). Although MMG has been described in horses it requires bulky equipment, which is not suitable for daily clinical practice. Mechanomyography measures force during isometric contraction; the limb should be fixed in position. The force generated after supramaximal nerve stimulation is recorded. Details on the MMG setup are described by Klein and colleagues.[40]

Electromyography (EMG) measures muscular cellular activation in response to nerve stimulation. Although an EMG monitor specifically designed to assess neuromuscular block is currently available, this technique is not widely distributed in equine anesthesia. **Fig. 2** shows an electromyographic tracing of a horse receiving cisatracurium. The EMG response recorded with this method does not depend on the movement produced, but on cellular activation. Hence, an advantage of EMG monitoring is that it is independent of position of the limb and type of movement. The hoof of a horse could be allowed to move freely, or it could be restrained and covered with surgical drapes during a procedure.

Acceleromyography (AMG) is possibly the most common objective monitor in current use, both for clinical use and research in humans and animals, including the horse (**Figs. 6** and **7**). Acceleromyography measures the acceleration of the evoked muscle twitch, which is closely related to force (force = mass × acceleration). Acceleration of the movement of the hoof is measured by attaching a small acceleration-sensitive transducer (or crystal) to the dorsal aspect of the hoof. The AMG monitor is a hand-held device, relatively affordable and simple in its use. A detailed description of this monitor has been published.[41] Acceleromyography, in contrast to MMG, measures the acceleration of the movement of the hoof rather than the isometric force of contraction. Hence, movement of the hoof should be free and unopposed. Changes in position or resistance added to the movement (as can be caused by drapes placed over the limb) can affect the results.

Although a recognized virtue of TOF stimulation is that the establishment of baseline values is not needed (each TOF acts as its own control), the AMG monitor might need to be calibrated before the relaxant is given in order to obtain accurate measurements. The current AMG monitors available (TOF Watch series) were designed to monitor neuromuscular block in people; the sensitivity of the acceleration crystal was set in accordance. When an uncalibrated AMG monitor was used in dogs, the movement

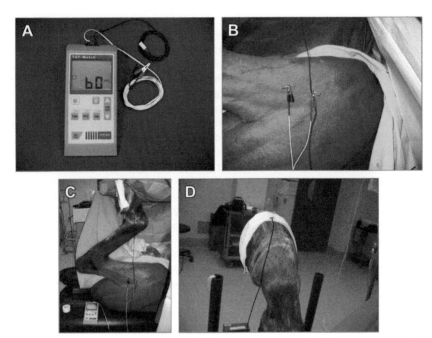

Fig. 6. (*A*) Acceleromyography monitor (TOF Watch, Organon). (*B–D*) Position of needles for peroneal nerve stimulation, and acceleration sensitive crystal taped to the dorsal aspect of the hoof in a horse in dorsal recumbency.

generated in response to nerve stimulation was too low to produce accurate results.[42] A similar problem occurred when the device was used in pediatric human patients.[43] Although no data have been published for horses, the author's experience using the AMG monitor without baseline calibration in horses is in accordance with that in dogs; lack of baseline calibration in this species may result in inaccurate results that do not provide information sufficient to determine whether recovery from neuromuscular block is complete.

Residual Neuromuscular Block

Residual neuromuscular block, or postoperative residual curarization (PORC) is a potential complication that can occur every time NMBA are included as part of the anesthesia protocol. The unidentified presence of even low levels of neuromuscular block during or after recovery from anesthesia is considered residual blockade. It has been demonstrated in humans that even a very low level of residual block can cause hypoxia and/or tracheal aspiration, and that this risk is decreased when objective monitoring of neuromuscular function is used intraoperatively.[44–46] Noteworthy is that residual blockade is a common complication in people, even when intermediate-acting agents are used. The incidence of residual curarization after atracurium, vecuronium, or rocuronium ranged between 45% and 62% in 2 different studies.[47,48]

Several factors are associated with a decrease in the incidence of postoperative residual block: the use of intermediate-acting agents, routine reversal of neuromuscular block, and intraoperative monitoring of neuromuscular depth. Indiscriminate pharmacologic reversal in horses has its own series of drawbacks. As discussed in the section on antagonism, reversal agents can be associated with cardiovascular changes. In addition, neuromuscular block cannot always be efficiently reversed, no

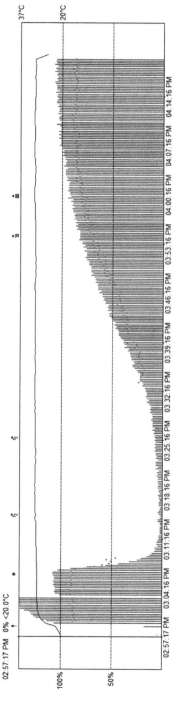

Fig. 7. Acceleromyographic TOF ratio (*red dots*) and height of the first twitch (T1) (*blue vertical lines*) in a horse after atracurium administration. TOF cannot be measured during the period of most profound blockade, when fewer than 4 responses to TOF can be obtained. The return of T2, T3, and TOF ratio of 70% and 80% are indicated above the trace.

matter the dose of reversal agent administered. Intraoperative monitoring, however, can potentially be used in every patient, as long as such a monitoring device is available. The combined use of monitoring and reversal decreased the incidence of residual block in people from 62% to 3%.[48]

It is unknown whether shallow levels of residual block will result in hypoxia, as occurs in people. Tracheal aspiration also occurs in people with mild degrees of residual block (eg, with a TOF ratio between 0.7 and 0.9). It is also not known whether shallow residual block could result in laryngeal dysfunction in horses, sufficient to cause a degree of upper airway collapse. Until that information becomes available, it is a safer approach to monitor neuromuscular block and document complete recovery of the TOF ratio before the patient is moved to the recovery stall. Although residual block has been overlooked in the veterinary literature, it is a potential complication that should be taken seriously when muscle relaxants are used. PORC was avoided in a few horses when longer than expected muscle relaxation occurred, likely thanks to the use of objective neuromuscular monitoring.[29,32]

Pharmacologic Antagonism of Neuromuscular Block

Antagonism of neuromuscular block may be necessary to accelerate recovery in those cases in where the surgical procedure is ending and residual block is still present. Because NMBA are competitive antagonists, reversal is possible by increasing the local concentration of ACh. For this purpose acetylcholinesterase inhibitors, such as edrophonium or neostigmine, are administered. These drugs block the action of the acetylcholinesterase enzyme responsible for the hydrolysis of ACh. As a result, the local concentration of ACh increases and competes with the NMBA at the NMJ.

Acetylcholinesterase inhibitors do not increase the production or release of ACh by the motor nerve cell; rather, they slow down the rate of hydrolysis. This characteristic has important clinical implications. First, there is a limit of local ACh concentration, which is dictated by the release of ACh from the presynaptic cell. In other words, once the activity of acetylcholinesterase has been inhibited, further administration of edrophonium or neostigmine cannot increase the local concentration of ACh. Second, the concentration of NMBA at the NMJ during profound block is high enough so that even complete inhibition of acetylcholinesterase activity does not result in a concentration of ACh sufficient to compete with the NMBA. As a consequence, profound relaxation cannot be effectively antagonized. Pharmacological antagonism with these agents is not attempted until some degree of spontaneous recovery has been established, which indicates that the concentration of NMBA at the site of action is decreasing. Typically at least 2 responses to TOF stimulation should be detected before antagonism begins. Reversal at a TOF count of 4 (ie, 4 responses visible after TOF stimulation) is likely to yield better results.

Because edrophonium and neostigmine can increase the levels of ACh, parasympathetic tone may increase; bradycardia and bronchospasm, as well as an increase in salivation, can occur. In other species, this is commonly prevented by the concomitant administration of atropine, but in horses this practice is typically avoided owing to the undesired effects of atropine on gastrointestinal function. Slow administration and the use of low doses typically prevent this problem. Doses of edrophonium ranging between 0.1 and 0.5 mg/kg have been commonly used in horses.[29] Neostigmine has also been used. Hildebrand and Howitt[49] studied the use of neostigmine, 0.04 mg/kg and edrophonium, 1 mg/kg in horses after pancuronium was given for relaxation. A transient increase in arterial blood pressure and a decrease in heart rate were seen following edrophonium, but no changes were seen after neostigmine administration. These drugs were given when twitch height had returned to only 10% of its baseline value, that is, during moderate levels of blockade. A much lower dose of neostigmine (0.007 mg/kg) was used to reverse mild rocuronium-induced blockade.[33,34]

A new reversal agent called sugammadex is now available (currently in Europe) to antagonize rocuronium-induced or vecuronium-induced block. Sugammadex is a modified γ-cyclodextrin, and represents a new concept for the reversal of NMBA; rather than increasing the local concentration of ACh, sugammadex forms a complex with rocuronium or vecuronium, encapsulating the agent and rendering it completely ineffective. The 3-dimensional conformation of sugammadex resembles that of a doughnut in which the NMBA can be contained. As defined in a recent review article, sugammadex is therefore the first selective relaxant binding agent.[18]

Sugammadex forms a tight complex with steroidal relaxants in a 1-to-1 ratio. The dissociation between host and guest is slow, making this complex stable, and virtually eliminating the risk of recurarization (ie, reestablishment of neuromuscular block). After sugammadex is injected it binds with free rocuronium in plasma, making the concentration of free rocuronium precipitate quite rapidly. Rocuronium then moves from the NMJ back into the plasma following a concentration gradient. The decrease in concentration of rocuronium at the NMJ reverses the neuromuscular block. Sugammadex does not increase the plasma levels of ACh, hence there is no need for administration of atropine. Sugammadex is excreted unchanged in the urine.[18]

Despite sugammadex being such a new agent, reports of its use in horses are already available. Mosing and colleagues[35] administered sugammadex, 4 mg/kg, 5 minutes after complete neuromuscular block had been established with rocuronium in ponies. Sugammadex quickly and effectively restored neuromuscular function (TOF ratio ≥ 0.9) in approximately 3.5 minutes. No side effects attributable to sugammadex were observed. Sugammadex therefore allows for quick, effective, and virtually side-effect–free reversal of rocuronium-induced and possibly vecuronium-induced block in horses, even when profound relaxation is present.

SUMMARY

In summary, NMBA produce muscle relaxation that may aid in providing optimal surgical conditions for selected procedures without the need to increase the dose of general anesthetics administered. This practice, in turn, may result in better hemodynamic stability. Atracurium and rocuronium are likely the best choices, given the current availability of agents at the time of writing.

Neuromuscular function should be monitored whenever these agents are used, to assess whether subsequent doses need to be administered and whether pharmacologic antagonism can be initiated (ie, neuromuscular block is not profound), and to exclude residual neuromuscular block at the end of the procedure.

Pharmacologic antagonism is possible by the administration of edrophonium or neostigmine, but neither drug is devoid of side effects, nor are they efficient for reversing intense neuromuscular block. The availability of sugammadex offers the possibility of reversing intense rocuronium-induced block, and should be available for use in the near future.

REFERENCES

1. Bergman IJ, Kluger MT, Short TG. Awareness during general anaesthesia: a review of 81 cases from the Anaesthetic Incident Monitoring Study. Anaesthesia 1954;57:549.
2. Griffith HR, Johnson GE. The use of curare in general anesthesia. Anesthesiology 1942;3:418.

3. Beecher TK, Todd DP. Study of deaths associated with anesthesia and surgery based on a study of 599 458 anesthesias in 10 institutions 1948-1952 inclusive. Ann Surg 1954;140:2.

4. Eger EI, Siadman LJ, Brandstater B. Minimum alveolar concentration: a standard of anesthetic potency. Anesthesiology 1965;26:756.

5. Quasha AL, Eger EI, Tinker JH. Determination and application of MAC. Anesthesiology 1980;53:315.

6. Seddighi R, Egger CM, Rohrbach BW, et al. The effect of midazolam on the end-tidal concentration of isoflurane necessary to prevent movement in dogs. Vet Anaesth Analg 2011;38:195.

7. Hildebrand SV, Holland M, Copland VS, et al. Clinical use of the neuromuscular blocking agents atracurium and pancuronium for equine anesthesia. J Am Vet Med Assoc 1989;195:212.

8. Martyn JA, Fagerlund MJ, Eriksson LI. Basic principles of neuromuscular transmission. Anaesthesia 2009;64:1.

9. Shear TD, Martyn JA. Physiology and biology of neuromuscular transmission in health and disease. J Crit Care 2009;24:5.

10. Fagerlund MJ, Eriksson LI. Current concepts in neuromuscular transmission. Br J Anaesth 2009;103:108.

11. Rich MM. The control of neuromuscular transmission in health and disease. Neuroscientist 2006;12:134.

12. Lien CA, Savarese JJ. Neuromuscular junction pharmacology. In: Hemmings HC Jr, Hopkins PM, editors. Foundations of anesthesia. Basic sciences for clinical practice. 2nd edition. Elsevier Mosby; 2006. p. 445–60.

13. McCoy EP, Mirakhur RK. Comparison of the effects of neostigmine and edrophonium on the duration of action of suxamethonium. Acta Anaesthesiol Scand 1995; 39:744.

14. Benson GJ, Hartsfield SM, Smetzer DL, et al. Physiologic effects of succinylcholine chloride in mechanically ventilated horses anesthetized with halothane in oxygen. Am J Vet Res 1979;40:1411.

15. Benson GJ, Manning JP, Hartsfield SM, et al. Intraocular tension of the horse: effects of succinylcholine and halothane anesthesia. Am J Vet Res 1981;42:1831.

16. Hildebrand SV, Howitt GA. Succinylcholine infusion associated with hyperthermia in ponies anesthetized with halothane. Am J Vet Res 1983;44:2280.

17. Himes JA, Edds GT, Kirkham WW, et al. Potentiation of succinylcholine by organophosphate compounds in horses. J Am Vet Med Assoc 1967;151:54.

18. Naguib M. Sugammadex: another milestone in clinical neuromuscular pharmacology. Anesth Analg 2007;104:575.

19. Jones RS, Knottenbelt DC. Disagree with use of muscle relaxant before euthanasia. J Am Vet Med Assoc 2001;218:1884.

20. Jonsson M, Gurley D, Dabrowski M, et al. Distinct pharmacologic properties of neuromuscular blocking agents on human neuronal nicotinic acetylcholine receptors: a possible explanation for the train-of-four fade. Anesthesiology 2006;105:521.

21. Smith LJ, Moon PF, Lukasik VM, et al. Duration of action and hemodynamic properties of mivacurium chloride in dogs anesthetized with halothane. Am J Vet Res 1999;60:1047.

22. Kopman AF, Lien CA, Naguib M. Determining the potency of neuromuscular blockers: are traditional methods flawed? Br J Anaesth 2010;104:705.

23. Donati F, Bevan DR. Neuromuscular blocking agents. In: Barash PG, Cullen BF, Stoelting RK, editors. Clinical anesthesia. 5th edition. Lippincott Williams & Wilkins; 2006. p. 421–52.

24. Hildebrand SV, Howitt GA, Arpin D. Neuromuscular and cardiovascular effects of atracurium in ponies anesthetized with halothane. Am J Vet Res 1986;47:1096.

25. Hildebrand SV, Arpin D. Neuromuscular and cardiovascular effects of atracurium administered to healthy horses anesthetized with halothane. Am J Vet Res 1988; 49:1066.

26. Hildebrand SV, Hill T 3rd. Effects of atracurium administered by continuous intravenous infusion in halothane-anesthetized horses. Am J Vet Res 1989;50:2124.

27. Martin-Flores M, Campoy L, Ludders JW, et al. Comparison between acceleromyography and visual assessment of train-of-four for monitoring neuromuscular blockade in horses undergoing surgery. Vet Anaesth Analg 2008;35:220.

28. Bardell D, Auer U, Mosing M. Reversal of vecuronium blockade with sugammadex in ponies. Vet Anaesth Analg 2010;37:17.

29. Gurney M, Mosing M. Prolonged neuromuscular blockade in a horse following concomitant use of vecuronium and atracurium. Vet Anaesth Analg 2012;39:119.

30. Martin-Flores M, Campoy L, Gleed RD. Further experiences with vecuronium in the horse. Vet Anaesth Analg 2012;38:218.

31. Fantoni DT, Alvarenga J, daSilva LC, et al. Controlled mechanical ventilation in horses under vecuronium blockage. Braz J Vet Res Anim Sci 1998;35:182.

32. Martin-Flores M, Pare MD, Adams W, et al. Observations of the potency and duration of vecuronium in isoflurane-anesthetized horses. Vet Anaesth Analg 2012;39: 385.

33. Auer U, Uray C, Mosing M. Observations on the muscle relaxant rocuronium bromide in horses—a dose-response study. Vet Anaesth Analg 2007;34:75.

34. Auer U, Moens Y. Neuromuscular blockade with rocuronium bromide for ophthalmic surgery in horses. Vet Ophthalmol 2011;14:244.

35. Mosing M, Auer U, Bardell D, et al. Reversal of profound rocuronium block monitored in three muscle groups with sugammadex in ponies. Br J Anaesth 2010;105:480.

36. Ali HH, Utting JE, Gray TC. Quantitative assessment of residual antidepolarizing block (part 1). Br J Anaesth 1971;43:473.

37. Engbaek J, Ostergaard D, Viby-Mogensen J. Double burst stimulation (DBS): a new pattern of nerve stimulation to identify residual neuromuscular block. Br J Anaesth 1989;62:274.

38. Viby-Mogensen J, Howardy-Hansen P, Chraemmer-Jorgensen B, et al. Posttetanic count (PTC): a new method of evaluating an intense nondepolarizing neuromuscular blockade. Anesthesiology 1981;55:458.

39. Kopman AF, Mallhi MU, Justo MD, et al. Antagonism of mivacurium-induced neuromuscular blockade in humans. Edrophonium dose requirements at threshold train-of-four count of 4. Anesthesiology 1994;81:1394.

40. Klein L, Hopkins J, Beck E, et al. Mechanical responses to peroneal nerve stimulation in halothane-anesthetized horses in the absence of neuromuscular block and during partial nondepolarizing blockade. Am J Vet Res 1983;44:781.

41. Fuchs-Buder T. Neuromuscular monitoring. Springer; 2010.

42. Martin-Flores M, Gleed RD, Basher KL, et al. TOF-Watch monitor: failure to calculate the train-of-four ratio in the absence of baseline calibration in anaesthetized dogs. Br J Anaesth 2012;108:240.

43. Driessen JJ, Robertson EN, Booij LH. Acceleromyography in neonates and small infants: baseline calibration and recovery of the response after neuromuscular blockade with rocuronium. Eur J Anaesthesiol 2005;22:11.

44. Eriksson L, Lennmarken C, Wyon N. Attenuated ventilatory response to hypoxaemia at vecuronium-induced partial neuromuscular block. Acta Anaesthesiol Scand 1992;36:710.

45. Eriksson L, Sundman E, Olsson R, et al. Functional assessment of the pharynx at rest and during swallowing in partially paralyzed humans: simultaneous video-manometry and mechanomyography of awake human volunteers. Anesthesiology 1997;87:1035.

46. Murphy GS, Szokol JW, Marymont JH. Intraoperative acceleromyographic monitoring reduces the risk of residual neuromuscular blockade and adverse respiratory events in the postanesthesia care unit. Anesthesiology 2008;109:389.

47. Debaene B, Plaud B, Dilly MP, et al. Residual paralysis in the PACU after a single intubating dose of nondepolarizing muscle relaxant with an intermediate duration of action. Anesthesiology 2003;98:1042.

48. Baillard C, Clec'h C, Catineau J, et al. Postoperative residual neuromuscular block: a survey of management. Br J Anaesth 2005;95:622.

49. Hildebrand SV, Howitt GA. Antagonism of pancuronium neuromuscular blockade in halothane-anesthetized ponies using neostigmine and edrophonium. Am J Vet Res 1984;45:2276.

Cardiac Output Monitoring in Horses

Andre Shih, DVM

KEYWORDS

- Cardiac output • Oxygen delivery • Hemodynamic monitoring
- Pulmonary thermodilution • Fick method oxygen extraction

KEY POINTS

- Cardiac output (CO) provides insight as to the adequacy of delivery of blood to the body as a whole.
- CO can be used to gauge fluid responsiveness and cardiovascular status of patients.
- Monitoring CO in horses is challenging due to patient size, temperament, and anatomic peculiarities.
- Pulmonary thermodilution (PAD), lithium dilution, echocardiogram, and the Fick method are capable of monitoring CO in both adult horses and foals.

DEFINITION

The function of the heart is to distribute essential oxygen, nutrients, and chemicals to all the cells of the body via the blood, thereby ensuring the cells' survival.[1,2] CO, defined as the volume of blood pumped out by the heart in the time interval of 1 minute,[3] indicates how well the heart is performing this function. CO is typically measured in either liters per minute (L/min) or dynes[3] per minute (dm^3/min). One dyne is the force required to accelerate a mass of 1 g at a rate of 1 cm per second squared.

There is significant variation in CO values, depending on patient size and age (**Table 1**). A normal value for neonatal foals is 6.7 L/min to 7.5 L/min, whereas a normal value for 400-kg to 500-kg adult horses is 32 L/min to 40 L/min.[4] To make a comparison between individuals, CO is, therefore, typically indexed to either body surface area (cardiac index = CO/surface area [m^2]) or body weight (BW) (COBW = CO/BW [kg]).[5]

CLINICAL USE OF CARDIAC OUTPUT MONITORING

CO is routinely measured in human medicine during general anesthesia and in critical care units and to study exercise physiology. With the advent of new technologies, this

Department of Large Animal Clinical Science, University of Florida College of Veterinary Medicine, 2015 Southwest 16th Avenue, Gainesville, FL 32610, USA
E-mail address: shih60@ufl.edu

Vet Clin Equine 29 (2013) 155–167
http://dx.doi.org/10.1016/j.cveq.2012.11.002
0749-0739/13/$ – see front matter © 2013 Elsevier Inc. All rights reserved.

Table 1
Changes in COBW according to age

Age	COBW (mL/kg/min)
Neonate, 2 h old	155.3 ± 8.1
Foal, 24 h old	197.3 ± 12
Foal, 14 d old	222.1 ± 21.6
Adult horse	72.2–99

is also becoming reality in veterinary medicine. Equine patients have intrinsic characteristics (body size, temperament, and unique anatomic changes) that makes monitoring CO a challenge.

Horses are well-adapted athletic animals with significant cardiac reserve capacity. The normal resting COBW for an adult horse is 72 mL/kg/min to 88 mL/kg/min.[6] During exercise, however, CO can increase to more than 8 times its resting value,[4] so evaluation of CO at rest does not determine if poor exercise performance is due to primary cardiac impairment. Knowledge of changes in CO and oxygen delivery (Do_2) over time is essential for understanding the physiology of exercise.[5]

CO not only is one of the most important factors to assess cardiovascular function[7] but also allows for calculation of many other cardiovascular parameters for more complete assessment of function. With knowledge of CO and heart rate (HR), stroke volume (SV) can be determined. In certain physiologic and pathophysiologic states, the body vascular resistance can change. Systemic vascular resistance (SVR) is calculated from the pressure in the vascular system (difference between mean arterial blood pressure [MAP] and right atrial pressure divided by CO). Knowledge of SVR allows for safer use of vasopressors and inotrope therapy.

CO, blood hemoglobin concentration, and oxygen saturation of hemoglobin are major factors in determination of global tissue Do_2.[3] Shock can be defined as an unbalance between Do_2 and consumption. The goal of most of the supportive care in critical care medicine is to improve Do_2. All therapies aimed to increase Do_2, however, also are associated with some degree of risk. By optimizing Do_2 (using CO monitoring), titrating therapy should be able to match the needs of patients, reducing the risk of overzealous treatment.[7]

Determination of CO also makes it possible for clinicians to determine important stress indicators, like intrapulmonary shunt, pulmonary vascular resistance, global oxygen consumption, and oxygen extraction ratio (**Box 1**).[7]

Cardiac Output Monitoring for Critically Ill Patients

A thorough physical examination, complemented by basic hemodynamic monitoring, is sufficient to direct the care of most patients.[7] There exists, however, a subset of patients for whom more direct assessment of CO (and its derivative parameters) is essential to proper case management.[7]

Knowledge of CO helps determine the different types/stages of shock in which a patient is presented. Hyperdynamic shock is characterized by supranormal CO and massive decrease in SVR, leading to evidence of poor microcirculation in tissue beds.[8] A classic example of hyperdynamic shock is the initial stages of septic shock. Hyperdynamic shock is a major cause of inadequate tissue perfusion in septic foals.[9] If not corrected, factors maintaining high CO are no longer active and hyperdynamic stage progresses to a hypodynamic stage.[8] Hypodynamic shock is characterized by decrease in CO with a decrease in SVR. An example of this stage is the later phase of septic shock,[8] also called unresponsive shock. Trauma, gastrointestinal disease,

---

Box 1
Equations

$CO = HR \times SV$

$Do_2 = Cao_2 \times CO$

$Cao_2 = 1.34\ Hb \times Sat + 0.003\ Pao_2$

$\dot{V}o_2 = Cao_2 - Cvo_2 \times CO$

$OER = \dot{V}o_2/Do_2$

$SVR = (MAP - CVP) \times 80/CO$

$PVR = (PAP - CVP) \times 80/CO$

Modified Stewart-Hamilton equation:

CO = amount of indicator/f (concentration indicator $\times$ time)

Abbreviations: Cao_2, oxygen content; Cvo_2, oxygen venous content; CVP, central venous pressure; Hb, hemoglobin; OER, oxygen extraction ratio; Pao_2, arterial oxygen tension; PAP, pulmonary arterial pressure; PVR, pulmonary vascular resistance; Sat, oxygen saturation; $\dot{V}o_2$, oxygen consumption.

---

and sepsis can all cause a sudden decrease in circulating blood volume, leading to lower venous return, causing hypovolemic shock. Hypovolemic shock is characterized by a decrease in CO and an increase in SVR. Sick horses can lose a fair amount of circulating volume due to third spacing into gastrointestinal track and due to vascular fluid leaking into interstitium and abdominal space as a result of capillary damage.[8]

Septic shock and hypovolemic shock represent a major cause of circulatory failure and mortality in horses.[8] As an important indicator of global macrocirculation, measurement of CO benefits the care of critically ill patients, more specifically animals with hypovolemic shock, septic shock, and systemic inflammatory response syndrome. Studies have shown that maintenance of appropriate CO and Do_2 is critical in preventing multiple organ ischemic injury and decreases morbidity and mortality in many clinical scenarios.[10–12]

Standard therapy for shock consists of aggressive fluid therapy and use of vasopressors to ensure adequate MAP.[13] Unfortunately, clinicians are unable to accurately assess the volume status of patients and replace the eventual deficit using these methods.[14] Another difficulty is that not all hypovolemic patients respond to volume loading; overzealous fluid administration can be harmful in a portion of the population.[15,16]

Variables traditionally used as indicators of preload to guide fluid resuscitation, such as central venous pressure, MAP, pulmonary capillary wedge pressure, blood lactate concentration, and urine output, have been repeatedly shown to be unreliable indicators of fluid status. Neither the absolute values of central venous pressure and pulmonary capillary wedge pressure nor their relative changes can consistently predict the hemodynamic response to a fluid challenge.[17–20]

This emphasizes the need for identification of variables that reliably estimate volume status and differentiate between patients who benefit from fluid resuscitation and patients who do not, a topic currently known as fluid responsiveness. Continuous evaluation of CO is a reliable indicator of fluid responsiveness and cardiovascular status.[3]

CO monitoring also has prognostic value. Studies revealed that the most commonly monitored indices (HR, body temperature, central venous pressure, and urine output) were the worst predictors of survival. At the same time, hemodynamic parameters, such as cardiac index, SVR, and $\dot{V}o_2$, showed good specificity and sensitivity with regards to predicting survival.[7] It was proposed that these values be incorporated as the goals of therapy for critically ill patients. This approach was termed, *goal-directed therapy*. Measurement of CO in critical care, therefore, helps guide therapy, allowing for rapid identification of a patient's potential responsiveness to fluid therapy and hopefully decreases morbidity.

Cardiac Output Monitoring During Anesthesia

Besides all the advantages discussed previously, CO monitoring is especially important during general anesthesia. Hypotension is one of the most commonly reported anesthetic complications. Typical treatment of hypotension during anesthesia consists of aggressive fluid therapy, inotropes, and vasopressors. Recently, however, there have been calls for a decrease in the volume of fluid administered to anesthetized patients and, as discussed previously, overzealous fluid administration can be harmful. Knowledge of CO in anesthetized animals aids optimal titration of fluid administration and vasopressor agents.[5]

All anesthetic agents significantly affect the cardiovascular system. Most anesthetic/sedative agents can cause direct change in SVR. Excessive vasoconstriction or vasodilatation makes arterial pressure an unreliable indicator of worsening cardiac performance. CO monitoring can be a much earlier indicator of deteriorating cardiovascular status than other commonly monitored cardiovascular variables, such as arterial blood pressure. All critically ill horses not responding to initial blood pressure intervention are potential candidates for CO monitoring.[9]

CO MEASUREMENT TECHNIQUES

Despite the significant advantages of CO monitoring, its use is limited in equine medicine. This is likely due to the invasive nature of many available methods[21] together with physical limitations due to the size and temperament of the equine patient. An excellent review of CO technologies as they pertain to horses was by Corley and colleagues in 2003[5]; however, newer methods for determination of CO have been established. When new monitoring techniques are introduced, comparative studies are needed to demonstrate that the measurements are meaningful in different clinical settings and over a wide physiologic range.

There are 4 basic methods of measuring CO: (1) indicator methods (such as PAD and lithium dilution techniques), (2) a derivation of the Fick principle, (3) arterial pulse wave analysis (pulse contour CO), and (4) imaging diagnostic techniques (transthoracic echocardiogram and thoracic bioimpedance).[1,2] The ways in which these methods obtain CO are described, together with their relevance to equine medicine.

Indicator Methods

Pulmonary thermodilution

PAD using a pulmonary arterial (PA) catheter (Swan-Ganz technique) remains the accepted clinical gold standard for CO measurement. PAD is one of the few methods capable of determining CO in adult horses. It remains a commonly used method for CO monitoring research in adult horses.

The Swan-Ganz PA catheter is a double-lumen, specially designed catheter with a thermistor monitor in the tip. The placement of a PA catheter in an adult horse is similar to that in other species. Briefly, the animal is sedated and maintained on standing position. The area over the distal jugular vein is clipped and aseptically cleaned. An introducer kit (8F) is placed over the jugular vein using a Seldinger technique. The Swan-Ganz catheter is fed though the introducer into the distal jugular. The proximal port can be connected to a pressure transducer and the clinician can use the pressure waveform to monitor the catheter advancement from jugular/right atrium to right ventricle and finally confirm placement in proximal PA. Most PA catheters have an inflatable balloon located near the tip of the catheter to facilitate passage from the ventricle to the pulmonary artery. Once positioned, the Swan-Ganz PA catheter proximal port should sit in the right atrial chamber and distal port should sit in PA. Placement of Swan-Ganz when the animal is on dorsal or lateral position is possible but more challenging. Regular Swan-Ganz catheters designed to fit a human heart dimension can be used for foals but should not be used in adult horses. A custom-made specially manufactured Swan-Ganz catheter (>110 cm length) has to be purchased to fit the heart size of an adult horse. An alternative, 2 introducers and 2 separate catheters, can be used, with the proximal catheter fed into the right atrium and the distal one (Edward Lifesciences, Irvine, California), fed into the pulmonary artery.[22]

The PAD method involves using thermal energy as an indicator. A small bolus of cold, isotonic solution (5% dextrose or 0.9% saline) is injected into the patient's blood proximal to the right ventricle (right atrium), and the dilution of the indicator is followed continuously at a point distal to the ventricle (the pulmonary artery). Plotting a graph of the concentration of the indicator against time produces a concentration-time curve, and the area under the curve (AUC) is calculated. CO is inversely proportional to the AUC and is determined by the Stewart-Hamilton principle (**Box 1**).

The PAD has several disadvantages. The use of a PA catheter carries significant risks, including arrhythmias, damage to the cardiac endothelium, infection, and pulmonary thromboembolism.[1,2,21,23] Although rare, the most devastating complication, PA rupture, has a mortality rate of approximately 50%. For those reasons, PAD is not routinely used in clinical veterinary medicine. There has, therefore, been growing interest in less-invasive techniques for CO measurement, such as trans-PAD, lithium dilution, and ultrasound velocity dilution (UD) techniques. These other indicator methods are, in principle, modifications of PAD and also follow the Stewart-Hamilton principle.

Lithium dilution

The lithium dilution method has demonstrated excellent agreement when compared with PAD in animal models.[12,22,24] It is capable of measuring CO in adult horses (including during exercise)[24] and is currently one of the most commonly used methods of determining CO in anesthetized foals.[5,25–27]

Lithium dilution technique (LiDCO, LiDCO, Lake Villa, Illinois) requires determination of hemoglobin concentration and serum sodium concentration, which can be obtained using a blood gas analyzer. Lithium chloride (0.003 mmol/kg) is injected via a central vein; then, arterial blood is withdrawn through a lithium sensor placed between the side port of a 3-way port and a metatarsal arterial catheter. Blood is collected through a peristaltic pump with a flow rate of 4 mL/min across the sensor. As with the PAD method, a graph is plotted of indicator (in this case lithium) concentration versus time, and CO is derived from this curve by Stewart-Hamilton principle.[25]

For an adult horse, blood removed for one LiDCO determination is minimal (20–40 mL per measurement) and should not be returned to the patient. Drawbacks associated with repeated LiDCO determinations include excessive blood loss[26] and potential accumulation of the indicator (lithium) in the body, leading to erroneous values and potential risk of other undesirable effects.[28] Lithium sensors can also react with some drugs commonly used during anesthesia, like neuromuscular blockers (ie, atracurium), resulting in unreliable readings.

Ultrasound velocity dilution

UD (COstatus, Transonic, Ithaca, New York) is a novel technique for determining CO that may resolve some of the disadvantages of previous CO determination methods.[29] UD COstatus is minimally invasive, does not involve blood loss, and uses a physiologic noncumulative signal (saline solution).[30,31] This technique has been used in anesthetized foals and juvenile horses with good success.[32,33] UD COstatus also allows clinicians to monitor other preload volumetric variables, such as total end-diastolic volume, which can have predictor value for patient fluid responsiveness **Fig. 1**.[33]

To determine CO using the UD COstatus technique, an arteriovenous loop is made by attaching tubing between metatarsal (peripheral) arterial and central venous catheters, creating an extracorporeal circuit.[30] Two ultrasound velocity sensors are attached to this circuit: a venous flow sensor is placed upstream from the venous catheter and an arterial flow sensor is placed downstream from the arterial catheter. A small bolus of isotonic saline (0.5–1 mL/kg) is injected into the venous circulation, creating a transient hemodilution and resulting in a change in the velocity of ultrasound in this blood.

CO is calculated as the product of the volume of isotonic saline and the consequent decrease in ultrasound velocity as the saline-diluted blood passes through an ultrasonic sensor. Ultrasound velocity in blood is normally 1560 m/s to 1590 m/s and mainly depends on the levels of red blood cells and protein.[34] Ultrasound velocity in isotonic saline is lower than in blood (1533 m/s). Injection of a saline bolus into the venous system, therefore, generates an UD curve due to transient dilution of blood proteins, which results in a decrease in ultrasound velocity in the arterial sample.[34–36]

For UD COstatus to be used in an adult horse, a large amount of fluid (0.5 mL/kg) to is required to be rapidly administered through the small arteriovenous loop. Due to the small diameter/high resistance of the current loop, the UD COstatus is not viable for use in animals larger than 250 kg.[33]

The Fick Method

The Fick technique is one of the oldest methods of measuring CO. In 1870, Adolph Fick derived this theoretic method and it was validated in horses in 1890.[5,37] For

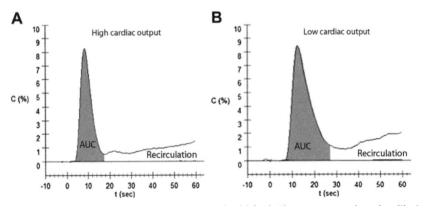

Fig. 1. CO indicator using UD curve in a 2-month-old foal. The computer plots the dilution curve (velocity over time) and determines the AUC. This is used for determination of CO by modified Stewart-Hamilton equation, where AUC is inversely proportion to CO. (A) Animal in a high CO state (low AUC) and (B) animal in a lower CO state (high AUC). After some time, the indictor recirculates through the blood flow and return back into the sensor (Recirculation). To properly calculate AUC, the computer detects the recirculation phase.

a substance that is taken up by a tissue (such as oxygen), the Fick principle simply states, "As long as there is no pulmonary and cardiac shunting, the oxygen uptake by the blood ($\dot{V}o_2$) is the product of the rate of blood flow through the lungs (CO) and the difference in oxygen content between pulmonary venous and PA blood." In other words, "What went in minus what came out must be equal to what was left behind."[7] Pulmonary venous oxygen content is equivalent to systemic oxygen content (Ca_{O2}), whereas blood collected at the pulmonary artery is known as mixed venous content (Cv_{O2}). According to the Fick principle: $\dot{V}o_2 = CO \times (Ca_{O2} - Cv_{O2})$. The equation can be rearranged as $CO = \dot{V}o_2/(Ca_{O2} - Cv_{O2})$ in order to determine CO when the other values are known. Although oxygen content analyzers are available to measure Ca_{O2}, it is more typical for clinicians to measure the oxygen partial pressure (P_{O2}), hemoglobin saturation (Sat), and hemoglobin concentration (Hb) with a gas analyzer and manually calculate systemic oxygen content using the formula: $Ca_{O2} = (1.34\ Hb \times Sat) + (0.003\ P_{O2})$.[8]

The Fick method has some drawbacks for modern clinical use. Mixed venous blood sampling (to measure Cv_{O2}) requires placement of a PA catheter, with complications (discussed previously), and blood samples from the right atrium and jugular vein are a poor substitute. Furthermore, the Fick method relies on patients maintaining a stable metabolic state throughout the period of gas collection; the less stable the patient, the less reliable this method becomes.[7] $\dot{V}o_2$ is calculated as $\dot{V}o_2 = \dot{V}E\ (F_{IO2} - F_{EO2})$, where $\dot{V}E$ is expired minute ventilation volume, F_{IO2} is fractional concentration of oxygen in inspired gas, and F_{EO2} is fractional concentration of oxygen in expired gas. Accurate determination of expired minute ventilation volume is difficult in conscious animals. It requires a specially designed tight fit mask and a cooperative horse.[24] In anesthetized ventilated foals, a commercial spirometer can easily be used to determine expired minute ventilation volume. In adult horses, however, methods for determining expired volume that are sufficiently accurate for the technique to be valid were not readily available.[5] A new large animal anesthesia ventilator with built-in spirometer specifically designed for horse anesthesia (Tafonius, Hallowell EMC, Pittsfield, Massachusetts) might fix this setback. To the author's knowledge, no validation of the Fick method has been performed using this machine.

To avoid some of these drawbacks, carbon dioxide (CO_2) production can be used instead of oxygen consumption in a modified Fick equation. The rate of CO_2 elimination by the lungs is the product of the CO and the difference in CO_2 content between pulmonary venous and PA blood. Mixed blood gas is substituted by having the animal rebreathe exhaled air until the CO_2 tension in the breathing circuit plateaus (NICO, Philips Respironics, Murrysville, Pennsylvania). This CO_2 tension is theoretically that of the mixed venous blood, therefore eliminating the need for a PA catheter.[2] This rebreathing technique has been validated in anesthetized foals and demonstrates good correlation when compared with the lithium dilution technique.[2,3] Unfortunately, however, the commercially available rebreathing circuits cannot be adapted for adult horses, making it a less than ideal technique for equine medicine (**Table 2**).

Pulse Contour Analysis

The concept of deriving CO based on the arterial pressure waveform is not new and can be traced back to 1904.[38] Early attempts, however, had limited success.[39,40] Calculation of CO based on the contour of the arterial pulse wave, if accurate, offers the advantages of minimally invasive, continuous, beat-to-beat CO. Current arterial wave analysis monitors also display preload volumetric variables, such as SV variation and pulse pressure variation. Both PPV and SSV have predictor value for patient fluid responsiveness.[41]

Table 2
Techniques for CO measurement and their application in equine anesthesia

CO Measurement Technique	Company Manufacturing Equipment	Use in Foals	Use in Adults	Use During Exercise	Accuracy	Observation
PAD	Edwards Lifesciences, Irvine, CA	Yes	Yes	Yes	Gold standard	Requires pulmonary artery catheter
Trans-PAD	Pulsion Medical Systems/Philips, Munich, Germany	Yes	No	No	Good correlation in foals	Requires central arterial catheter
Lithium dilution	LiDCO, Lake Villa, IL	Yes	Yes	Yes	Good correlation	Requires peripheral arterial catheter
UD	Transonic, Ithaca, NY	Yes	No	No	Good correlation in foals	Requires peripheral arterial catheter
Fick principle		Yes	No	Yes	Good correlation	Requires pulmonary artery catheter
Rebreathing CO_2	NiCO, Philips Respironics, Murrysville, PA	Yes	No	No	Good correlation in foals	Requires mechanical ventilation
Pulse contour CO		Yes	Yes	?	Weak correlation	Requires calibration when changes in hemodynamic status occurs
TEB		Yes (?)	Yes (?)	?	?	Data not yet validated for horses
Echocardiogram		Yes	Yes	No	Moderate correlation	Difficult to determine in adult horses under anesthesia

The arterial waveform is a product of the SV force (arterial peak before the dicrotic notch) and the elastic component of the arteries or Windkessel effect (area after the dicrotic notch).[42] The SV correlates well with the area of the arterial wave before the dicrotic notch; however, the arterial pressure waveform depends on multiple factors, including changes in aortic impedance, SVR, and waveform damping, all of which prevent this from being a straightforward relationship.[39,43]

To adjust for this, most of the available pulse contour CO monitors use a second, more reliable, method to determine true CO, involving a calibration factor. Pulse contour CO monitors that do not have a calibration factor typically use built-in algorithms based on healthy human values, making them less useful in veterinary medicine. Currently, 2 pulse contour CO monitors have been evaluated in animals: the lithium dilution arterial waveform analysis monitor (PulseCO, LiDCO, Lake Villa, Illinois) and the transpulmonary pulse contour analysis monitor (PiCCO, Pulsion Medical Systems, Munich, Germany). The PulseCO uses the lithium chloride dilution technique for calibration whereas the PiCCO uses cold saline trans-PAD for calibration (see indicator methods described previously).[44]

Investigators have compared PulseCO and PiCCO with lithium and thermodilution indicator methods in foals and juvenile horses. In anesthetized neonatal foals, both PiCCO and PulseCO methods are able to monitor CO changes in the same direction (ie, pulse wave–derived CO increases as CO increases and vice versa).[25] With significant changes in SVR and volemic state of the patient, however, pulse contour technology is less accurate, making the clinical usefulness of both these monitors limited in the presence of severe arrhythmias, severe vasoconstriction, and hemodynamically unstable patients. Furthermore, the manufacturer of the PiCCO device recommends that the arterial catheter be placed in the femoral artery with the catheter tip located in the aorta (central catheterization) to detect central aortic blood pressure. Such central arterial catheterization is not commonly performed in equine medicine, and this method requiring femoral catheterization makes it less clinically applicable for adult horses.[25]

Imaging Techniques

Echocardiogram
Lithium dilution, UD, and pulse contour analysis are all less-invasive methods than PAD, but they still require placement of both venous and arterial catheters. In contrast, the echocardiogram is one of the truly noninvasive techniques available for measurement of CO in both juvenile and adult horses.[23]

Measurement of blood velocity (using Doppler ultrasound) and aortic diameter allows estimates of SV and, therefore, CO. Determining the aorta Doppler velocity can be challenging in adult horses. Another alternative to estimate CO is using the modified Simpson formula (**Fig. 2**). In this method, a 2-D view of left ventricle in its widest cross section is acquired, making sure the endocardial borders are well visualized. Using the geometric assumption that the left ventricular cavity represents a cylinder/cone configuration, the biplane Simpson divides the outline of ventricular chamber into slices. Each slice volume can then be calculated and, using an algorithm, total ventricular volume (during systole and diastole) estimated. End-diastolic volume minus end-systolic volume equals SV. CO can be derived from SV and HR. The Simpson method has some built-in error and some variability is expected in the result.[45] Although CO by echocardiogram represents significantly less risk to patients than other methods of CO determination, this method requires highly trained personnel and expensive equipment. Transthoracic echocardiogram is also more challenging in adult horses once an animal is anesthetized and placed in lateral or dorsal position.

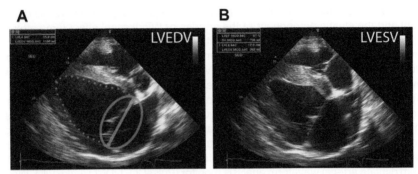

Fig. 2. Determination of CO by Simpson method. CO equals (*A*) left-ventricular volume at the end of diastolic phase (LVEDV) minus the (*B*) left-ventricular volume at the end of systolic phase (LVESV)—by underlining endocardium, the computer makes an assumption that the left ventricle has a cone-shaped appearance and uses an algorithm to determine chamber volume.

Repeated CO estimation is routinely performed in human anesthesia transesophageal echocardiogram. This technique is a great option for foals but currently there is no commercially available probe that is long enough for an adult horse transesophageal echocardiogram. A modified echocardiogram probe can be custom made for use in the horse adapted from a 160-cm colonoscope.[45,46]

Transthoracic electrical bioimpedance

Transthoracic electrical bioimpedance (TEB) is a noninvasive method of evaluating changes in the conductivity of the thorax resulting from pulsatile flow of blood within the thoracic cavity.[7] If proved accurate, TEB would be an ideal CO method for horses. TEB is noninvasive, able to fit adult and pediatric horses, and capable of CO monitoring during anesthesia and during exercise.

Determination of CO by this method involves placement of sets of electrodes around a patient's chest. By applying a small, known voltage to the patient and measuring what proportion of the initial voltage reaches distal electrodes, the conductivity (and, therefore, impedance) of the thorax can be calculated. Changes in thoracic blood volume over time (CO) lead to changes in the bioimpedance.[7]

In humans, TEB had good correlation and good directional tracking but values were not interchangeable (not complete agreement) to Pulmonary arterial pressure (PAP) or the Fick method.[47] Although as yet little used, TEB method holds promise and a special bioimpedance belt is being designed for the equine thorax.

SUMMARY

In conclusion, frequent and accurate monitoring of CO can be useful to guide therapy and improve clinical outcome. In critically ill patients, it can be used to gauge fluid responsiveness and more accurately determine cardiovascular status and, therefore, appropriate therapy.[8] In anesthetized patients, it can be used to detect deteriorating cardiovascular status earlier than is possible with other, more commonly monitored variables. To successfully use CO to monitor cardiovascular status, it is important to understand that although CO provides insight as to the adequacy of delivery of blood to the body as a whole, it does not have a direct relationship with adequacy of microcirculation. A good CO, therefore, does not indicate good tissue perfusion. CO value should always be interpreted together with a thorough physical examination and other auxiliary microcirculatory monitoring parameters.

Although there is increasing research into clinically useful methods of monitoring CO in equine patients, there are limitations to the available methods. PAD, although still the gold standard and commonly used in adult horse research, is typically too invasive for routine clinical use. Currently, one of the most commonly used methods in anesthetized foals is lithium dilution. UD method and echocardiogram may be valuable options for sick and anesthetized foals. The noninvasive method, thoracic bioimpedance, is perhaps the most promising for clinical equine use in the future.

REFERENCES

1. Hoffman GM, Ghanayem NS, Tweddell JS. Noninvasive assessment of cardiac output. Semin Thorac Cardiovasc Surg Pediatr Card Surg Annu 2005;12:12–21.
2. Giguere S, Bucki E, Adin DB, et al. Cardiac output measurement by partial carbon dioxide rebreathing, 2-dimensional echocardiography, and lithium-dilution method in anesthetized neonatal foals. J Vet Intern Med 2005;19:737–43.
3. Valverde A, Giguere S, Sanchez LC, et al. Effects of dobutamine, norepinephrine, and vasopressin on cardiovascular function in anesthetized neonatal foals with induced hypotension. Am J Vet Res 2006;67:1730–7.
4. Evans DL. Cardiovascular adaptations to exercise and training. Vet Clin North Am Equine Pract 1985;1:513–31.
5. Corley KT, Donaldson LL, Durando MM, et al. Cardiac output technologies with special reference to the horse. J Vet Intern Med 2003;17:262–72.
6. Bonagura J, Reef V. Cardiovascualar diseases. In: Reed S, WM B, editors. Equine internal medicine. 1st edition. Philadelphia: WB Saunders; 1998. p. 290–370.
7. Mellema M. Cardiac output monitoring. In: Silverstein D, Hopper K, editors. Small animal critical care medicine. Misouri: Saunders Elsevier; 2009. p. 894–8.
8. Corley KT. Inotropes and vasopressors in adult and foals. Vet Clin North Am Equine Pract 2004;20:77–106.
9. Magdesian KG. Monitoring the critically ill equine patient. Vet Clin North Am Equine Pract 2004;20:11–39.
10. Tantalean JA, Leon RJ, Santos AA, et al. Multiple organ dysfunction syndrome in children. Pediatr Crit Care Med 2003;4:181–5.
11. Hatherill M, Waggie Z, Purves L, et al. Mortality and the nature of metabolic acidosis in children with shock. Intensive Care Med 2003;29:286–91.
12. Kim JJ, Dreyer WJ, Chang AC, et al. Arterial pulse wave analysis: an accurate means of determining cardiac output in children. Pediatr Crit Care Med 2006;7:532–5.
13. Perel A. Bench-to-bedside review: the initial hemodynamic resuscitation of the septic patient according to surviving sepsis campaign guidelines—does one size fit all? Crit Care 2008;12:223.
14. Geeraedts LM Jr, Kaasjager HA, van Vugt AB, et al. Exsanguination in trauma: a review of diagnostics and treatment options. Injury 2009;40:11–20.
15. Durairaj L, Schmidt GA. Fluid therapy in resuscitated sepsis: less is more. Chest 2008;133:252–63.
16. Wiedemann HP, Wheeler AP, Bernard GR, et al. Comparison of two fluid-management strategies in acute lung injury. N Engl J Med 2006;354:2564–75.
17. Shippy CR, Appel PL, Shoemaker WC. Reliability of clinical monitoring to assess blood volume in critically ill patients. Crit Care Med 1984;12:107–12.
18. Godje O, Peyerl M, Seebauer T, et al. Central venous pressure, pulmonary capillary wedge pressure and intrathoracic blood volumes as preload indicators in cardiac surgery patients. Eur J Cardiothorac Surg 1998;13:533–9 [discussion: 539–40].

19. Marik PE, Baram M, Vahid B. Does central venous pressure predict fluid responsiveness? A systematic review of the literature and the tale of seven mares. Chest 2008;134:172–8.
20. Kumar A, Anel R, Bunnell E, et al. Pulmonary artery occlusion pressure and central venous pressure fail to predict ventricular filling volume, cardiac performance, or the response to volume infusion in normal subjects. Crit Care Med 2004;32:691–9.
21. Tibby SM, Murdoch IA. Monitoring cardiac function in intensive care. Arch Dis Child 2003;88:46–52.
22. Linton RA, Jonas MM, Tibby SM, et al. Cardiac output measured by lithium dilution and transpulmonary thermodilution in patients in a paediatric intensive care unit. Intensive Care Med 2000;26:1507–11.
23. Connors AF Jr, Speroff T, Dawson NV, et al. The effectiveness of right heart catheterization in the initial care of critically ill patients. SUPPORT Investigators. JAMA 1996;276:889–97.
24. Durando MM, Corley KT, Boston RC, et al. Cardiac output determination by use of lithium dilution during exercise in horse. Am J Vet Res 2008;8:1054–62.
25. Shih AC, Giguere S, Sanchez LC, et al. Determination of cardiac output in anesthetized neonatal foals by use of two pulse wave analysis methods. Am J Vet Res 2009;70:334–9.
26. Corley KT, Donaldson LL, Furr MO. Comparison of lithium dilution and thermodilution cardiac output measurements in anaesthetised neonatal foals. Equine Vet J 2002;34:598–601.
27. Linton RA, Band DM, Haire KM. A new method of measuring cardiac output in man using lithium dilution. Br J Anaesth 1993;71:262–6.
28. Beaulieu JM, Sotnikova TD, Yao WD, et al. Lithium antagonizes dopamine-dependent behaviors mediated by an AKT/glycogen synthase kinase 3 signaling cascade. Proc Natl Acad Sci U S A 2004;101:5099–104.
29. Shih A, Giguere S, Vigani A, et al. Determination of cardiac output by ultrasound velocity dilution in normovolemia and hypovolemia in dogs. Vet Anaesth Analg 2011;38:279–85.
30. Eremenko A, Balykov I, Chaus N, et al. Use of an extracorporeal arteriovenous tubing loop to measure cardiac output in intensive care unit patients by ultrasound velocity dilution. ASAIO J 1998;44:M462–4.
31. Kitzler TM, Sergeyeva O, Morris A, et al. Noninvasive measurement of cardiac output in hemodialysis patients by task force monitor: a comparison with the Transonic System. ASAIO J 2007;53:561–5.
32. Shih A, Giguere S, Sanchez LC, et al. Determination of cardiac output in neonatal foals by ultrasound velocity dilution and its comparison to the lithium dilution method. J Vet Emerg Crit Care (San Antonio) 2009;19:438–43.
33. Vigani A, Shih A, Queiroz P, et al. Quantitative response of volumetric variables measured by a new ultrasound dilution method in a juvenile model of hemorrhagic shock and resuscitation. Resuscitation 2012;83:1031–7.
34. Veal N, Moal F, Wang J, et al. New method of cardiac output measurement using ultrasound velocity dilution in rats. J Appl Physiol 2001;91:1274–82.
35. Melchior R, Darling E, Terry B, et al. A novel method of measuring cardiac output in infants following extracorporeal procedures: preliminary validation in a swine model. Perfusion 2005;20:323–7.
36. Krivitski NM. Theory and validation of access flow measurement by dilution technique during hemodialysis. Kidney Int 1995;48:244–50.
37. Zuntz N, Hagemann O. Untersuchunger uber den Stoffwechsel des Pferdes bei ruhe und Arbeit. Landwirtsch Jahrb 1894;27:284–301.

38. Graves CL, Stauffer WM, Klein RL, et al. Aortic pulse contour calculation of cardiac output. Anesthesiology 1968;29:580–4.
39. Chen HC, Sinclair MD, Dyson DH, et al. Comparison of arterial pressure waveform analysis with the lithium dilution technique to monitor cardiac output in anesthetized dogs. Am J Vet Res 2005;66:1430–6.
40. van Lieshout JJ, Wesseling KH. Continuous cardiac output by pulse contour analysis? Br J Anaesth 2001;86:467–9.
41. Cannesson M, le Manach P, Hofen CK, et al. Assessing the diagnostic accuracy of pulse pressure variation for the prediction of fluid responsiveness. Anesthesiology 2011;115:231–41.
42. Guyton AC, Hall JE. In: Guyton AC, Hall JE, editors. Text book of medical physiology. 10th edition. Philadelphia: W.B. Saunders; 1996. p. 210–22.
43. Cooper ES, Muir WW. Continuous cardiac output monitoring via arterial pressure waveform analysis following severe hemorrhagic shock in dogs. Crit Care Med 2007;35:1724–9.
44. Orme RM, Pigott DW, Mihm FG. Measurement of cardiac output by transpulmonary arterial thermodilution using a long radial artery catheter. A comparison with intermittent pulmonary artery thermodilution. Anaesthesia 2004;59:590–4.
45. Marr CM, Patteson MW. Echocardiogram. In: Marr CM, Bowen M, editors. Cardiology of the horse. 2nd edition. Philadelphia: Saunders Elsevier; 1999. p. 105–24.
46. Young LE, Blissit KJ, Clutton RE. Feasibility of transoesophageal echocardiography for evaluation of left ventricular performance in anesthetized horses. Equine Vet J 1995;19(Suppl 1):63–70.
47. Engoren M, Barbee D. Comparison of cardiac output determination by bioimpedance, thermodilution and the Fick's method. Am J Crit Care 2005;14:40–5.

General Anesthesia in Horses on Fluid and Electrolyte Therapy

Lindsey B.C. Snyder, DVM, MS*, Erin Wendt-Hornickle, DVM

KEYWORDS

- Crystalloids • Colloids • Hypertonic • Saline • Calcium • Potassium

KEY POINTS

- Hypotension is linked to myopathies in horses, with prolonged hypotension (defined as mean arterial pressure of 55–65 mm Hg) resulting in a significantly increased risk of post-anesthetic myopathy.
- Maintaining a colloid oncotic pressure (COP) above 20 mm Hg has been suggested to prevent tissue and intestinal edema. Reducing the COP below 20 mm Hg with fluid therapy in humans is associated with an increase in the interstitial fluid volume in relation to the plasma volume.
- The Starling-Landis equation dictates the body's fluid dynamics.
- Balanced electrolyte solutions are most commonly used for fluid therapy during anesthesia; however, colloid solutions will maintain the vascular volume.
- The colloid osmotic pressure is the primary force opposing the leakage of fluid from blood vessels.
- Electrolyte imbalances can play an important role in fluid therapy, and can be greatly influenced by the fluids administered.

RATIONALE FOR FLUID THERAPY

General anesthesia of horses is not without complications, with morbidity and mortality rates higher than those for other species (0.12%–0.90%).[1] Morbidity, even in horses that are systemically healthy, can include hypotension and subsequent neuropathies, as well as postoperative tissue and pulmonary edema. Horses, because of their large body mass, are especially prone to anesthesia-related myopathies.[2] One of the most common complications in equine inhalant anesthesia is hypotension. Hypotension is linked to myopathies in horses, with prolonged hypotension (defined as mean arterial pressure of 55–65 mm Hg), resulting in a significantly increased risk of postanesthetic myopathy.[3] Hypotension can be treated various ways. One

Anesthesia & Pain Management, Department of Surgical Sciences, University of Wisconsin-Madison School of Veterinary Medicine, 2015 Linden Drive, Madison, WI 53706, USA
* Corresponding author.
E-mail address: culpl@svm.vetmed.wisc.edu

recognized therapy to limit hypotension is to administer intravenous (IV) fluids in an effort to maintain or even increase intravascular volume.[1] The type of IV fluids chosen can affect fluid shifts between the vascular and interstitial spaces, therefore contributing to or limiting the development of tissue and pulmonary edema.

Further evidence for fluid therapy includes the fact that general anesthesia with inhalant anesthetics has been shown to decrease myocardial contractility and mean arterial pressure in horses.[2] Inhalant anesthetics decrease myocardial functioning.[4] One way to limit anesthetic-induced myopathies in horses is to prevent myocardial depression and maintain tissue blood flow.[2] Fluid loading, the administration of high volumes of IV fluids over a short duration, is one way to accomplish this goal. Fluid loading counteracts the hypovolemia induced by preoperative fasting and ongoing losses from urinary output.[5] The need for intraoperative fluid therapy is all the more important in cases with existing comorbidities. In horses with strangulating-type colic, the morbidity rate is high because of the pathologic changes, including hypotension, that endotoxemia causes secondary to translocation of toxins across the gut.[6]

BACKGROUND

A horse's adult body weight is approximately 60% water, located in various compartments throughout the body.[7,8] Body fluids are divided into the intracellular and extracellular fluid (ECF) compartments. The extracellular compartment is further divided into the interstitial, intravascular, and transcellular compartments. Dehydration causes a decrease in the ECF secondary to a decrease in total body water and is characterized by an increase in packed cell volume (PCV) and total protein (TP). Hypovolemia, on the other hand, is a decrease in fluid in the intravascular compartment. Physical examination and clinical pathology laboratory results (PCV, TP) can aid in determining the degree of dehydration or hypovolemia. In extreme losses, heart rate may also become elevated and the pulse quality will be decreased. A blood pressure measurement can assist in quantitating the degree of hypovolemia or dehydration. In either case, dehydration or hypovolemia, fluid therapy is critical in the face of inhalant anesthetics. In the case of dehydration, fluid deficits should ideally be replaced slowly to allow for fluid equilibriums to be reestablished between intravascular, interstitial, and intracellular compartments. Under anesthesia, however, the need for fluid support outweighs the slow equilibration process. Hypovolemia can be treated much more rapidly by filling the vascular compartment to improve tissue perfusion. The standard intraoperative fluid rate of 10 mL/kg/h in anesthetized patients may need to be increased in a dehydrated or hypovolemic horse to fill the vascular and interstitial spaces and prevent ischemia of the tissues.[7] In any case, the goal in anesthetic fluid therapy should be to optimize cardiac preload.[5]

FLUID DYNAMICS

The colloid oncotic pressure (COP), is the osmotic pressure exerted by proteins in plasma that draw water into the vascular system. Proteins are the only substances that do not readily diffuse through the capillary membrane.[9] Numerous studies have evaluated the effects of fluid administration on the COP. In healthy awake horses, COP and TP decrease in a linear fashion when 40 mL/kg/h of IV crystalloids are administered[10] and 11 mL/kg/h when anesthetized.[11] The linear relationship has also been demonstrated in horses given 15 to 25 mL/kg/h IV crystalloids during colic surgery.[12] Additionally, healthy anesthetized dogs had a decrease in COP of 5 mm Hg when administered 9.4 ± 4.6 mL/kg/h of crystalloids. The administration of fluids did not change the fact that anesthetized, healthy dogs that did not receive IV fluids had a similar decrease in COP. The volume of crystalloids administered did not reliably predict the decrease in COP.[13] In hypoproteinemic, unanesthetized horses, however, COP increases when hydroxyethyl starch (HES) is administered at a rate of 8 to 10 mL/kg over 4 hours[9] in addition to clinically normal, unanesthetized ponies at a rate of 10 or 20 mL/kg over 2 hours.[10] Plasma contains endogenous colloids that are large molecular weight particles. The major contributors to COP are proteins. Plasma proteins play a major role in the maintenance of intravascular fluid volume.[8] Proteins within plasma exert the COP, and maintain fluid within the vascular space.[9,14] More specifically, COP is made of albumin, globulins,[14] and fibrinogen.[15] All of these proteins (TP) together make up 70.5% of COP and are important in shaping the fluid distribution between the vascular and interstitial spaces.[11]

There are 4 main forces at the level of the capillary that regulate fluid distribution: intravascular COP, interstitial and intravascular hydrostatic pressure, and interstitial oncotic pressure.[15] It is the interaction between these forces that influence fluid shifts between the capillary and the interstitial space. *The colloid osmotic pressure is the primary force opposing the leakage of fluid from blood vessels.* The capillary COP supports retention of fluid within the vasculature.[9] Albumin and other plasma proteins are responsible for producing the COP.[14] The interaction of hydrostatic and osmotic forces across capillary walls is a determining factor in the fluid movement between the interstitium and the intravascular space.[14] Transcapillary fluid exchange and subsequent distribution of bodily fluids is described by the Starling-Landis equation.[9] The Starling-Landis equation further describes the relationship between the oncotic pressure and the capillary hydrostatic pressure,[16,17]

$$Q = \kappa S[(P_c - P_i) - \sigma(\pi_c - \pi_i)]$$

where Q is the net transcapillary fluid exchange, κ is the net permeability of the capillary wall, S is capillary surface area, P_c is capillary hydrostatic pressure, P_i is interstitial hydrostatic pressure, σ is the capillary reflection coefficient, π_c is the capillary COP, and π_i refers to the interstitial COP.

Based on the Starling-Landis equation, anything that causes the oncotic pressure within the capillaries to decrease will result in the net filtration of fluids into the interstitium. Transcapillary movement of fluid across the endothelium is most likely attributable to a local difference in COP and hydrostatic pressure across the endothelial surface glycocalyx instead of a difference in the hydrostatic and oncotic pressure between the intravascular and interstitial spaces.[5] Regardless, a decrease in the COP is an important factor in the development of tissue edema and hypotension secondary to fluid leaving the vascular space. Decreases in COP have been found to be responsible for morbidity in patients, such as edema.[14] The Starling-Landis equilibrium and COP are required to maintain capillary fluid dynamics in the lung, myocardium, and gut.[9] Reducing the amount of crystalloid administered during intestinal surgeries in horses might reduce the degree of postoperative ileus that results secondary to intestinal edema.[18] Nevertheless, it may also be possible to prevent the development of intestinal edema by administering colloids to increase the COP. In humans, after the COP drops to 15 mm Hg or below, intestinal edema becomes apparent intraoperatively; however, 10% HES or albumin administration can prevent intestinal edema development in these patients.[19,20] It should be noted that anesthesia alone can cause a decrease in the COP and TP. Dogs that are not administered crystalloids during anesthesia had a similar drop in their COP and TP as dogs administered crystalloids during anesthesia.[21] Maintaining a COP above 20 mm Hg has been suggested to prevent tissue and intestinal edema.[22,23] Reducing the COP below 20 mm Hg with fluid therapy in humans is associated with an increase in the interstitial fluid volume in relation to the plasma volume.[9]

Disease processes that cause a loss of intravascular fluid and proteins can result in a hypovolemic, hypo-oncotic condition. Administration of crystalloid fluid solutions can further dilute the plasma proteins and increase the interstitial fluid volume secondary to the decrease in COP.[9] Postanesthetic pulmonary edema in horses, although not common, has been reported as a source of increased morbidity.[24] Despite the risk of morbidity, perioperative fluid overload is considered a minor problem despite evidence of fluid accumulation in tissues.[5]

SELECTION OF FLUIDS

Selecting the proper fluids for a particular case should be done following evaluation of the patient's physical examination, clinical pathology laboratory results (with emphasis on the PCV, TP, and electrolyte status), and assessment of the horse's hemodynamic state. Consideration should be given to the horse's hydration status and any hypovolemia present. Thought should also be given to the reason for fluid therapy (eg, intraoperative fluid therapy vs maintenance fluids). Additionally, the relative ease of administration should be taken into account (eg, 1-L bags vs 5-L bags). The type of fluid to be used can then be chosen based on these considerations.

Crystalloids

Crystalloids are the most commonly used fluid solutions used in horses. Routinely used crystalloid solutions include balanced electrolyte solutions and physiologic saline. Balanced electrolyte solutions are the fluid of choice in the anesthetized horse to maintain near normal electrolyte concentrations and provide a means of base replacement. Balanced electrolyte solutions (BESs) contain a bicarbonate precursor (lactate, acetate, or gluconate) as a buffer and are isotonic solutions, osmotically similar to plasma, that can transiently fill the vascular space when administered IV. The down side to crystalloid solutions is that they leave the vascular compartment and redistribute into the interstitial space relatively rapidly. Within 1 hour of administration, it is estimated that 75% of the BES administered has left the vascular compartment. BESs have been shown to decrease the COP and TP in a linear fashion throughout general anesthesia of horses[11,25]; however, the volume of BES administered could not accurately predict the changes in COP.[13,25]

Saline has no buffer and therefore can be an acidifying solution. Saline consists of 154 mEq/L of sodium and 154 mEq/L of chloride.[7] The determining factor for fluid therapy is often the availability of reasonably sized bags for rapid delivery in the anesthetized patient. Again, BESs are the most commonly used fluid solution in horses under general anesthesia.

Hypertonic Saline

Hypertonic saline (7.2%), in contrast to crystalloid fluid solutions, is approximately 8 times the tonicity of plasma.[7] The use of hypertonic saline in animals has been demonstrated to be associated with significant increases in serum sodium and serum chloride as well as osmolality.[26] Hypertonic saline is used in the emergency situation to rapidly, but transiently, expand the vascular volume while additional, longer lasting, fluids can be administered. In the horse, administration of hypertonic saline has been shown to expand the plasma volume.[26] Hypertonic saline will rapidly expand the vascular volume by drawing in fluid from the interstitial and intracellular compartments. Each liter of hypertonic saline administered will expand the plasma volume by 3.0 to 4.5 L.[7] Hypertonic saline administration is associated with a decrease in the PCV, hemoglobin concentrations, and TP concentrations. These changes are thought to be secondary to the hemodilution associated with the volume expansion that comes with the use of hypertonic saline.[26] Hemodynamics can, therefore, rapidly be improved with hypertonic administration. Cardiac output, mean systemic arterial blood pressure, cardiac contractility, and a decrease in total peripheral resistance have all been observed, in experimental models of hemorrhagic shock, following the administration of hypertonic saline in dogs, sheep, and pigs.[26] The effect is very transient, however, as sodium is not contained in the vascular space and instead will be distributed to the interstitial compartment. Hypertonic saline will not correct underlying fluid deficits, so additional fluids must be administered. The effect may be amplified by combining with colloid fluid therapy. Hypertonic saline solution administration has been shown to cause temporary increases in cardiac contractility and cardiac output, to reduce endothelial and tissue edema, and to increase microcirculation, oxygen transport, and blood viscosity.[6]

Colloids

Colloids are fluid solutions that include molecules, like HESs, which are too large to cross the capillary wall, thus remaining in the vascular compartment. HES solutions are fluid solutions composed of artificial colloids that are used for increasing the COP and for plasma volume expansion.[27] Administration of fluid solutions containing large oncotically active molecules will maintain COP, thereby resulting in plasma volume expansion and limiting transcapillary fluid movement.[9] Intravenously administered synthetic colloids are frequently given to patients with hypoproteinemia to prevent fluids from leaving the vascular compartment and developing tissue edema. Colloids are also administered to hypovolemic animals as an element of resuscitation efforts.

One of the most commonly administered synthetic colloids is 6% HES, a synthetic polymer of glucose (amylopectin).[9,28] HESs are crystalloid solutions containing large starch polymers and are classified by their mean molecular weight.[27] HES solutions are also classified by their degree of substitution, which is the number of hydroxyethyl groups per glucose unit within the branched chain glucose polymer,[27] as well as the pattern of hydroxyethlyation (C2:C6 ratio). Veterinary medicine has many commercial formulations of HES available. For instance, HES 450/0.7 has an average molecular weight of 450 kDa and a molar substitution ratio of 7 hydroxyethyl groups per 10 molecules of glucose.[28] With a COP of 29 to 32 mm Hg,[29,30] HES can increase the plasma volume in human and canine patients by the volume given.[31,32] Therefore, 1 L of hetastarch has the effect of expanding the vascular volume by 2 L. In some cases, the plasma expansion can be even greater, expanding by more than the volume given.[31,32] In dogs given 450 mL HES IV, within 30 minutes of administration, plasma volume increased by greater than 650 mL.[32] In clinical studies, HES and albumin had similar volume-expanding effects.[9] Administering 5 to 10 mL/kg of 6% hetastarch improves hemodynamic effects for 18 to 24 hours.[7,10]

In experimentally induced hypoproteinemic states, in comparison with crystalloid solutions, HES supports capillary COP and increases the capillary-to-interstitial oncotic gradient (Starling-Landis equation).[9] A linear decreasing COP was observed during administration of lactated Ringer solution (LRS) over the duration of the anesthetic period[11,25]; however, the addition of 6% HES to the fluid therapy for a total of 2.5 mL/kg HES administered over 1 hour did not attenuate this decrease.[25] This appears to be an anesthetic effect, as a similar rate of HES administration (2.0–2.5 mL/kg/h) was given to unanesthetized, hypoproteinemic horses and HES raised COP significantly for 6 hours after administration.[10] Again, the horses in this study were not anesthetized and were hypoproteinemic before HES administration.

The use of colloids is not without complication. Side effects of HES solutions, in humans, include impeding platelet function both in vitro and in vivo. Some human patients appear to have a greater rate of postoperative blood loss after administration of HES. In dogs, 20 mL/kg of HES (mw 670/ds 0.75) prolongs clotting times (CT) for 5 hours following administration. Hetastarch solutions are classified by their molecular weight (MW) and the average number of hydroxyethyl groups per glucose unit within the branched-chain glucose polymer (DS). Volume expansion causing a dilutional effect is thought to contribute to the prolonged CT in patients following HES administration.[27] Plasma expansion may also decrease the total protein concentration because of a dilutional effect. Ponies given HES had a more substantial reduction in TP when compared with ponies that were administered only saline[10]; however, smaller volumes of HES administration (2.5 mL/kg total dose) did not cause a sufficient volume expansion to dilute TP.[25]

Recently, a veterinary-labeled product, VetStarch (Abbott Laboratories, North Chicago, IL, USA) has been introduced to the market. Vetstarch is a synthetic colloid, a 6% hydroxyethyl starch in 0.9% sodium chloride, with an average molecular weight of 130 kDa, a molar substitution rate of 0.4 and a pattern of hydroxyethyl substitution (C2:C6 ratio) of 9:1.[33] The low molar substitution is the main pharmacologic determinant for the beneficial effects including faster metabolism without plasma accumulation and reduced postoperative effects on coagulation and renal function.[34] Currently there are no published reports on its use in canine and feline patients; however, in rats and humans there are few studies supporting the use of Vetstarch.[34,35]

Electrolytes and Osmolality

Transcellular fluid homeostasis is influenced by osmolality. Osmolality (OSM) is also useful in assessing the impact of fluid administration on electrolyte concentrations and hemodilution.[25] For example, except for the sodium concentration, volume expansion associated with the administration of hypertonic saline would decrease the existing electrolyte concentrations.[26] Osmolality is the number of osmoles per kilogram of solvent. In physiologic fluids, substances that add to osmolality include sodium, potassium, chloride, bicarbonate, and glucose.[15] The concentration of each of these substances in the intracellular and extracellular spaces will control the fluid dynamics in each of these spaces.[15] In horses administered LRS and HES, serum OSM did not change over the course of anesthesia[25]; however, in horses administered LRS alone, OSM was significantly higher postanesthesia when compared with preanesthesia values.[25] The increase in OSM was proposed to be secondary to xylazine administration. In dogs administered xylazine, osmolality was increased 2 to 5 hours postadministration.[36] The exact mechanism for this phenomenon is unknown, but likely has multiple factors. Increased serum glucose concentrations, in part, have been proposed as causes in horses as well as in other species.[36,37]

When measuring electrolytes, only the electrolytes in the ECF can be easily measured. The true electrolyte status may not be represented by the ECF. For example, only 2% of total body potassium is located in the ECF.[7]

Calcium

Calcium is important in muscular contractions, including the myocardium, neuromuscular function, and hemostasis. Fifty percent of the total serum calcium concentration is bound to plasma proteins, most importantly albumin; 40% of the remaining calcium in plasma is in the ionized, active form.[8] Inhalant anesthetics can influence total calcium concentration. Volatile anesthetics have direct effects on normal calcium activity. Isoflurane and halothane have both been shown to cause significant decreases in the serum ionized and total calcium concentrations.[2] Inhalants decrease the rate of influx of calcium ions into cardiac cells through the slow calcium channels, they depress calcium ion release by the sarcoplasmic reticulum, and they decrease the responsiveness of contractile proteins to calcium.[2] Inhalant anesthetics reduce the entry of calcium through the calcium selective channels in the myocardium as well as decreasing the uptake and release of calcium from the sarcoplasmic reticulum.[4] Alterations in normal cellular calcium ion activity associated with the use of inhalant anesthetics are, in part, responsible for the dose-dependent depression of myocardial contractility.[2] Calcium ions are necessary for normal myocardial contraction.[4] Because the ionized form is the active form, ionized calcium should be preferentially measured. A decrease in the total plasma concentration of calcium, without a change in the ionized calcium concentration, has been demonstrated in halothane-anesthetized ponies 30 minutes following anesthetic induction.[4]

Intraoperative hypocalcemia can also, in part, be a result of aggressive fluid therapy causing a dilutional effect of the total plasma calcium concentration. Intraoperative signs of hypocalcemia can include prolonged QT and ST segments due to prolonged myocardial action potentials.[8] In addition to cardiac changes and alterations in hemodynamics, postanesthetic myopathy in horses has been associated with intraoperative hypocalcemia.[2] Treating hypocalcemia can reverse the myocardial contractility depression associated with inhalant anesthetics.[2] Hypocalcemia can be treated with either 10% calcium chloride or calcium gluconate, depending on the level of hypocalcemia to be treated. Ten percent calcium chloride contains 1.4 mEq/mL of calcium, and calcium gluconate contains 0.45 mEq/mL of calcium.[8] The administration of calcium gluconate in isoflurane anesthetized horses caused an increase in the myocardial contractility.[2] Careful monitoring of the electrocardiogram (ECG) should be performed while administering calcium infusion, as calcium administration has been associated with sinus arrest, first-degree AV block, and atrial fibrillation.[2]

Potassium

Only 2% of the body's total content of potassium is located in the extracellular fluid. As a result, serum potassium monitoring may not accurately depict potassium alterations within the body. Additionally, serum potassium concentrations are easily altered by disease states, acid-base status, and serum pH. It is, therefore, essential to evaluate potassium levels in the perioperative period.

Serum potassium levels greater than 6.5 mmol/L are associated with the development of abnormal clinical signs. Clinical signs of hyperkalemia include a decrease in myocardial contractility, bradycardia, and ECG changes, including absent P-waves and tall, tented T-waves. At serum levels of 8.0 mmol/L and higher, fatal arrhythmias can result.[8] Correction of hyperkalemia is, therefore, imperative before anesthesia. Several methods have been described to decrease serum potassium levels.[8] Dextrose 5% can be administered at 0.5 mL/kg to assist in driving potassium into the cells and thus decreasing the extracellular concentration. Insulin can be added to the therapy at 0.1 IU/kg with dextrose to aid in pushing potassium intracellularly if dextrose by itself is unsuccessful. Sodium bicarbonate can be administered at 1 mEq/kg to decrease acidemia and cause more potassium to move intracellularly. In the face of the cardiac changes caused by elevated potassium levels, calcium gluconate at 4 mg/kg can be administered slowly to stabilize the cardiac membrane and decrease the hyperkalemic effects on the myocardium.[8]

Anesthesia can have a direct effect on potassium levels. In ponies, xylazine has been shown to increase the urinary clearance of potassium, sodium, and chloride.[37,38] Administration of detomidine to horses before gas anesthesia was associated with an increase in serum potassium concentrations.[4,38] In horses with hyperkalemic periodic paralysis (HYPP), potassium can be exceptionally critical to monitor. General anesthesia and recovery from general anesthesia have been identified as causative factors for episodes of HYPP in horses.[39] HYPP episodes are associated with elevated serum potassium concentrations of 5.1 to 12.3 mEq/L and clinical signs secondary to the elevated potassium, such as facial muscle spasms and electrocardiographic changes.[39] In horses suspected of HYPP, monitoring potassium should be done throughout anesthesia to prevent a critical situation.

Sodium

Concentrations of sodium can be effected by the electrolyte itself as well as fluid concentrations. Alterations in sodium concentrations can, therefore, be greatly influenced by fluids administered. In a model of hemorrhagic shock in anesthetized horses, it was found that low-volume hypertonic saline administration significantly increased the plasma sodium and chloride ion concentrations. Both sodium and chloride exceeded normal values immediately following administration but gradually returned to normal values over time.[26] Drugs also have an influence on sodium concentrations. In ponies, xylazine has been shown to increase the urinary clearance of sodium.[37,38]

REFERENCES

1. Wagner AE. Complications in equine anesthesia. Vet Clin North Am Equine Pract 2008;24:735–52.
2. Grubb TL, Benson GJ, Foreman JH, et al. Hemodynamic effects of ionized calcium in horses anesthetized with halothane or isoflurane. Am J Vet Res 1999;60:1430–5.
3. Grandy JL, Steffey EP, Hodgson DS, et al. Arterial hypotension and the development of postanesthetic myopathy in halothane-anesthetized horses. Am J Vet Res 1987;48(2):192–7.
4. Gasthuys F, De Moor A, Parmentier D. Cardiovascular effects of low dose calcium chloride infusions during halothane anaesthesia in dorsally recumbent ventilated ponies. J Am Vet Med Assoc 1991;38:728–36.
5. Chappell D, Jacob M, Hofmann-Kiefer K, et al. A rational approach to perioperative fluid management. Anesthesiology 2008;109:723–40.
6. Pantaleon LG, Furr MO, McKenzie HC, et al. Cardiovascular and pulmonary effects of hetastarch plus hypertonic saline solutions during experimental endotoxemia in anesthetized horses. J Vet Intern Med 2006;20:1422–8.
7. Hardy J. Venous and arterial catheterization and fluid therapy. In: Muir WW, Hubbell JA, editors. Equine anesthesia: monitoring and emergency therapy. 2nd edition. St Louis (MO): Elsevier Inc; 2009. p. 131–47.
8. Seeler DC. Fluid, electrolyte, and blood component therapy. In: Tranquilli WJ, Thurmon JC, Grimm KA, editors. Lumb & Jones' veterinary anesthesia and analgesia. 4th edition. Ames (IA): Blackwell; 2007. p. 185–201.
9. Jones PA, Bain FT, Byars TD, et al. Effect of hydroxyethyl starch infusion on colloid oncotic pressure in hypoproteinemic horses. J Am Vet Med Assoc 2001;218:1130–5.

10. Jones PA, Tomasic M, Gentry PA. Oncotic, hemodilutional, and hemostatic effects of isotonic saline and hydroxyethyl starch solutions in clinically normal ponies. Am J Vet Res 1997;58:541–8.
11. Boscan P, Watson Z, Steffey EP. Plasma colloid osmotic pressure and total protein trends in horses during anesthesia. Vet Anaesth Analg 2007;34:275–83.
12. Boscan P, Steffey EP. Plasma colloid osmotic pressure and total protein in horses during colic surgery. Vet Anaesth Analg 2007;34:408–15.
13. Dismukes DI, Thomovsky EJ, Mann FA, et al. Effects of general anesthesia on plasma colloid oncotic pressure in dogs. J Am Vet Med Assoc 2010;236:309–11.
14. Thomas LA, Brown SA. Relationship between colloid osmotic pressure and plasma protein concentration in cattle, horses, dogs, and cats. Am J Vet Res 1992;53:2241–4.
15. DiBartola SP, Kohn CW, Wellman ML. Applied physiology of body fluids in dogs and cats. In: Fathman L, Stringer S, editors. Fluid, electrolyte and acid-base disorders in small animal practice. 3rd edition. St Louis (MO): Elsevier Inc; 2006. p. 3–25.
16. Starling EH. On the absorption of fluids from the connective tissue spaces. J Physiol 1896;19:312–26.
17. Landis EM, Pappenheimer JR. Exchange of substances through capillary walls. In: Hamilton WF, editor. Handbook of physiology. Washington, DC: Am Physiol Soc; 1963. p. 961–1034.
18. Doherty TJ. Postoperative ileus: pathogenesis and treatment. Vet Clin North Am Equine Pract 2009;25:351–62.
19. Prien T, Backhaus N, Pelster F, et al. Effect of intraoperative fluid administration and colloid osmotic pressure on the formation of intestinal edema during gastro-intestinal surgery. J Clin Anesth 1990;2:317–23.
20. Haynes GR, Navickis RJ, Wilkes MM. Albumin administration—what is the evidence of clinical benefit? A systematic review of randomized controlled trials. Eur J Anaesthesiol 2003;20:771–93.
21. Wright BD, Hopkins A. Changes in colloid osmotic pressure as a function of anesthesia and surgery in the presence and absence of isotonic fluid administration in dogs. Vet Anaesth Analg 2008;35:282–8.
22. Schüpbach P, Pappova E, Schlit W. Perfusate oncotic pressure during cardiopulmonary bypass. Optimum level as determined by metabolic acidosis, tissue edema, and renal function. Vox Sang 1978;35:332–44.
23. Lundsgaard-Hansen P, Pappova E. Colloids versus crystalloids as volume substitutes: clinical relevance of the serum oncotic pressure. Ann Clin Res 1981;13:5–17.
24. Kaartinen MJ, Pang DS, Cuvelliez SG. Post-anesthetic pulmonary edema in two horses. Vet Anaesth Analg 2010;37:136–43.
25. Wendt-Hornickle EL, Snyder LB, Tang R, et al. The effects of lactated Ringer's solution (LRS) or LRS and 6% hetastarch on the colloid osmotic pressure, total protein and osmolality in healthy horses under general anesthesia. Vet Anaesth Analg 2011;38:336–43.
26. Schmall LM, Muir WW, Robertson JT. Haematological, serum electrolyte and blood gas effects of small volume hypertonic saline in experimentally induced haemorrhagic shock. Equine Vet J 1990;22:278–83.
27. Smart L, Jandrey KE, Kass PH, et al. The effect of Hetastarch (670/0.75) in vivo on platelet closure time in the dog. J Vet Emerg Crit Care (San Antonio) 2009;19:444–9.
28. Bateman S, DiBartola SP. Introduction to fluid therapy. In: Fathman L, Stringer S, editors. Fluid, electrolyte and acid-base disorders in small animal practice. 3rd edition. St Louis (MO): Elsevier Inc; 2006. p. 325–43.

29. Posner LP, Moon PF, Bliss SP, et al. Colloid osmotic pressure after hemorrhage and replenishment with oxyglobin solution, hetastarch, or whole blood in pregnant sheep. Vet Anaesth Analg 2003;30:30–6.
30. Pascoe PJ. Perioperative management of fluid therapy. In: Fathman L, Stringer S, editors. Fluid, electrolyte and acid-base disorders in small animal practice. 3rd edition. St Louis (MO): Elsevier Inc; 2006. p. 391–419.
31. Smiley LE. The use of hetastarch for plasma expansion. Probl Vet Med 1992;4: 652–67.
32. Silverstein DC, Aldrich J, Haskins SC, et al. Assessment of changes in blood volume in response to resuscitative fluid administration in dogs. J Vet Emerg Crit Care 2005;15:185–92.
33. VetStarch North Chicago (IL): Abbott Laboratories; 2011.
34. Neff TA, Doelberg M, Jengheinrich C, et al. Repetitive large-dose infusion of the novel hydroxyethyl starch 130/0.4 in patients with severe head injury. Anesth Analg 2003;96:1453–9.
35. Leuschner J, Opitz J, Winkler A, et al. Tissue storage of 14C-labeled hydroxyethyl starch (HES) 130/0.4 and HES 200/0.5 after repeated intravenous administration to rats. Drugs R D 2003;6:331–8.
36. Talukder H, Hikasa Y, Matsuu A, et al. Antagonistic effects of atipamezole and yohimbine on xylazine-induced diuresis in healthy dogs. Vet Med Sci 2009;71: 539–48.
37. Trim CM, Hanson RR. Effects of xylazine on renal function and plasma glucose in ponies. Vet Rec 1986;118:65–7.
38. Greene S, Keegan R, Brown J, et al. Effect of furosemide and hypertonic saline on electrolytes during post exercise anaesthesia. Equine Vet J Suppl 1999;30:434–7.
39. Bailey JE, Pablo L, Hubbell JA. Hyperkalemic periodic paralysis episode during halothane anesthesia in a horse. J Am Vet Med Assoc 1996;208:1859–65.

Anesthesia for Ophthalmic Procedures in the Standing Horse

Amber L. Labelle, DVM, MS*, Stuart C. Clark-Price, DVM, MS

KEYWORDS

- Local anesthesia • Eye • Standing surgery • Analgesia • Horse

KEY POINTS

- A working knowledge of regional anatomy is essential for the accurate delivery of local anesthetics to peripheral nerves.
- Standing sedation and analgesia may be provided with bolus injections of an α2-agonist for a short procedure or a constant-rate infusion for longer procedures.
- Local anesthesia may be used to facilitate ocular examination, diagnostic procedures, therapeutic techniques, and surgery of the equine eye.
- Local anesthetics may be delivered by a topical or injectable route.

INTRODUCTION

As safe, effective, and economical agents for chemical restraint become more commonly used by equine practitioners, standing ocular surgery is increasing in frequency. The effective delivery of local anesthesia is critical to the success of standing surgical procedures in the horse. Local anesthesia can be used to facilitate examination of the fragile or painful eye. It can also be used to obtain diagnostic samples (such as corneal cytology, conjunctival biopsy or aqueocentesis), facilitate therapeutic interventions (such as subpalpebral lavage tube placement), and provide surgical anesthesia for procedures involving the adnexa, ocular surface, globe, and orbit. Requisite to the successful delivery of local and regional anesthesia is an understanding of clinically relevant anatomy and approaches for blocking sensory and motor nerves.

LOCAL ANESTHETIC DRUGS

Local anesthetics are one of the few categories of drugs that actually provide "true" anesthesia, the condition of having sensation, including the feeling of pain, blocked

Department of Veterinary Clinical Medicine, College of Veterinary Medicine, University of Illinois Urbana-Champaign, 1008 West Hazelwood Drive, Urbana, IL 61802, USA
* Corresponding author.
E-mail address: alabelle@illinois.edu

Vet Clin Equine 29 (2013) 179–191
http://dx.doi.org/10.1016/j.cveq.2012.12.001
0749-0739/13/$ – see front matter © 2013 Elsevier Inc. All rights reserved.

or temporarily taken away. In fact, the mechanism of action by which local anesthetics work is to reversibly bind to sodium channels in nerve cell membranes, preventing neural impulses, or messages, from conducting to the next nerve cell or target cell. This impulse disruption results in blockade of sensory, motor, and autonomic functions of the targeted area. Removal or metabolism of the local anesthetic from the site results in complete return of nerve conduction and function with no permanent effects.[1]

In veterinary medicine, lidocaine is by far the most commonly used local anesthetic agent. Other local anesthetics used in veterinary procedures include mepivacaine, bupivacaine, ropivacaine, proparacaine, and tetracaine. The onset and duration of action varies and is related to the individual drug's lipid solubility and protein binding within the target cell's membrane (Table 1). The selection of which local anesthetic drug to use depends on several factors, including the area to be anesthetized, the volume of drug needed, the onset of action and the duration of action desired, cost, and availability. Lidocaine is often selected because of its speed of onset, its relatively low cost, and its abundant availability. However, for procedures that may require a prolonged time or cause a significant amount of tissue damage, an agent with a longer duration of action may be more suitable. For practitioners wishing for an agent with a quicker onset but a longer duration of action, 2 local anesthetics may be combined. The use of a mixture of lidocaine and bupivacaine may result in a quicker onset from lidocaine and a prolonged duration of action from bupivacaine.

Toxicity and Side Effects

Toxicity and side effects of local anesthetics are mostly related to systemic absorption and elevated plasma levels of the drug. In horses, toxic effects of the nervous and cardiovascular systems can be seen clinically. Toxic effects of the nervous system are seen initially as subtle muscle twitching and progress to obvious muscle tremors, ataxia, stumbling and falling, and seizures. Cardiovascular toxic effects result in vasodilation, reduced cardiac contractility, cardiac dysrhythmias (bradyarrhythmias), and full cardiovascular collapse. Lidocaine tends to be the least toxic of the local anesthetics used in horses owing to its short half-life, but agents such as bupivacaine can result in prolonged neurologic and cardiovascular side effects that warrant treatment. In adult average-sized horses, overdose and toxicity with local anesthetics is probably a rare occurrence, as the sheer volume necessary to cause toxicity when performing local infiltration or nerve blocks is not approached. However, even small volumes when administered directly into a blood vessel can result in signs of toxicity. To this end it is important to always aspirate with a syringe before injecting a local anesthetic, to minimize administration into an artery or vein.

Table 1
Onset and duration of action of local anesthetic drugs used for equine ophthalmic procedures

Drug	Onset of Action (min)	Duration of Action (min)	Use
Lidocaine	5–15	60–120	Local infiltration, direct nerve blockade
Mepivicaine	5–30	90–180	Local infiltration, direct nerve blockade
Bupivacaine	15–45	180–480	Local infiltration, direct nerve blockade
Ropivacaine	15–45	180–480	Local infiltration, direct nerve blockade
Proparacaine	<1	5–25	Topical for anesthesia of the cornea
Tetracaine	<1	5–30	Topical for anesthesia of the cornea

Adjuvant Drugs

Adjuvant drugs can be added to local anesthetics to enhance their duration of action, increase the area of blockade, or supplement the anesthetic effects. Vasoactive agents such as epinephrine or phenylephrine may be added to cause constriction of the blood vessels of the area to be blocked. This addition decreases the systemic uptake and metabolism of the local anesthetic and thus prolongs its duration of action by increasing its resident time. Epinephrine may be added to lidocaine at a dose of 5 µg epinephrine per milliliter of lidocaine. The use of phenylephrine does not appear to have any advantage over epinephrine.

Similar to epinephrine, the addition of an α2-agonist drug such as dexmedetomidine or detomidine can enhance the duration of action of local anesthetics through vasoconstriction. Other interactions between the 2 classes of drugs as well as local anesthetic effects of the α2-agonist drugs themselves probably occur, but have not been well elucidated.

Hyaluronidase, an enzyme that disrupts cell-to-cell adhesion, has been added to local anesthetics to improve the spread of the agents such as lidocaine. This addition results in a wider and deeper area of anesthesia of local infiltration. Hyaluronidase at a dose of 3.75 IU per milliliter of lidocaine has been used for retrobulbar anesthesia.[2] The use of the hyaluronidase results in a more effective but shorter duration of retrobulbar anesthesia.

Drugs for Standing Sedation

In many cases, the use of local anesthetics may not allow a practitioner to perform an ocular procedure because of pain, patient apprehension, anxiety, and movement. The addition of sedative and systemic analgesic medications may be necessary. For short procedures, single injection of standard doses of an α2-agonist such as xylazine, romifidine, or detomidine is often sufficient. For longer procedures, constant-rate infusions (CRI) may be advantageous over repeated bolus injections to provide a consistent level of sedation.

α2-Agonists are the most commonly used sedative agent in horses, exerting their sedative and analgesic effects through centrally located α2 receptors. However, because of a wide distribution of α2 receptors, this class of drugs has many other effects including initial hypertension followed by hypotension, decreased cardiac output, hyperglycemia, and increased urine output. The use of a CRI of detomidine has been described for longer, standing surgical procedures.[3] An initial bolus of 8.4 µg/kg is followed by an infusion of 0.5 µg/kg/min for 15 minutes, then reduced to 0.3 µg/kg/min for 15 minutes and then 0.15 µg/kg/min for the duration of the procedure. Infusions with romifidine have also been described, which may impart sedation with less ataxia.[4] A loading dose of 80 µg/kg is followed by an infusion of 30 µg/kg/h.

In some cases, additional systemic analgesia and sedation is desired in horses receiving an α2-agonist CRI. The opioid butorphanol has also been described for use in horses as a CRI and may be used as an adjunctive drug.[5] A loading dose of butorphanol of 17.8 µg/kg is administered and is followed by an infusion of 0.38 µg/kg/min.

TECHNIQUES FOR EXAMINATION, DIAGNOSTIC SAMPLING, AND THERAPEUTIC INTERVENTION

Local anesthesia for examination of the equine eye has 2 purposes: first, to provide akinesia (inhibition of voluntary movement) of the mobile eyelids and second, to provide anesthesia to the adnexa and ocular surface.[6] In a nonpainful eye, akinesia alone may be sufficient to facilitate complete examination; however, a painful eye may require both akinesia and anesthesia. Excessive digital pressure should be avoided in fragile eyes, such as those with full-thickness lacerations or deep corneal ulcers, making nerve blocks essential for safe examination of these cases.

Auriculopalpebral Nerve Block

The most commonly used and important nerve block is the auriculopalpebral (AP).[7] A branch of cranial nerve VII, the AP nerve provides motor innervation to the orbicularis oculi muscle that closes the eyelids. The powerful orbicularis oculi muscle is a significant impediment to examination of the eye in horses, and akinesia of this muscle greatly facilitates examination, particularly in painful eyes. The AP nerve emerges from beneath the parotid salivary gland near the temporomandibular joint and courses superficially over the temporalis muscle and dorsal orbit. The palpebral branch of the AP nerve is easily palpated as it travels horizontally over the zygomatic process of the temporal bone. Although the AP nerve can be blocked at other sites, this location is the easiest to identify and avoids inadvertent contact with the ears during injection, which some horses find objectionable.

To perform an AP nerve block, the skin overlying the nerve is gently tented, a 25-gauge 1 inch (2.54 cm) needle is inserted subcutaneously, a syringe is attached to the needle, gentle aspiration is applied, and 1 to 2 mL of local anesthetic is injected (**Figs. 1** and **2**). Care should be taken to insert the needle with the tip pointing toward the ground; if the horse suddenly moves its head, the needle is more likely to remain in the correct location and not be tossed away. Onset and duration of akinesia is determined by the local anesthetic agent used for the block. Agents with shorter duration (ie, lidocaine) should be used for most routine examinations. When akinesia is desirable as part of a therapeutic or surgical procedure, agents of longer duration are

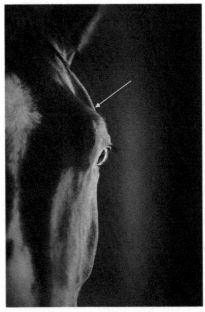

Fig. 1. The frontal view of a normal horse shows the site for performing an auriculopalpebral nerve block, marked by an arrow.

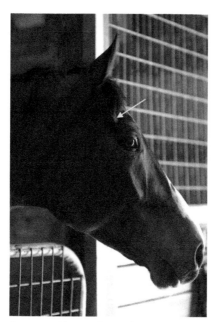

Fig. 2. The lateral view of a normal horse shows the site for performing an auriculopalpebral nerve block, marked by an arrow.

preferred. An effective AP nerve block results in ptosis, decreased resistance to manipulation of the eyelid, and an impaired or incomplete blink reflex. When longer-duration local anesthetic agents are used, a lubricating ointment should be applied to the ocular surface to protect the cornea from desiccation until a normal blink reflex returns.

Frontal Nerve Block

The frontal nerve is a branch of the ophthalmic branch of cranial nerve V. It provides sensory input to the central portion of the upper eyelid but has no motor function. A frontal nerve block is useful when an AP block alone does not provide sufficient compliance of the upper eyelid to manipulation or when sensory anesthesia is necessary, such as is required for placement of a subpalpebral lavage tube.[8] The frontal nerve is most easily blocked as it courses through the supraorbital foramen located in the dorsolateral orbital rim. To locate the supraorbital foramen, place the thumb under the ventral aspect of the dorsolateral orbital rim and use the index finger to palpate a distinct depression in the frontal bone. A 25-gauge 0.5 to 1-inch needle can be inserted directly into the foramen and 1 to 2 mL local anesthetic injected after aspirating to confirm extravascular needle location (**Fig. 3**). Alternatively, 1 to 2 mL of local anesthetic may be injected subcutaneously overlying the foramen, followed by gentle digital massage of the site. Similarly to the AP block, the duration of effect is determined by the duration of action of the local anesthetic agent used. An effective frontal nerve block results in denervation of the central upper eyelid.

Topical Anesthetics

Topical anesthetic agents cause temporary reductions in corneal and conjunctival sensitivity. This situation is advantageous when examining a painful eye, collecting

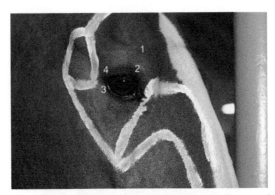

Fig. 3. Markings with white paint round a normal horse's right eye delineate the areas innervated by branches of cranial nerve V. The numbers are placed in the corresponding location where each nerve should be blocked. 1, frontal nerve; 2, infraorbital nerve; 3, zygomatic nerve; 4, lacrimal nerve.

diagnostic specimens such as during cytology of the cornea or conjunctiva, and when performing diagnostic procedures such as tonometry (the measurement of intraocular pressure). Commercially available preparations include proparacaine hydrochloride 0.5% solution, tetracaine hydrochloride 0.5% solution, and tetracaine hydrochloride 1% solution. All 3 formulations have been shown to be safe and effective for use in the horse.[9,10] The duration of effect of a single drop of proparacaine is approximately 25 minutes, with the maximum anesthetic effect occurring 5 minutes after administration.[9] A single drop of tetracaine has a 30-minute duration of effect, with the maximum anesthetic effect also occurring 5 minutes after administration.[11] Using 2 different local anesthetics increases the time to maximum anesthetic effect for both drugs, and thus is not recommended. Adding a second drop of topical anesthetic does prolong the duration of effect but does not affect the maximal anesthetic effect.[11] In some horses, corneal sensation is not completely eliminated, which may necessitate multiple doses of topical anesthetic agent to achieve maximum anesthetic effect.[9] Topical anesthetics should never be used for long-term therapeutic purposes, as they are associated with corneal epithelial toxicity, exposure keratopathy, secondary infection, and corneal perforation.[12]

In humans, proparacaine is associated with less ocular discomfort on administration than tetracaine.[13] No such evaluation has been conducted in horses, but investigators have not noted adverse ocular effects or signs of ocular discomfort with the use of 0.5% and 1% tetracaine.[10,11] Both proparacaine and tetracaine appear to be suitable for clinical use in equine patients.

TECHNIQUES FOR SURGICAL ANESTHESIA AND ANALGESIA

The goal of local anesthesia for standing surgical procedures is the complete abolition of sensation, such that the patient does not perceive pain during the procedure. Effective nerve-block techniques accomplish this goal through the precise application of local anesthetic agents to the appropriate anatomic location. Quality, rather than quantity, is the key to successful local anesthesia.

Anesthesia of the Eyelids and Third Eyelid

Akinesia of the eyelids has already been discussed (see the section on auriculopalpebral nerve block). Four nerves provide sensation to the upper and lower eyelids: the frontal, lacrimal, infratrochlear (all branches of the ophthalmic branch of cranial nerve V) and the zygomatic (a branch of the maxillary branch of cranial nerve V) (**Fig. 4**). All 4 nerves must be blocked to provide complete anesthesia of the eyelids. One technique is to perform a ring block, encircling the palpebral fissure with a continuous line of local anesthetic. Using a 22-gauge 1-inch (2.54 cm) needle, 10 to 20 mL of local anesthetic is placed subcutaneously at approximately the level of the orbital rim, creating a complete circle around the palpebral fissure. This technique has the disadvantage of being less precise, requiring a larger volume of local anesthetic and providing incomplete or patchy anesthesia of the eyelids. It can be useful to augment regional anesthesia in selected cases, particularly those whereby alternative techniques have failed to provide adequate anesthesia, or for those cases whereby distortion of the tissue by injection of local anesthetic agent may interfere with the surgical procedure, such as may be the case with an eyelid laceration or transpalpebral enucleation.

An alternative technique for providing eyelid anesthesia is to block each nerve individually using a 25-gauge 0.5 to 1-inch needle. The technique for anesthesia of the frontal nerve has already been discussed (see the section on frontal nerve block). The lacrimal nerve can be anesthetized by injecting 1 to 2 mL of local anesthetic slightly medial to the lateral canthus, aiming medially beneath the orbital rim. The infratrochlear nerve can be anesthetized by injecting 1 to 2 mL of local anesthetic caudally and rostrally beneath the orbital into the infratrochlear notch, which can be palpated on the cranial surface of the dorsomedial orbital rim (**Fig. 3**). The zygomatic nerve can be anesthetized by injecting 1 to 2 mL of local anesthetic along the ventrolateral orbital rim (see **Fig. 3**).

The infratrochlear nerve provides sensation to the third eyelid, thus anesthetizing this nerve as already described may be effective. An alternative technique is to inject 5 to 10 mL of local anesthetic into the base of the third eyelid, fanning the injection across the base (see **Fig. 3**).[14] This technique can augment or replace the infratrochlear nerve block and is particularly useful when resection of the third eyelid is being performed.

Topical anesthetic agents do not provide any anesthesia of the periocular skin, but do allow anesthesia of their conjunctival surfaces. Use of a topical anesthetic agent may be a useful adjunctive technique when repairing full-thickness eyelid lacerations

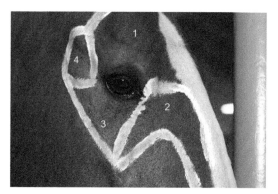

Fig. 4. Markings with white paint round a normal horse's right eye delineate the areas innervated by branches of cranial nerve V. Each region is marked with a number corresponding to the nerve innervating the delineated area. 1, frontal nerve; 2, infraorbital nerve; 3, zygomatic nerve; 4, lacrimal nerve.

or creating full-thickness wounds, as may be necessary for resecting a lesion on the eyelid margin. It is prudent to remember that reapplication of the topical anesthetic may be necessary.[11]

Anesthesia of the Globe

Anesthesia of the globe includes the ocular surface (cornea and conjunctiva), the globe, and intraocular and orbital contents, which include the extraocular muscles, the optic nerve, orbital fat, and orbital fascia. Corneal/conjunctival anesthesia may be accomplished with the administration of topical or injectable anesthetics. Short procedures or procedures that do not require immobility of the globe are best suited to topical anesthesia, including obtaining samples for cytology, corneal debridement, or biopsy of superficial conjunctival lesions. More complex surgical procedures such as keratectomy, intracameral injection, or corneal suturing require anesthesia of the ocular surface and akinesia of the extraocular muscles. Local anesthesia for advanced ocular surface procedures, surgery of the globe, and surgery of the orbit is best accomplished by retrobulbar block.

A retrobulbar block provides anesthesia to the sensory (cranial nerves II, V) and motor nerves (cranial nerves III, IV, VI) of the globe and orbit. Anesthesia of the eyelids is not routinely provided by a retrobulbar block. These nerves are located within the orbital cone, consisting of extraocular muscles, fat, and fascia. Although several approaches to the retrobulbar space have been described, including a 4-point block and a modified Peterson block, the most effective technique is direct injection into the orbital cone using a dorsal and/or lateral approach.[15–18] A recent study suggests the utility of ultrasound guidance for confirming accurate deposition of local anesthesia in the orbital cone.[18] Accurate needle placement is essential for avoiding complications associated with a retrobulbar block, including inadvertent penetration of the optic nerve or globe, hemorrhage and hematoma formation, orbital abscess/cellulitis, intrameningeal injection leading to central nervous system signs, and sudden death.[19,20] These complications are rare, and largely preventable by using accurate needle-placement techniques, appropriate patient restraint, and adequate preparation of the injection site.

There are 2 ways to approach the retrobulbar space: dorsally and laterally. Either site should first be clipped with a #40 blade and aseptically prepared using a dilute povidone-iodine solution. The periocular use of surgical scrubs should be avoided, as they are associated with significant ocular surface irritation and corneal ulceration.[21] A 20-gauge 3.5-inch (8.9 cm) spinal needle is used for either approach. For the dorsal approach, the needle is placed caudal to the center of the dorsal orbital rim, with the needle dropped down into the retrobulbar space perpendicular to the plane of the skull (**Figs. 5** and **6**). A resistance is felt as the needle touches the extraocular muscle cone, with a slight "pop" as the needle advances through the cone. The eye can be observed to rotate dorsally as the needle presses against the cone, with the globe returning centrally as the needle enters the cone. Aspirating before injecting 10 to 12 mL of local anesthetic is strongly advised to avoid inadvertent intraocular, intra-arterial, or intrameningeal administration.

The lateral approach to the retrobulbar space occurs from the lateral aspect of the orbit. The needle is placed cranial to the ramus of the mandible and ventral to the ventral border of the zygomatic bone, just ventral to the facial crest (**Figs. 7–11**). The needle is aimed slightly caudally and slowly advanced. The needle should be inserted nearly to the level of the hub. Any resistance met after advancing the needle less than 1 inch (2.54 cm) is likely the result of excessive caudal direction causing contact with the ramus of the mandible, and the needle should be redirected more cranially/rostrally.

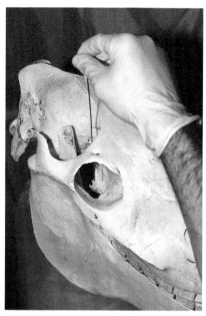

Fig. 5. Demonstration, using an equine skull, of correct placement of a 20-gauge 3.5-inch (8.9 cm) spinal needle for the dorsal approach to a retrobulbar block. The needle is placed caudal to the most caudal border of the central orbital rim perpendicular to the plane of the skull.

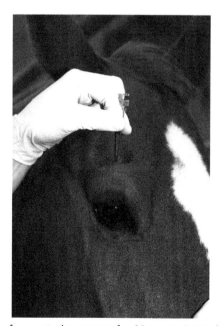

Fig. 6. Demonstration of correct placement of a 20-gauge 3.5-inch spinal needle for the dorsal approach to a retrobulbar block. The needle is placed caudal to the most caudal border of the central orbital rim perpendicular to the plane of the skull.

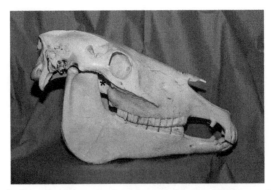

Fig. 7. Equine skull demonstrating the location of the lateral approach to a retrobulbar block. An asterisk marks the anatomic location of the needle placement.

The dorsal and lateral approaches may be combined in the same patient for faster onset and more complete anesthesia.[22] An effective retrobulbar block results in mild exophthalmos of the globe, mydriasis, immobility of the globe, and complete anesthesia of the ocular surface. The time to maximal anesthetic effect and duration of effect varies with the local anesthetic agent used. Exposure keratopathy and corneal ulceration may be consequences of long-acting agents, as corneal sensation is reduced and the blink reflex is impaired. Generous lubrication of the cornea or temporary tarsorrhaphy is necessary to ensure the cornea remains lubricated and protected during this recovery phase. Complete or partial visual impairment may accompany retrobulbar anesthesia; therefore bilateral administration is not recommended, to prevent sudden loss of vision and patient disorientation.

In addition to being a useful technique for local anesthesia, retrobulbar anesthesia can also be an adjunctive analgesic technique for surgical procedures performed under general anesthesia. Retrobulbar anesthesia may be performed before enucleation or exenteration for intraoperative and postoperative analgesia.

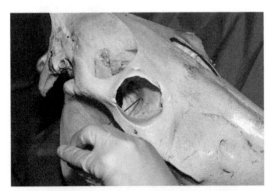

Fig. 8. Demonstration, using an equine skull, of correct placement of a 20-gauge 3.5-inch spinal needle for the lateral approach to a retrobulbar block. The needle is placed cranial to the ramus of the mandible and ventral to the ventral border of the zygomatic bone, just ventral to the facial crest.

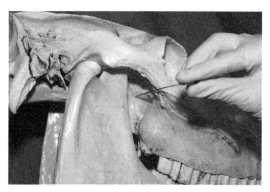

Fig. 9. Demonstration, using an equine skull, of correct placement of a 20-gauge 3.5-inch spinal needle for the lateral approach to a retrobulbar block. The needle is placed cranial to the ramus of the mandible and ventral to the ventral border of the zygomatic bone, just ventral to the facial crest.

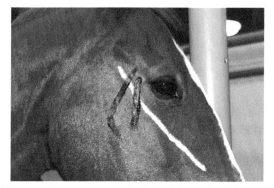

Fig. 10. A normal horse's right eye marked with white and black paint to delineate the anatomic landmarks important for the lateral approach to a retrobulbar block. The straight white line represents the facial crest. The straight black line represents the caudal border of the dorsal orbital rim. The curved black line represents the ramus of the mandible. The needle should be placed in the location marked by the asterisk in **Fig. 7**.

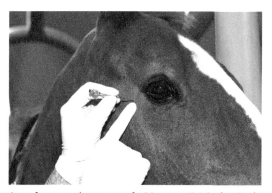

Fig. 11. Demonstration of correct placement of a 20-gauge 3.5-inch spinal needle for the lateral approach to a retrobulbar block. The needle is placed cranial to the ramus of the mandible and ventral to the ventral border of the zygomatic bone, just ventral to the facial crest.

REFERENCES

1. Stolting RK, Hillier SC. Local anesthetics. In: Stolting RK, Hillier SC, editors. Pharmacology and physiology in anesthetic practice. 4th edition. Philadelphia: Lippincott Williams & Wilkins; 2006. p. 197–207.
2. Skarda RT, Tranquilli WJ. Local anesthetics. In: Tranquilli WJ, Thurmon JC, Grimm KA, editors. Lumb and Jones veterinary anesthesia and analgesia. 4th edition. Ames (IA): Blackwell Publishing; 2007. p. 395–418.
3. Goodrich LR, Clark-Price SC, Ludders J. How to attain effective and consistent sedation for standing procedures in the horse using constant rate infusion. Proceedings of the 50th annual convention of the American Association of Equine Practitioners. 2004. p. 229–32.
4. Ringer SK, Portier K, Torgerson PR, et al. The effects of a loading dose followed by constant rate infusion of xylazine compared with romifidine on sedation, ataxia and response to stimuli in horses. Vet Anaesth Analg 2012. [Epub ahead of print].
5. Sellon DC, Monroe VL, Roberts MC, et al. Pharmacokinetics and adverse effects of butorphanol administered by single intravenous injection or continuous intravenous infusion in horses. Am J Vet Res 2001;62:183–9.
6. Cooley PL. Normal equine ocular anatomy and eye examination. Vet Clin North Am Equine Pract 1992;8:427–49.
7. Rubin LF. Auriculopalpebral nerve block as an adjunct to the diagnosis and treatment of ocular inflammation in the horse. J Am Vet Med Assoc 1964;144:1387–8.
8. Manning JP, St Clair LE. Palpebral, frontal, and zygomatic nerve blocks for examination of the equine eye. Vet Med Small Anim Clin 1976;71:187–9.
9. Kalf KL, Utter ME, Wotman KL. Evaluation of duration of corneal anesthesia induced with ophthalmic 0.5% proparacaine hydrochloride by use of a Cochet-Bonnet anesthesiometer in clinically normal horses. Am J Vet Res 2008;69:1655–8.
10. Monclin SJ, Farnir F, Grauwels M. Determination of tear break-up time reference values and ocular tolerance of tetracaine hydrochloride eyedrops in healthy horses. Equine Vet J 2011;43:74–7.
11. Monclin SJ, Farnir F, Grauwels M. Duration of corneal anaesthesia following multiple doses and two concentrations of tetracaine hydrochloride eyedrops on the normal equine cornea. Equine Vet J 2011;43:69–73.
12. McGee HT, Fraunfelder FW. Toxicities of topical ophthalmic anesthetics. Expert Opin Drug Saf 2007;6:637–40.
13. Bartfield JM, Holmes TJ, Raccio-Robak N. A comparison of proparacaine and tetracaine eye anesthetics. Acad Emerg Med 1994;1:364–7.
14. Labelle AL, Metzler AG, Wilkie DA. Nictitating membrane resection in the horse: a comparison of long-term outcomes using local vs. general anaesthesia. Equine Vet J Suppl 2011;43(Suppl 40):42–5.
15. Gilger BC, Stoppini R. Equine ocular examination: routine and advanced diagnostic techniques. In: Gilger BC, editor. Equine ophthalmology. 2nd edition. Maryland Heights (MO): Elsevier Saunders; 2011. p. 1–51.
16. Hewes CA, Keoughan GC, Gutierrez-Nibeyro S. Standing enucleation in the horse: a report of 5 cases. Can Vet J 2007;48:512–4.
17. Pollock PJ, Russell T, Hughes TK, et al. Transpalpebral eye enucleation in 40 standing horses. Vet Surg 2008;37:306–9.
18. Morath U, Luyet C, Spadavecchia C, et al. Ultrasound-guided retrobulbar nerve block in horses: a cadaveric study. Vet Anaesth Analg 2012. [Epub ahead of print].

19. Robertson SA. Standing sedation and pain management for ophthalmic patients. Vet Clin North Am Equine Pract 2004;20:485–97.
20. Raffe MR, Bistner SI, Crimi AJ, et al. Retrobulbar block in combination with general anesthesia for equine ophthalmic surgery. Vet Surg 1986;15:139–41.
21. Mac Rae SM, Brown B, Edelhauser HF. The corneal toxicity of presurgical skin antiseptics. Am J Ophthalmol 1984;97:221–32.
22. Labelle AL, Clark-Price SC, Breaux CB, et al. Local anesthesia for standing enucleation in the horse. Lexington (KY): International Equine Ophthalmology Consortium; 2009.

Anesthesia for the Horse with Colic

Jordyn M. Boesch, DVM

KEYWORDS

- Anesthesia • Colic • Endotoxemia • Equine • Exploratory laparotomy • Horse

KEY POINTS

- Hemodynamic, acid-base, and electrolyte disturbances should be corrected to the greatest extent possible before anesthetic induction; early goal-directed therapy, a concept shown to reduce mortality in septic humans that involves resuscitation to achieve specific macrovascular and microvascular end points, may be important in horses with colic.
- The optimal fluid type (isotonic crystalloids, hypertonic crystalloids, colloids) for resuscitation is still controversial, and it is likely that a combination that provides the advantages of each should be used.
- Horses with severe colonic gas distension, which can lead to life-threatening hypoxemia and cardiovascular impairment, may benefit from colonic gas decompression before anesthetic induction.
- Cardiovascular depression under general anesthesia should be treated by minimizing inhalant requirements via a balanced anesthetic technique and by administering antiendotoxemic therapies, intravenous fluids, positive inotropic drugs and, possibly, vasopressors.
- The anesthetist must attempt to strike a balance between maintaining cardiovascular function, which is depressed by positive-pressure ventilation, and instituting ventilatory strategies that maintain arterial partial pressure of oxygen greater than 60 mm Hg. Alveolar recruiting maneuvers combined with positive end-expiratory pressure instituted soon after induction may improve oxygenation in horses with venous admixture.
- Analgesia is of paramount importance and may decrease morbidity. Options include nonsteroidal anti-inflammatory drugs, opioids, α_2-agonists, ketamine, and lidocaine. Ketamine may have beneficial immunomodulatory properties, and strong evidence exists for lidocaine's promotility and anti-inflammatory/immunomodulatory effects.

INTRODUCTION

Horses requiring surgery for colic caused by acute disease of the gastrointestinal (GI) tract can be some of the most intensive anesthetic patients encountered; this holds especially true for horses in which intestinal ischemia has resulted in endotoxemia

Funding sources: None.
Conflict of interest: None.
Department of Clinical Sciences, Cornell University College of Veterinary Medicine, Ithaca, NY 14850, USA
E-mail address: jmb264@cornell.edu

Vet Clin Equine 29 (2013) 193–214
http://dx.doi.org/10.1016/j.cveq.2012.11.005
0749-0739/13/$ – see front matter © 2013 Elsevier Inc. All rights reserved.

or horses with severe abdominal distension. Surgical patients with colic are not only critically ill, with multiple hemodynamic, blood gas, acid-base, and electrolyte disturbances, but can also be in extreme pain and, therefore, anxious, fractious, and potentially dangerous. These animals usually cannot be completely stabilized before inducing general anesthesia, predisposing them to multiple anesthetic complications; recovery of patients with colic that survive anesthesia and surgery can also be fraught with problems. Many individuals may be involved in a colic case, and the atmosphere can rapidly become loud and hectic if order is not maintained; furthermore, the anesthetist must work quickly because the time between the onset of intestinal ischemia and surgical correction is critical and must be minimized. These factors can create the potential for anesthetic errors to occur.

The ways in which veterinarians manage these sickest of equine anesthetic patients is, unfortunately, still largely empiric rather than evidence-based, because of a relative paucity of randomized, controlled, clinical trials and meta-analyses of these trials. This situation has arisen mostly because of the smaller number of clinical patients available to us and the expense involved in conducting such studies in our profession. However, exciting new information arises every year. This update on anesthesia for colic addresses how to provide the safest anesthesia and most effective analgesia for this high-risk surgical population, focusing on new developments in these areas.

PREANESTHETIC PREPARATION
Preparation of the Clinic

Preparation for these horses should begin before they ever enter the hospital. An induction station or room can be designated as an emergency area that can be used for patients with colic and, if possible, should be distinct from the area used for orthopedic cases to prevent contamination. This area can be set up ahead of time with everything needed for anesthetizing patients with colic, saving valuable time (**Fig. 1**). The anesthesia machine should undergo a complete checkout procedure daily before it is used for any cases, with certain steps repeated for each case. The Food and Drug Administration (FDA) developed a pre-use checkout procedure in 1986 that was modified in 1993.[1] However, some steps will not apply to all equine anesthesia machines.

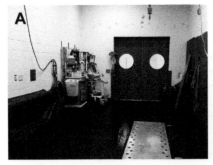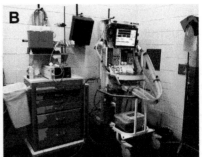

Fig. 1. (A) Induction room prepared ahead of time for a horse with colic. (B) Close-up view of the upper left-hand corner of (A) showing anesthesia machine/ventilator; roller cabinet with multiple labeled drawers for supplies and monitoring equipment (ie, electrocardiograph, arterial blood pressure transducer setup) on top; and fluid pole with intravenous fluids and bag of dobutamine attached.

Anamnesis

A thorough history should be taken for every patient with colic and should include but not be limited to:

- Duration of signs of colic
- Treatments administered for the current problem, including dose, route, frequency, the time all doses were given, and response
- Comorbidities (eg, laryngeal paralysis, hyperkalemic periodic paralysis [HYPP], recurrent airway obstruction [RAO], orthopedic disease), and any medications administered chronically for these. This part of the history is sometimes overlooked in the rush to work up and stabilize the horse, but is crucial because unknown problems can create unexpected anesthetic complications
- Any prior surgeries or problems under general anesthesia if this information is available

Physical Examination

A complete physical examination should be performed by the anesthetist, even if other clinicians have already performed their own examinations, with particular attention paid to certain aspects (**Box 1**).

Minimum Database

A blood sample should be collected before administering intravenous fluids. The minimum database required for general anesthesia is

- Complete blood count or, at a minimum, packed cell volume (PCV)
- Total protein (TP) or total solids (TS)

Box 1
Aspects of the preanesthetic physical examination of particular importance in the horse with colic

- Vital signs, including degree of pain
- Body condition score
- Mentation or level of sedation
- Degree of dehydration
- Mucous membrane color and capillary refill time
- Auscultation of the heart over all 4 heart valves, listening for heart murmurs and transient heart sounds
- Intensity of heart sounds
- Heart rhythm
- Peripheral pulse quality and synchronicity with heart beat
- Respiratory character
- Auscultation of the lungs over all fields
- Gut sounds
- Presence and severity of abdominal distension
- Rectal palpation
- Any obvious neurologic deficits or orthopedic problems

- Acid-base status, including lactate
- Creatinine
- Electrolytes (Na^+, K^+, Cl^-, and ionized Ca^{2+} [iCa^{2+}])
- Blood glucose (BG)

A point-of-care analyzer such as the VetScan i-STAT 1 Handheld Analyzer (Abaxis, Union City, CA) or the Stat Profile Critical Care Xpress (NOVA Biomedical, Waltham, MA) is useful for obtaining many of these values (**Fig. 2**).

An increased PCV from hemoconcentration is common with acute gastrointestinal disease that causes severe inflammation and dehydration. The TP may be increased from hemoconcentration, or decreased (eg, from loss through the ischemic gastrointestinal tract). Interpretation of PCV and TP together is important; for instance, if the PCV is increased but the TP is normal, fluid administration may unmask hypoproteinemia.

The clinician anesthetizing horses with colic should have at least a basic understanding of arterial blood gas and acid-base physiology, which is reviewed elsewhere.[2,3] A jugular venous sample can be used for preoperative assessment of acid-base status, but only an arterial blood sample can be used to evaluate oxygen exchange in the lungs (ie, arterial partial pressure of oxygen [Pao_2]); however, this is not yet routinely done during the preanesthetic workup. Normal values for horses have been published.[2] Venous blood pH will be slightly lower and partial pressure of carbon dioxide (Pco_2) and HCO_3^- concentration slightly higher than in arterial blood.[4] Horses with colic can suffer mild to severe disturbances of the respiratory or the metabolic (or nonrespiratory) component of the acid-base system, or both (ie, mixed disturbances). Little is known about respiratory or metabolic compensation for acid-base disorders in horses. For further discussion of acid-base abnormalities in horses with colic and their treatment, refer to the section on complications.

Electrolyte imbalances are also common. Causes and treatment of such imbalances are also discussed in the section on complications.

Coagulation panels are not yet routinely performed preoperatively, as they often are in septic small companion animals, but coagulopathies (eg, disseminated intravascular coagulation [DIC]) do occur in horses with colic (and are most severe in those

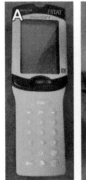
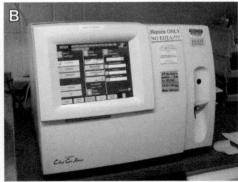

Fig. 2. (A) VetScan i-STAT 1 Handheld Analyzer, a portable point-of-care analyzer that can be used with a variety of cartridges to measure different analytes. (B) Stat Profile Critical Care Xpress, used at the University of Illinois Veterinary Teaching Hospital to analyze pH, blood gases, and acid-base status (including lactate), hematocrit, electrolytes, glucose, blood urea nitrogen, and creatinine. Both provide results in 2 minutes.

with massive intestinal ischemia/inflammation).[5,6] Diagnosis and treatment have been reviewed.[6] In the future, it is likely that thromboprophylaxis (eg, early administration of heparin in horses at risk for DIC) will receive more attention in these patients.

Other Diagnostic Tests

The anesthetist, if not the same person performing the colic workup, should be aware of the results of nasogastric tubing (also a therapeutic procedure to prevent gastric rupture), abdominal ultrasonography, and abdominocentesis/peritoneal fluid analysis. The author also recommends thoracic ultrasonography to check for diaphragmatic hernia, which can be an unexpected finding during exploratory laparotomy. It may be difficult to detect decreased lung sounds, and the absence of gut sounds in the thorax does not rule out the presence of diaphragmatic hernia. Horses with diaphragmatic hernias may have higher heart rates and a history of trauma.[7]

Stabilization

The patient with colic should be stabilized as much as possible before general anesthesia. Stabilization involves:

- Initiation of correction of fluid, acid-base, and electrolyte derangements
- Therapies to address endotoxemia (these were recently reviewed[8] and are not discussed in detail here)
- Analgesia (see later discussion)
- Decompression of the colon if gas distension is severe and is impairing cardiovascular function and ventilation. The author knows of one horse with massive abdominal distension that was not decompressed, which developed presumptive severe hypoxemia and ventricular tachycardia following induction, then arrested. The technique for percutaneous decompression of the colon has been described elsewhere.[2]

After blood is collected, a minimum of 1 large-gauge jugular catheter (10–14 gauge, depending on the horse's size and the rapidity with which intravenous fluids must be administered) is placed. The author prefers to have a catheter in each jugular vein before induction, and in severe cases has placed additional catheters in other vessels after induction to permit administration of large volumes of fluids and other drugs. Guidelines for fluid therapy are listed in **Box 2**.

Assessment of the degree of dehydration is subjective at best, but a table has been published that correlates physical and clinicopathologic findings with degree of dehydration.[2] Administering a fraction of the deficit (eg, one-quarter), then reevaluating the horse and repeating the process (rather than just administering the entire calculated deficit), can help to avoid overhydration; dilution of important substances such as erythrocytes, platelets, albumin, and coagulation factors; and tissue edema. What, precisely, should be evaluated? In humans and in small companion animals, the concept of early goal-directed therapy (EGDT) has gained attention.[10,11] EGDT, first introduced in human medicine in 2001 at which time it was shown to significantly reduce in-hospital mortality, is the stepwise administration of therapies aimed at achieving specific "resuscitation end points" to better match tissue oxygen delivery (D_{O_2}) to consumption as soon as sepsis is diagnosed.[10] In the original study, these end points include normalization of not only conventionally assessed "macrovascular" variables (eg, central venous pressure [CVP], mean arterial pressure [MAP], urine output) but also central venous oxygen saturation ($S_{CV}O_2$, the percentage of hemoglobin saturated with oxygen in blood sampled from a central vein, such as the jugular vein). The latter is one of multiple microvascular variables that are measured after blood

---

Box 2
General guidelines for designing a fluid therapy plan in horses with colic

1. Calculate and replace as much of the fluid deficit as possible before anesthesia.

Multiply the horse's weight in kilograms by the percentage of dehydration (eg, 500-kg horse, 12% dehydrated: 500 × 0.12 = 60 L fluid deficit). The type of fluid used to replace the deficit is controversial (see text). The appropriate rate of replacement is dependent on many factors. It is usually not possible to completely correct the deficit before general anesthesia; replacing it over 6 to 12 hours is a more reasonable goal. Slower rates are recommended in horses with suspected capillary leak secondary to endotoxemia while monitoring for tissue edema.

2. Add maintenance requirements each hour.

Maintenance fluid requirement for the horse has been estimated at 60 mL/kg/d (or 2.5 mL/kg/h), which is likely an overestimation in the healthy, resting horse.[2] A rate of 10 mL/kg/h (approximately 5 L/h in the average adult horse, or one 5-L bag run "wide open") of an isotonic crystalloid is arbitrarily used as "anesthetic maintenance rate" in the healthy horse undergoing general anesthesia. This rate is based on studies in humans undergoing major abdominal surgery, and is meant to replace insensible fluid losses (eg, from the respiratory tract and surgical site) and to counteract the negative hemodynamic effects of anesthesia.[9] The exact maintenance rate needed in healthy horses, let alone horses with colic, is difficult to define; however, this is the minimum rate the author uses once the fluid deficit has been replaced.

3. Account for ongoing losses each hour.

Fluid losses may occur in the horse with colic that do not occur in the healthy horse (eg, nasogastric reflux, emptying of colonic contents). It is possible that the maintenance fluid rate (see above) will cover these losses, but if losses are massive, higher rates may be required.

---

flows through capillary beds, and may better assess tissue oxygenation; others include pH, base excess (BE), and lactate. $S_{CV}O_2$ monitoring is not yet routine in horses with colic but likely will be in the future. Equine practitioners do rely on a combination of other macrovascular and microvascular variables such as mucous-membrane color, capillary refill time (CRT), vital signs (including MAP), PCV, TS, creatinine, pH, BE, and lactate. Bolusing fluids to achieve a normal CVP is the recommended first step in EGDT, and CVP monitoring to better guide fluid therapy, though also not yet routinely done, may be beneficial in these horses.[10]

There exists an ongoing controversy in human medicine regarding which fluid type (crystalloids vs colloids) should be used for resuscitation. Guidelines set forth by the Surviving Sepsis Campaign in 2008 do not recommend one type over another in humans.[12] Small (also known as limited) volume fluid resuscitation, a term first coined in 1984, was initially defined as resuscitation from hemorrhagic shock using hypertonic saline solution (HSS; usually 7.2%–7.5%) and later came to indicate resuscitation with both HSS and a colloid.[13,14] The rationale behind this technique is as follows. The high osmolality of HSS (>2400 mOsm/L, which is more than about 8 times that of plasma) draws extravascular fluid (including that which may have accumulated abnormally in endothelial cells secondary to inflammation) into the intravascular space to rapidly restore intravascular volume, not only increasing preload but also blood vessel lumen diameter, decreasing afterload and improving microcirculation.[13,15] HSS may also interfere with neutrophil-endothelial cell interactions in other species.[13] The rapidity with which HSS expands intravascular volume (within 20 minutes) is beneficial in horses requiring emergent anesthesia.[15] However, being a crystalloid, the HSS will eventually redistribute extravascularly, making its effects short-lived (60–120 minutes).[16] The addition of a colloid is intended to increase colloid oncotic pressure (COP) and to help prevent the HSS from redistributing out of the vasculature; this is in contrast to the larger volume of isotonic crystalloids alone that would be necessary to resuscitate a horse. Concern has been expressed that isotonic crystalloids alone may not have the same beneficial effects on the microcirculation and, because the majority of an isotonic crystalloid bolus redistributes out of the intravascular space shortly after administration, may result in tissue edema in patients with capillary leak secondary to endotoxemia. HSS and colloids have indeed been shown to be effective in resuscitating horses, but it is still unclear as to whether they are superior to isotonic crystalloids alone.[15,17] One early study using an equine hemorrhagic shock model compared administration of 2 L of HSS with 2 L of isotonic saline (a volume of isotonic saline considered to be totally inadequate for resuscitation), virtually guaranteeing that the cardiovascular status of the horses receiving HSS would be better.[15] More recently, a small study (ie, 6 horses/group) comparing resuscitation during experimental endotoxemia with a small volume of crystalloid (15 mL/kg), a large volume of crystalloid (60 mL/kg), and a combination of HSS (5 mL/kg) and hydroxyethyl starch (HES) (Hetastarch, 10 mL/kg) also did not demonstrate superiority of one treatment over another.[18] Peripheral edema was noted in 2 horses receiving the large volume of crystalloid.[18] A study comparing HSS and HES in client-owned horses undergoing surgery for colic found that patients receiving preoperative HES had a higher cardiac index (CI, or cardiac output [CO] indexed to body size) than those receiving preoperative HSS; however, the investigators admitted that baseline hemodynamic data could not be collected preoperatively for practical reasons and might have been significantly different between groups.[19] Furthermore, the study was not large enough to investigate effects on mortality.[19] It is likely that a combination of fluid types is appropriate for resuscitation of hypovolemic horses. The author rarely uses one fluid type alone but rather administers 2 to 4 mL/kg of HSS (1–2 L per average 450-kg horse) as rapidly as possible (before induction of general anesthesia if feasible) before or along with crystalloids, then adds colloids (HES and/or plasma) if TP and COP are low.

The type of isotonic crystalloid used is also important, and is discussed in the section on complications.

PREMEDICATION

There is still no one "correct" protocol for anesthesia of horses with colic. An α_2-agonist (eg, xylazine, detomidine) with or without an opioid is almost universally used for premedication. Some horses' pain is refractory to any analgesic drugs, and continuing to give boluses of α_2-agonists to these horses will only further depress cardiovascular function. The administration of opioids to horses, especially those with colic, is still highly controversial. Although it is known that opioids decrease GI motility, there are still either insufficient or conflicting data on the analgesic efficacy and clinical GI effects of opioids in horses with naturally occurring colic. The reader is referred to an excellent recent review on opioids in horses.[20] The author usually uses 1 to 2 low doses of either butorphanol (0.01–0.02 mg/kg intravenously) or a full μ-agonist (morphine or methadone, 0.1 mg/kg intravenously) perioperatively.

INDUCTION AND INTUBATION

Immediate induction of anesthesia may be necessary to prevent a severely painful horse from inflicting injury to itself and personnel. If enough assistance is available and the horse is showing evidence of severe cardiovascular compromise, fluids and/or dobutamine can be infused during the induction.

A benzodiazepine (midazolam or diazepam, 0.05–0.1 mg/kg) plus ketamine (2.2 mg/kg) can be administered intravenously to induce general anesthesia. Guaifenesin, a centrally acting muscle relaxant, has been used in lieu of a benzodiazepine; however, it has been shown to decrease arterial blood pressure, so the minimum amount necessary should be used, especially in severely cardiovascularly compromised horses.[21] Thiopental is no longer available in the United States but is still used for equine induction in other countries. Again, the minimum amount of thiopental necessary should be administered, as barbiturates cause dose-dependent cardiovascular depression.

Adequate preoxygenation is difficult in a horse with colic; however, nasal insufflation with 100% oxygen before induction can be performed and is the standard of practice in some hospitals. The trachea must be rapidly intubated with the largest cuffed endotracheal tube possible (usually 26 mm in the average 450-kg horse) immediately after the horse becomes recumbent. The cuff should be lightly coated with sterile water-based lubricant; this permits a better seal with the trachea at a lower cuff-inflation pressure. The next priority is to attach the breathing circuit to provide 100% oxygen. Only then should the endotracheal tube be secured in place and the cuff inflated. Once the airway is secured, the anesthetist should quickly palpate for the presence of a pulse (as horses with colic can arrest on induction) and obtain a general sense of rate and character. Intermittent positive-pressure ventilation (IPPV) is advised, and the author begins IPPV before hoisting the horse into dorsal recumbency, as many horses become apneic and severely hypoxemic on induction. Ventilation is discussed in more detail later.

MAINTENANCE
Monitoring

Every 5 minutes, the anesthetist should evaluate:

- Depth of anesthesia
- Mucous-membrane color/CRT
- Heart rate (HR)
- Ventilator settings (tidal volume [V_T], respiratory rate [RR], inspiratory to expiratory ratio [I:E], and peak inspiratory pressure [PIP])
- Electrocardiography
- Invasive (ie, via an arterial catheter) blood pressure (systolic/diastolic/mean)

Pulse oximetry and capnography can be used to monitor oxygenation and ventilation in between blood gas analyses, but the limitations of these monitoring devices should be understood. The pulse oximeter must detect a pulse to function and may not work if peripheral perfusion is abnormal (eg, vasoconstriction, venous congestion). Pulse oximetry may underestimate arterial hemoglobin saturation with oxygen (Sao_2) in horses with colic.[22] Although partial pressure of end-tidal carbon dioxide ($P_{ET}co_2$) can be much lower than the partial pressure of arterial carbon dioxide ($Paco_2$) (ie, wide $P_{a-ET}co_2$) in horses owing to ventilation/perfusion (V/Q) mismatching and alveolar dead space,[22] once the $P_{a-ET}co_2$ is known, if all else remains the same, changes in $Paco_2$ can be estimated from changes in $P_{ET}co_2$ and trends can be followed. Furthermore, the shape of the waveform provides abundant valuable information about everything from anesthesia-machine malfunction to endotracheal tube problems to the horse's upper and lower respiratory system. The Website www.capnography.com is an excellent exhaustive resource for those wishing to learn more about this monitoring device.

PCV/TS, blood gases/acid-base status (including lactate), and electrolyte and BG concentrations should be evaluated intermittently as well, with frequency dependent on the patient's condition. Reassessment as frequently as every 30 minutes may be necessary.

Preemptive Analgesia and Reduction in Inhalant Requirements

Constant rate infusions (CRIs) have long been used to provide preemptive analgesia and to decrease inhalant requirements in an effort to minimize cardiovascular depression, both of which are crucial in patients with colic. The reader is referred to the article on balanced anesthesia and CRIs written by Valverde and colleagues elsewhere in this issue for more information and doses.

Ketamine is well known for its ability to reduce inhalant requirements and stimulate the sympathetic nervous system.[23] The use of ketamine as an analgesic in horses was recently reviewed.[24] Best known as an N-methyl-D-aspartate receptor antagonist, ketamine has also been shown to have a myriad of other effects that may account for its analgesic properties.[24] Although it has been difficult to demonstrate its acute antinociceptive effects in conscious horses, ketamine does appear to have antihyperalgesic effects in this species that may be useful in patients with colic.[25–27] In humans, there is strong evidence in favor of ketamine's opioid-sparing effects in the first 24 hours after surgery.[28] The potential immunomodulatory effects of ketamine in septic patients have also gained attention. One study failed to demonstrate any clinical or immunologic benefit of administering a loading dose followed by a CRI to mares during endotoxin injection, but ketamine did inhibit tumor necrosis factor (TNF)-α and interleukin (IL)-6 in a dose-dependent fashion in an equine macrophage cell line.[29,30] More extensive research in other species has been promising. In rat models of endotoxemia, ketamine suppressed the endotoxin-induced increase in pulmonary and intestinal TNF-α and IL-6 production, nuclear factor κB activity, and toll-like receptor (TLR)2 and TLR4 expression; inhibited hypotension and metabolic acidosis dose-dependently; and decreased mortality.[31–33] In dogs, ketamine blunted the endotoxin-induced increase in plasma TNF-α.[34] More research on ketamine administration in endotoxemic horses, including at other doses, is clearly indicated.

A recent meta-analysis showed that perioperative intravenous lidocaine in humans reduced postoperative pain, opioid requirement, ileus recovery time, length of stay in hospital, and nausea/vomiting, with the greatest benefit seen in abdominal surgery patients.[35] Proposed mechanisms of action and potential therapeutic benefits of lidocaine in horses were recently reviewed.[36] Studies in anesthetized horses not undergoing surgical stimulation have shown that, despite its ability to reduce sevoflurane requirements in a dose-dependent fashion, the addition of a lidocaine CRI did not improve cardiovascular performance provided anesthetic depth was maintained constant.[37,38] However, the anesthetic-sparing effects of lidocaine were supported in a blinded study, which showed that horses that received a lidocaine CRI during exploratory laparotomy required significantly less isoflurane and needed significantly less dobutamine and phenylephrine to maintain normal MAP.[39] Somatic antinociception (assessed using a thermal stimulus) but, surprisingly, not visceral antinociception (assessed using duodenal and colorectal distension), was demonstrated in conscious horses in one study; however, the investigators pointed out that horses with normal, not inflamed, GI tracts were used and that an insufficient dose of lidocaine or study methodology may have been responsible for the failure to demonstrate antinociception.[40] Lidocaine is commonly used to treat postoperative ileus (POI), and several studies support its use in this way, including at least 2 prospective, blinded, placebo-controlled, randomized studies in clinical patients.[41–44] In one study comparing lidocaine with placebo in horses with a diagnosis of POI or enteritis, significantly more horses in the lidocaine group than in the placebo group stopped refluxing within

30 hours, and those horses that responded to lidocaine passed feces within 16 hours; lidocaine administration also resulted in shorter hospitalization time for survivors.[42] Finally, lidocaine appears to have anti-inflammatory effects. Studies have shown that in horses with ischemia-injured jejunum, lidocaine ameliorated the decrease in transepithelial resistance and increase in permeability to lipopolysaccharide (LPS) caused by flunixin, reduced prostaglandin E_2 metabolite concentration and mucosal cyclooxygenase-2 expression, and ameliorated the flunixin-induced increase in neutrophil counts.[45,46] Lidocaine also resulted in lower concentrations of peritoneal fluid TNF-α in comparison with saline after experimental intraperitoneal LPS injection.[47]

COMPLICATIONS
Hypotension

For a more exhaustive discussion of cardiovascular support, the reader is referred to the relevant article Schauvliege and colleagues elsewhere in this issue. Many horses with colic are hypotensive to some extent, and for at least some of the time under general anesthesia. It is generally accepted that MAP must be greater than 70 to 80 mm Hg under general anesthesia to adequately perfuse not only the vital organs but the large, heavy skeletal muscles, to decrease the risk of postanesthetic myoneuropathy. Treating hypotension effectively involves addressing decreases in HR, stroke volume (SV), and systemic vascular resistance (SVR) because of the role they play in arterial blood pressure, as depicted by the following equations.

Arterial blood pressure (ABP) = CO × SVR

CO = SV × HR

Bradycardia can be treated by:

- Decreasing the concentration of inhalant used if the horse is at too deep a plane of anesthesia
- Administering atropine (0.01–0.02 mg/kg) or glycopyrrolate (0.005–0.01 mg/kg) intravenously

Decreased SV can be due to decreased left ventricular preload and/or decreased myocardial contractility. The Frank-Starling law states that decreased cardiac preload caused by hypovolemia results in decreased affinity of cardiac myofilaments for Ca^{2+} and, thus, lesser force of contraction. IPPV worsens left ventricular preload and SV, especially in hypovolemic horses, by decreasing right ventricular preload and SV and increasing pulmonary vascular resistance (PVR); this may be manifested by dramatic cyclical variation in ABP during IPPV. IPPV may also decrease CO_2 too much, eliminating the stimulatory effects of CO_2 on the sympathetic nervous system, which increases myocardial contractility. Decreased myocardial contractility can also result from anesthetic drugs (eg, inhalants), electrolyte disorders (eg, hypocalcemia), and endotoxemia. Myocardial dysfunction is a well-known complication of sepsis in humans and is apparently multifactorial. Substances including cytokines (TNF-α, IL-1β, and IL-6), lysozyme C, and endothelin-1, overproduction of nitric oxide and superoxide, reductions in cytosolic calcium levels, and apoptosis have all been shown to play a role in myocardial dysfunction in septic humans and animals.[48] Decreased systolic function and even myocardial damage, as evidenced by increased cardiac troponin I, have been documented in horses with colic.[49,50] Myocardial contractility can be improved in the horse by:

- Optimizing preload
- Minimizing the concentration of inhalant used by assessing anesthetic depth frequently and using a balanced anesthetic technique
- Using positive inotropic drugs (eg, dobutamine, ephedrine, Ca^{2+})
- Administering therapies for endotoxemia

Dobutamine is the most commonly used inotropic drug because of its efficacy, titratability, and rapid onset of action. A synthetic catecholamine that acts primarily as a β_1-agonist, dobutamine increases CO and, thus, ABP, while its β_2-agonist effects are responsible for vasodilation and decreased SVR.[51,52] Both effects likely contribute to improvement in tissue perfusion. Improvement in skeletal muscle blood flow is well known, and improvement in splanchnic blood flow has been noted in other species and may also occur in the horse.[51–53] Rapid metabolism dictates its administration as a CRI. The higher the dose, the more likely is the occurrence of tachycardia.[51] An alternative drug must be used if the dose of dobutamine required to improve ABP causes tachycardia. Ephedrine is a synthetic noncatecholamine that acts as an α- and β-agonist and also induces release of norepinephrine presynaptially.[52] SV, CO, and ABP increase, and SVR decreases.[54,55] Because HR can also increase, ephedrine should be used cautiously in horses that are already tachycardic.[55] Calcium can be used as an inotropic drug and has been shown to attenuate the cardiovascular depression caused by isoflurane; it may be particularly effective if the horse is hypocalcemic.[56] The use of Ca^{2+} solutions is discussed later.

Horses with endotoxemia may suffer vasodilation and decreased SVR.[57] Isoflurane is also a vasodilator. Lack of improvement in ABP in response to the aforementioned interventions may indicate a need for vasopressors. Excessive vasoconstriction can decrease CO, so these drugs should be titrated carefully via CRI and while continuing administration of intravenous fluids and inotropic drugs. Norepinephrine is often recommended as a first-line vasopressor because although primarily an α-agonist it also has some β_1-agonist activity, which theoretically should partially offset the negative effects of the increased vasoconstriction on cardiac output (unless the dose is inappropriately high).[53] In healthy, normotensive, neonatal foals, norepinephrine and dobutamine increased ABP to a greater extent than norepinephrine alone; however, CI decreased.[58] In neonatal foals with isoflurane-induced hypotension, however, norepinephrine did increase CI.[59] In normal horses under halothane anesthesia, phenylephrine, a pure α-agonist, increased MAP by virtue of an increase in SVR; however, it decreased SV, CO, and femoral arterial blood flow and did not improve intramuscular blood flow.[51] Vasopressin is unique in that it causes vasoconstriction via interaction with V1a receptors and other mechanisms of action.[53] Horses with colic have been shown to already have increased circulating concentrations of vasopressin, calling into question the rationale of its use in horses with colic.[60] None of the vasopressors, however, have been studied in horses with endotoxemia-mediated vasodilation under general anesthesia, in which they may be beneficial if a dose is used that improves SVR without impairing cardiac output. The effects of various vasopressors on GI perfusion is being studied in humans but as yet has received little attention in horses.

Doses of drugs used to treat hypotension are listed in **Table 1**.

Hypoxemia and Hypoventilation

Hypoxemia and hypoventilation are common complications in horses with colic, especially those with severe abdominal distension. Even healthy horses are at risk for hypoxemia and hypoventilation under general anesthesia; horses with colic have reason to be at even greater risk (**Box 3**).

Table 1
Doses of some drugs used to treat hypotension in horses with colic

Drug	Dose
Dobutamine	0.5–5 μg/kg/min[61]
Ephedrine	0.05–0.2 mg/kg[54,55]
Ca^{2+}	5–10 mL/100 kg (10% $CaCl_2$)[61]
	20 mL/100 kg (10% Ca^{2+} gluconate)[61]
	2 mg/kg/h (approximately 50 mL of 23% Ca^{2+} borogluconate added to a 5 L of intravenous fluids and given to a 500-kg horse over 1 h)[62]
Norepinephrine	0.01–1 μg/kg/min[53,59]
Phenylephrine	0.25–2 μg/kg/min[51]
Vasopressin	0.25–1 mU/kg/min[53,59]

As previously stated, horses with severe colonic gas distension may be trocarized before induction to relieve abdominal pressure. If this is impossible while the horse is conscious, the horse should be induced, rapidly intubated, and given 100% oxygen, then decompressed. Some investigators advocate waiting until the horse's colon can be decompressed before beginning IPPV (or the abdomen can be surgically opened), and initial ABP can be measured to avoid the combined negative cardiovascular effects of increased intrathoracic and intra-abdominal pressure. However, if a horse is apneic, hemoglobin saturation decreases rapidly and IPPV will be necessary.[64] Airway pressures of greater than 60 mm Hg may be generated by a volume-targeted ventilator delivering a V_T of less than 10 mL/kg and may severely depress

Box 3
Causes of hypoventilation and hypoxemia in horses with colic anesthetized for exploratory laparotomy

Hypoventilation

- Decreased V_T due to decreased compliance of the thorax secondary to the cranial displacement of the diaphragm by a severely distended abdomen
- Decreased functional residual capacity due to cranial displacement of the diaphragm
- Respiratory muscle fatigue

Hypoxemia

- Hypoventilation (see above)
- Venous admixture caused by 1 or more of the following:
  - Diffusion impairment: Lung damage is a well-known complication of endotoxemia in humans and dogs and is an expanding area of research in horses.[63] Inflammation, including interstitial and/or alveolar edema, can increase the diffusion path for oxygen from the alveolus to the pulmonary capillary.
  - V:Q mismatch: Large numbers of alveoli with decreased V:Q ratios (V:Q<1) are an important cause of hypoxemia and can occur because of atelectasis or alveolar edema. Complete shunting of blood past totally unventilated alveoli is an extreme form of V:Q mismatch (V:Q = 0). Large numbers of alveoli with increased V:Q ratios (V:Q>1) contribute to alveolar dead space and are a result of poor perfusion of parts of the lungs; this may come about because of low pulmonary artery pressure, poor CO, or pulmonary thromboembolism in horses in DIC.

CO and/or damage alveoli; even at such high pressures, hypoxemia, which is generally regarded as a Pa_{O_2} <80 mm Hg, may be present. Delivering a low RR (eg, 2 breaths per minute) and minimizing the time until the colon can be decompressed can help reduce some of the side effects of high airway pressure. The clinician should attempt to strike a balance between ventilating to achieve a Pa_{O_2} of at least 60 mm Hg, which will correspond to approximately 90% saturated hemoglobin,[22] and maintaining MAP above 70 to 80 mm Hg.

A summary of techniques that may be beneficial in increasing Pa_{O_2} is listed in **Box 4**.

Note that increasing V_T, adding positive end-expiratory pressure (PEEP), using an inverse I:E, and performing an alveolar recruitment maneuver (ARM) can all significantly depress cardiovascular function, especially in the hypovolemic horse.

In 2011, Hopster and colleagues[67] compared 2 different ventilatory strategies in horses undergoing exploratory laparotomy in dorsal recumbency for acute colic: conventional IPPV without PEEP or an ARM (n = 12) versus IPPV with constant PEEP and an ARM (n = 12). In both groups, PIP was maintained between 35 and 45 cm H_2O, and the RR was adjusted to keep Pa_{CO_2} between 35 and 45 mm Hg. Arterial blood gas analysis was conducted every 20 minutes. Immediately after the first arterial blood gas measurement at 20 minutes postinduction in the treatment group, an ARM was performed if the Pa_{O_2} was less than 400 mm Hg. This maneuver consisted of increasing the PIP to 60 to 80 cm H_2O for 3 consecutive breaths and holding it there for 10 to 12 seconds. If a Pa_{O_2} of 400 mm Hg was not attained 20 minutes later, or if it decreased to less than 400 mm Hg on subsequent measurements, the ARM was repeated. PEEP was also increased between 10 and 12 to 15 cm H_2O if 5 ARMs failed. These investigators were able to demonstrate a 2- to 3-fold higher Pa_{O_2} in the treatment group; however, a median of 3 ARMs (and as many as 8 ARMs) were required, and in 2 horses (both suffering from severe abdominal distension) the target Pa_{O_2} was never reached. These results suggest that either the ARM was insufficient to open the lungs or the level of PEEP was insufficient to keep them open, or both. The treatment group had a significantly higher Pa_{O_2} at the first

---

Box 4
Treatments to address venous admixture and hypoxemia under general anesthesia

- Increase V_T (eg, decompress colon, surgically open abdomen, increase V_T on ventilator).

- Add PEEP (a ventilatory strategy whereby airway pressure is maintained above atmospheric pressure at the end of exhalation via mechanical impedance, usually a valve, within the breathing circuit to increase the volume of gas remaining in the lungs at end-expiration and thus prevent atelectasis and shunting of blood).

- Increase I:E or use inverse I:E (ie, 1:1 or higher); this is done so that inspiratory time equals or exceeds expiratory time, thus improving gas distribution in the lung and increasing mean airway pressure. RR should be set rapidly enough that the patient does not exhale completely before the next breath, resulting in some gas remaining in the lung at end-expiration.

- Perform alveolar recruiting maneuver (a sustained increase in PIP, eg, 40 cm H_2O for 40 seconds, to open collapsed lung units, which is usually followed by PEEP to keep them open).

- Administer aerosolized albuterol (2 μg/kg) via endotracheal tube.[65]

- Increase ABP to improve lung perfusion (eg, intravenous fluids, inotropic drugs).

- Position horse in sternal recumbency in recovery.[66]

measurement of arterial blood gas, suggesting that a low level of PEEP (10 cm H_2O) applied from the very beginning of anesthesia is beneficial. This finding was encouraging, given that past studies have demonstrated that higher PEEP (20–30 cm H_2O) was needed to improve oxygenation and caused CO to decrease.[68] Surprisingly, the effects of the ARM on MAP in this study were mild and transient, although CO was not measured and thus Do_2 could not be calculated. There were no statistically significant differences in MAP or amount of fluids or dobutamine administered between the groups. The author has empirically found low PEEP (10 cm H_2O) to be beneficial (even if not started on induction and used with an ARM) in some horses, and will at least attempt it as a means of improving Pao_2 if MAP can be supported with fluids and inotropes.

Variables such as pH, BE, and lactate can be monitored to estimate whether hypoxemia is contributing to anaerobic metabolism.

Hypoproteinemia and Decreased COP

The COP (which is mainly determined by proteins such as albumin) of healthy horses and horses with colic that are administered isotonic crystalloids decreases under general anesthesia.[69,70] COP in mm Hg in unanesthetized healthy horses is typically somewhere in the low 20s but may be lower in horses with colic even before anesthesia, possibly owing to causes such as protein loss into the diseased GI tract lumen.[69–71] TP concentration lower than 3.5 to 4 g/dL and subsequently, decreased COP, may result in tissue edema. Synthetic colloids such as 6% HES (Hetastarch), which has a higher COP than plasma (29–32 mm Hg), do not replace plasma protein but are administered to increase COP.[69] HES has been shown to increase COP in unanesthetized healthy ponies and hypoproteinemic horses.[72,73] Wendt-Hornickle and colleagues[69] compared the trend in COP in two groups of healthy anesthetized horses both receiving the same rate of isotonic crystalloid administration; one group also received an infusion of 2.5 mL/kg of HES administered over an hour. The HES failed to attenuate the decrease in COP seen during anesthesia, but the investigators pointed out that the dose of HES used was lower than that in other studies demonstrating increased COP and may have been insufficient.[69] The maximum daily dose of HES is typically 10 to 20 mL/kg/d. It can be bolused rapidly before or during general anesthesia, using pressure bags if needed. The increased COP persists for up to 24 hours in the horse.[73] Coagulation abnormalities (ie, a trend toward significantly increased cutaneous bleeding time associated with marked reduction in activity of von Willebrand factor antigen) have been seen in ponies at the 20 mL/kg dose.[72]

Plasma, a natural colloid, is sometimes included in the treatment regime for endotoxemia and is also administered to address coagulopathies. However, the COP is not as high as that of HES. Furthermore, large volumes are often needed to increase TP, adding considerably to treatment expense.

Acid-Base and Electrolyte Abnormalities

Acid-base and electrolyte abnormalities are common in horses with colic. Simple acid-base disturbances and their causes and treatments specific to horses with colic are listed in **Table 2**.

Mixed metabolic (ie, metabolic acidosis and metabolic alkalosis) or metabolic-respiratory (ie, metabolic acidosis or alkalosis and respiratory acidosis or alkalosis) disorders exist and can have additive or neutralizing effects on pH. Even triple disorders exist (ie, mixed metabolic disorder with a respiratory disorder).

If metabolic acidemia remains severe (pH <7.2) despite adequate fluid resuscitation, sodium bicarbonate ($NaHCO_3$) supplementation is indicated. The guidelines for

Table 2
Simple acid-base disturbances and their causes in horses with colic

Disturbance	Cause	Treatment
Metabolic acidosis	Dehydration, decreased tissue perfusion, and inadequate tissue Do_2, with subsequent anaerobic metabolism and lactate production	Correct underlying cause, administer intravenous balanced electrolyte solutions (eg, LRS, Plasmalyte A, Normosol-R), supplement oxygen, provide inotropic support
Metabolic alkalosis	Loss of H^+ and Cl^- with high-volume nasogastric reflux Loss of Cl^- in sweat	Correct underlying cause, administer 0.9% NaCl (HS along with a balanced electrolyte solution can be effective in lieu of 0.9% saline)
Respiratory acidosis	Alveolar hypoventilation Colonic distension Diaphragmatic hernia Respiratory muscle fatigue	Correct underlying cause, decompress colon, administer IPPV
Respiratory alkalosis	Alveolar hyperventilation Hypoxemia Pain or fear	Correct underlying cause, supplement oxygen, provide analgesia/sedation

Abbreviations: HS, hypertonic saline; IPPV, intermittent positive-pressure ventilation; LRS, lactated Ringer solution.

$NaHCO_3$ supplementation are listed in **Box 5**. $NaHCO_3$ must be administered cautiously because Pco_2 increases in blood and cerebrospinal fluid (CSF) following its administration; plasma HCO_3^- enters CSF slowly, and a paradoxic CSF acidosis may result. Horses must be ventilated to eliminate the excess CO_2 produced. An overdose can cause hyperosmolarity, as this solution is hypertonic (1500 mOsm/L); hypernatremia and hypokalemia may also result, but in the author's experience are not severe if the correct dose is calculated and administered slowly.

Electrolyte disturbances and their causes specific to horses with colic are listed in **Box 6**.

Disturbances of Na^+ and Cl^- are usually corrected by administering the appropriate type of intravenous crystalloid. The rate of supplemental KCl administration should always be calculated to ensure it does not exceed 0.5 mEq/kg/h. Doses of Ca^{2+} solutions for treatment of ionized hypocalcemia are listed in **Table 1**.

Hypoglycemia and Hyperglycemia

Dysglycemia is common in horses with acute abdominal disease.[74] The production of inflammatory cytokines in endotoxemia promotes hyperglycemia; pain and anxiety

Box 5
Guidelines for administering $NaHCO_3$

$NaHCO_3$ (mEq) = 0.3 × body weight (kg) × base deficit

This equation assumes that normal base deficit in the horse is 0. In reality, the base deficit in horses is slightly positive.[4]

eg, 500-kg horse, base deficit = −12

0.3 × 500 × 12 = 1800 mEq × 1 mEq/ml = 1800 mL

Give half of the calculated dose over 20 to 30 minutes, then reassess acid-base status before administering the second half, as overcorrection will cause metabolic alkalosis.

Box 6
Some electrolyte disturbances and possible causes in horses with colic

Sodium

- Hypernatremia
  - In the hypovolemic horse, implies hypotonic fluid loss
  - Overzealous hypertonic saline or $NaHCO_3$ administration
- Hyponatremia
  - In the hypovolemic horse, implies hypertonic fluid loss

Chloride

- Hyperchloremia
  - Hypotonic fluid loss (if increases in proportion to Na^+ concentration)
  - Excessive gain of Cl^- relative to Na^+ (eg, excessive administration of 0.9% NaCl, HSS, KCl-supplemented fluids)
- Hypochloremia
  - Hypertonic fluid loss (if decreases in proportion to Na^+ concentration)
  - Excessive loss of Cl^- relative to Na^+ (eg, nasogastric reflux)

Potassium

- Hyperkalemia
  - Uncommon but may be seen in horses suffering from severe muscle damage or in horses with HYPP
- Hypokalemia
  - Administration of large volumes of K^+-deficient fluids
  - Translocation into cells (eg, alkalemia, catecholamines, hyperglycemia)
  - Gastrointestinal losses

Ionized Calcium

- Ionized hypocalcemia
  - Administration of large volumes of Ca^{2+}-deficient fluids or $NaHCO_3$
  - Transfusion of blood products containing citrated anticoagulant
  - Endotoxemia

---

cause release of catecholamines, cortisol, and glucagon, leading to insulin resistance, glycogenolysis, and gluconeogenesis.[75] The α_2-agonists also cause hyperglycemia by interfering with insulin release from the pancreas. Hypoglycemia can result from decreased intake of food, decreased hepatic function, and increased glucose consumption induced by inflammatory mediators or anaerobic glycolysis, and severe hypoglycemia leads to neuronal cell death.[76,77]

In adult humans, there is no consensus on the definition of hypoglycemia and when dextrose should be supplemented in septic patients. Hyperglycemia may increase morbidity and mortality in critically ill humans, and intravenous insulin therapy adjusted to maintain BG concentration within narrow limits is currently the subject of intense research.[12] Hypoglycemia and hyperglycemia have been associated with decreased survival in critically ill foals, whereas hyperglycemia has been associated with decreased survival in adult horses with acute abdominal disease.[74,78] There are no strict guidelines on the range within which BG should be kept in horses, nor do recommendations regarding insulin therapy for hyperglycemia in patients with colic exist. The author attempts to maintain BG concentration above 70 mg/dL (the lower limit of normal at the University of Illinois Veterinary Teaching Hospital) while avoiding iatrogenic hyperglycemia (>130 mg/dL) by oversupplementation of dextrose or unnecessary boluses of α_2-agonists.

Clinical signs of hypoglycemia may not be apparent in the anesthetized horse. A bolus of 0.1 to 0.5 g/kg of 50% dextrose/kg diluted 1:2 to 1:4 can be given over 5 minutes for severe hypoglycemia. A 2.5% to 5% dextrose solution can be made by adding the appropriate amount of 50% dextrose to isotonic crystalloids.

Arrhythmias (Dysrhythmias)

The heart rhythm can often be improved or normalized by correcting underlying abnormalities. Sinus tachycardia is probably the most common arrhythmia in horses with colic, and treatment involves correcting the underlying problem(s) (eg, hypovolemia, endotoxemia, pain, hypercapnia, hypoxemia, anemia). Atrial fibrillation can occur, but if it does not abate on correction of systemic abnormalities it is often treated with "benign neglect" because the ventricular rate is rarely rapid enough to impair ABP and tissue perfusion. Ventricular premature contractions (VPCs) and ventricular tachycardia can result from sympathomimetic drugs, myocardial ischemia (due to hypovolemia or hypoxemia), inflammatory mediators released because of endotoxemia, acid-base disturbances, and electrolyte disturbances (eg, hypokalemia, hypomagnesemia). If VPCs are frequent or polymorphic (ie, 2 or more different abnormal QRS-T configurations can be identified), if the HR is fast enough that diastolic filling time and CO seem to be suffering (eg, pale mucous membranes, prolonged CRT, hypotension), or if the R-on-T phenomenon (the VPC overlaps the T wave of the previous P-QRS-T complex) occurs, lidocaine should be administered. An intravenous dose of 0.25 to 0.5 mg/kg is given slowly and can be repeated in 5 to 10 minutes. The total dose given as a bolus should not exceed 1.5 to 2 mg/kg, as overdose can produce cardiovascular and neurologic side effects. If the anesthetist finds that boluses are required frequently, a CRI at 0.05 mg/kg/min can be started. Ventricular tachycardia and fibrillation are often terminal rhythms. Atropine (0.01–0.02 mg/kg intravenously) or glycopyrrolate (0.005 mg/kg intravenously) are used to treat bradyarrhythmias such as sinus bradycardia, high-grade second-degree atrioventricular (AV) block (more than 2 consecutive nonconducted P waves), or third-degree AV block, but these are uncommon in these patients.

RECOVERY

The recovery stall should be clean and dry. Horses should be turned from dorsal to lateral recumbency very slowly while monitoring peripheral pulses because horses, especially if hypovolemic, can suffer cardiac arrest on turning. In general, patients with colic require intensive care during recovery, with the intensity of monitoring and supportive care dependent on how ill the horse is. These horses should never be left unattended or unmonitored; they usually take longer than healthy horses to begin to move (although signs of arousal from anesthesia should be present), and during this time hemodynamic, blood gas, acid-base, and electrolyte derangements can develop or worsen. Horses that were severely hypoxemic during surgery should be positive-pressure ventilated with 100% oxygen during transport to the recovery stall and in the recovery stall until they begin ventilating spontaneously. Positioning horses in sternal recumbency, if possible, has been shown to improve oxygenation.[66] When they begin to ventilate spontaneously, they can inspire 100% oxygen using a demand valve. When the horse can swallow, it can be extubated. Following extubation, a nasal cannula can be passed into the pharynx or trachea to insufflate 100% oxygen at 5 to 15 L/min; the catheter can be withdrawn when the horse tries to stand. A pulse oximeter can be used to monitor the efficacy of O_2 supplementation in between sampling of arterial blood for blood gas analysis. Fluid administration with supplemental K^+ and/or Ca^{2+} can be continued if needed until the horse tries to stand. Blood pressure can be monitored noninvasively or even invasively if necessary and supported using fluid therapy, inotropes, and/or vasopressors as the case dictates, until the horse begins to move. Horses should have their rectal temperature monitored. Horses are usually hypothermic after anesthesia and should be dried off if wet, then covered with blankets; forced warm air (eg, from a Bair hugger) can then be pumped under the blankets. The nasal mucosa can be decongested using 0.15% phenylephrine.

No more than light sedation, if any, is usually necessary because these horses are commonly so exhausted that they usually sleep until the majority of inhalant has been exhaled, although exceptions occur. Judicious doses of α_2-agonists can be given for sedation in the uncommon cases of premature attempts to rise and will provide analgesia. The author usually does not administer acepromazine to patients with colic recovering from surgery because of its lack of analgesic benefits, relatively long duration of action, lack of commercially available antagonist, and potential to increase the time it takes for the horse to rouse. Acepromazine can also cause hypotension by virtue of its α_1-agonist effects.

Postoperative analgesia is of paramount importance in critically ill patients. Nonsteroidal anti-inflammatory drugs (eg, flunixin) are commonly given. One blinded study showed that horses treated with a butorphanol CRI (13 µg/kg/h) after exploratory laparotomy had lower plasma cortisol concentrations, lost less weight during hospitalization, appeared less painful as judged by a pain-scoring system, and were discharged from the hospital earlier; time to first passage of manure, however, was delayed.[79] Peripheral opioid antagonists such as methylnaltrexone may be used in the future in horses with colic to reverse the decreased GI motility caused by opioids while retaining the analgesic effects. Other options for analgesia include CRIs of lidocaine, ketamine, or α_2-agonists. The α_2-agonists do decrease GI motility and should be used judiciously in these patients.

Attempts to stand can be weak and uncoordinated. The author has seen some horses stand on their first attempt completely unassisted; however, it is recommended that assistance be provided if a horse is geriatric, has concurrent orthopedic disease (eg, osteoarthritis), was showing signs of colic for a long time before surgery, or is critically ill and therefore, weak. Horses that do not stand within 2 to 4 hours after surgery should be reassessed and encouraged to stand, but in severe cases can be bedded down in the recovery stall and have postoperative care administered there for a period of time.

REFERENCES

1. Dorsch JA, Dorsch SE. The anesthesia machine. In: Understanding anesthesia equipment. 5th edition. Philadelphia: Lippincott Williams & Wilkins; 2008. p. 83–120.
2. Hardy J. Critical care. In: Reed SM, Bayley WM, Sellon DC, editors. Equine internal medicine. 3rd edition. St Louis (MO): Saunders Elsevier; 2010. p. 246–79.
3. Hubbell JA, Muir WW. Monitoring anesthesia. In: Muir WW, Hubbell JA, editors. Equine anesthesia: monitoring and emergency therapy. 2nd edition. St Louis (MO): Saunders Elsevier; 2009. p. 149–70.

4. Estepa C, Hernandez M, Garfia B, et al. Comparative study of the acid-base state of arterial and venous blood of healthy horses. Med Vet 2000;17:222–8.
5. Dallap BL, Dolente B, Boston R. Coagulation profiles in 27 horses with large colon volvulus. J Vet Emerg Crit Care 2003;13:215–25.
6. Monreal L, Cesarini C. Coagulopathies in horses with colic. Vet Clin North Am Equine Pract 2009;25:247–58.
7. Ludders JW, Gleed RD, Campoy L, et al. Indicators of diaphragmatic hernia in horses presenting with colic: a retrospective matched, case-control study. In: Proceedings of the 14th International Veterinary Emergency and Critical Care Symposium. Phoenix (AZ): 2008. p. 853.
8. Kelmer G. Update on treatments for endotoxemia. Vet Clin North Am Equine Pract 2009;25:259–70.
9. Pascoe PJ. Perioperative management of fluid therapy. In: Dibartola SP, editor. Fluid therapy in small animal practice. 2nd edition. Philadelphia: W.B. Saunders; 2000. p. 307–29.
10. Rivers E, Nguyen B, Haystad S, et al. Early goal-directed therapy in the treatment of severe sepsis and septic shock. N Engl J Med 2001;345:1368–77.
11. Butler AL. Goal-directed therapy in small animal critical illness. Vet Clin North Am Small Anim Pract 2011;41:817–38.
12. Dellinger RP, Levy MM, Carlet JM, et al. Surviving sepsis campaign: international guidelines for management of severe sepsis and septic shock: 2008. Crit Care Med 2008;36:296–327.
13. Kreimeier U, Messmer K. Small-volume resuscitation: from experimental evidence to clinical routine. Advantages and disadvantages of hypertonic solutions. Acta Anaesthesiol Scand 2002;46:625–38.
14. Nakayama S, Sibley L, Gunther RA, et al. Small-volume resuscitation with hypertonic saline (2,400 mosm/liter) during hemorrhagic shock. Circ Shock 1984;13:149–59.
15. Schmall LM, Muir WW, Robertson JT. Haemodynamic effects of small volume hypertonic saline in experimentally induced haemorrhagic shock. Equine Vet J 1990;22:273–7.
16. Arden WA, Reisdorff E, Loeffler BS, et al. Effect of hypertonic saline on cardiopulmonary function on endotoxemic anesthetized ponies. Vet Surg 1991;20:329.
17. Arden WA, Reisdorff E, Loeffler BS, et al. Effect of hypertonic-hyperoncotic fluid resuscitation on cardiopulmonary function during colon torsion shock in ponies. Vet Surg 1991;20:329.
18. Pantaleon LG, Furr MO, McKenzie HC, et al. Cardiovascular and pulmonary effects of Hetastarch plus hypertonic saline solutions during experimental endotoxemia in anesthetized horses. J Vet Intern Med 2011;20:1422–8.
19. Hallowell GD, Corley KT. Preoperative administration of hydroxyethyl starch or hypertonic saline to horses with colic. J Vet Intern Med 2006;20:980–6.
20. Clutton RE. Opioid analgesia in horses. Vet Clin North Am Equine Pract 2010;26:493–514.
21. Hubbell JAE, Muir WW, Sams RA. Guaifenesin: cardiopulmonary effects and plasma concentrations in horses. Am J Vet Res 1980;41:1751–5.
22. Koenig J, McDonell W, Valverde A. Accuracy of pulse oximetry and capnography in healthy and compromised horses during spontaneous and controlled ventilation. Can J Vet Res 2003;67:169–74.
23. Muir WW, Sams R. Effects of ketamine infusion on halothane minimal alveolar concentration in horses. Am J Vet Res 1992;53:1802–6.
24. Muir WW. NMDA receptor antagonists and pain: ketamine. Vet Clin North Am Equine Pract 2010;26:565–78.

25. Fielding CL, Brumbaugh GW, Matthews NS. Pharmacokinetics and clinical effects of a subanesthetic continuous rate infusion of ketamine in awake horses. Am J Vet Res 2006;67:1484–90.

26. Peterbauer C, Larenza PM, Knobloch M. Effects of a low dose infusion of racemic and S-ketamine on the nociceptive withdrawal reflex in standing ponies. Vet Anaesth Analg 2008;35:414–23.

27. Redua MA, Valadao CA, Duque JC, et al. The preemptive effect of epidural ketamine on wound sensitivity tested by using von Frey filaments. Vet Anaesth Analg 2002;29:200–6.

28. Bell RF, Dahl JB, Moore RA, et al. Perioperative ketamine for acute postoperative pain. Cochrane Database Syst Rev 2006;(1):CD004603.

29. Alcott CJ, Sponseller BA, Wong DM, et al. Clinical and immunomodulating effects of ketamine in horses with experimental endotoxemia. J Vet Intern Med 2011;25:934–43.

30. Lankveld DP, Bull S, van Dijk P, et al. Ketamine inhibits LPS-induced tumour necrosis factor-alpha and interleukin-6 in an equine macrophage cell line. Vet Res 2005;36:257–62.

31. Yu M, Shao D, Liu J, et al. Effects of ketamine on levels of cytokines, NF-kappaB and TLRs in rat intestine during CLP-induced sepsis. Int Immunopharmacol 2007;7:1076–82.

32. Yu M, Shao D, Yang R, et al. Effects of ketamine on pulmonary inflammatory responses and survival in rats exposed to polymicrobial sepsis. J Pharm Pharm Sci 2007;10:434–42.

33. Taniguchi T, Takemoto Y, Kanakura H, et al. The dose-related effects of ketamine on mortality and cytokine responses to endotoxin-induced shock in rats. Anesth Analg 2003;97:1769–72.

34. DeClue AE, Cohn LA, Lechner ES, et al. Effects of subanesthetic doses of ketamine on hemodynamic and immunologic variables in dogs with experimentally induced endotoxemia. Am J Vet Res 2008;69:228–32.

35. Vigneault L, Turgeon AF, Côté D, et al. Perioperative intravenous lidocaine infusion for postoperative pain control: a meta-analysis of randomized controlled trials. Can J Anaesth 2011;58:22–37.

36. Doherty TJ, Seddighi MR. Local anesthetics as pain therapy in horses. Vet Clin North Am Equine Pract 2010;26:533–49.

37. Rezende ML, Wagner AE, Mama KR, et al. Effect of intravenous administration of lidocaine on the minimum alveolar concentration of sevoflurane in horses. Am J Vet Res 2011;72:446–51.

38. Wagner AE, Mama KR, Steffey EP, et al. Comparison of the cardiovascular effects of equipotent anesthetic doses of sevoflurane alone and sevoflurane plus an intravenous infusion of lidocaine in horses. Am J Vet Res 2011;72:452–60.

39. Bubb L, Driessen B, Staffieri F, et al. The isoflurane-sparing effect of intravenous lidocaine administered to horses undergoing exploratory celiotomy [abstract]. In: 14th International Veterinary Emergency & Critical Care—Annual Symposium of the American College of Veterinary Anesthesiologists. Phoenix (AZ): 2008. p. 853–4.

40. Robertson SA, Sanchez LC, Merritt AM, et al. Effect of systemic lidocaine on visceral and somatic nociception in conscious horses. Equine Vet J 2005;37:122–7.

41. Brianceau P, Chevalier H, Karas A, et al. Intravenous lidocaine and small-intestinal size, abdominal fluid, and outcome after colic surgery in horses. J Vet Intern Med 2002;16:736–41.

42. Malone E, Ensink J, Turner T, et al. Intravenous continuous infusion of lidocaine for treatment of equine ileus. Vet Surg 2006;35:60–6.

43. Torfs S, Delesalle C, Dewulf J, et al. Risk factors for equine postoperative ileus and effectiveness of prophylactic lidocaine. J Vet Intern Med 2009;23:606–11.

44. Guschlbauer M, Hoppe S, Geburek F, et al. In vitro effects of lidocaine on the contractility of equine jejuna smooth muscle challenged by ischaemia-reperfusion injury. Equine Vet J 2010;42:53–8.

45. Cook VL, Jones Shultz J, McDowell M, et al. Attenuation of ischaemic injury in the equine jejunum by administration of systemic lidocaine. Equine Vet J 2008;40:353–7.

46. Cook VL, Neuder LE, Blikslager AT, et al. The effect of lidocaine on in vitro adhesion and migration of equine neutrophils. Vet Immunol Immunopathol 2009;129:137–42.

47. Peiro JR, Barnabe PA, Cadioli FA, et al. Effects of lidocaine infusion during experimental endotoxemia in horses. J Vet Intern Med 2010;24:940–8.

48. Zanotti-Cavazzoni SL, Hollenburg SM. Cardiac dysfunction in severe sepsis and septic shock. Curr Opin Crit Care 2009;15:392–7.

49. Borde L, Amory H, Leroux AA, et al. Echocardiographic assessment of left ventricular systolic function in colic horses. J Equine Vet Sci 2011;31:481–7.

50. Radcliffe RM, Divers TJ, Fletcher DJ, et al. Evaluation of L-lactate and cardiac troponin I in horses undergoing emergency abdominal surgery. J Vet Emerg Crit Care 2012;22:313–9.

51. Lee YH, Clarke KW, Alibhai HI, et al. Effects of dopamine, dobutamine, dopexamine, phenylephrine, and saline solution on intramuscular blood flow and other cardiopulmonary variables in halothane-anesthetized ponies. Am J Vet Res 1998;59:1463–72.

52. Raisis AL. Skeletal muscle blood flow in anaesthetized horses. Part II: effects of anaesthetics and vasoactive agents. Vet Anaesth Analg 2005;32:331–7.

53. Corley KT. Inotropes and vasopressors in adults and foals. Vet Clin North Am Equine Pract 2004;20:77–106.

54. Grandy JL, Hodgson DS, Dunlop CI, et al. Cardiopulmonary effects of ephedrine in halothane-anesthetized horses. J Vet Pharmacol Ther 1989;12:389–96.

55. Lee YH, Clarke KW, Alibhai HI, et al. The effects of ephedrine on intramuscular blood flow and other cardiopulmonary parameters on cardiopulmonary parameters in halothane-anesthetized ponies. Vet Anaesth Analg 2002;29:171–81.

56. Grubb TL, Benson GJ, Foreman JH, et al. Hemodynamic effects of ionized calcium in horses anesthetized with halothane or isoflurane. Am J Vet Res 1999;60:1430–5.

57. Trim CM, Moore JN, Hardee MM, et al. Effects of an infusion of dopamine on the cardiopulmonary effects of *Escherichia coli* endotoxin in anesthetized horses. Res Vet Sci 1991;50:54–63.

58. Hollis AR, Ousey JC, Palmer L, et al. Effects of norepinephrine and a combined norepinephrine and dobutamine infusion on systemic hemodynamics and indices of renal function in normotensive neonatal Thoroughbred foals. J Vet Intern Med 2006;20:1437–42.

59. Valverde A, Giguere S, Sanchez LC, et al. Effects of dobutamine, norepinephrine, and vasopressin on cardiovascular function in anesthetized neonatal foals with induced hypotension. Am J Vet Res 2006;67:1730–7.

60. Ludders JW, Palos HM, Erb HN, et al. Plasma arginine vasopressin concentration in horses undergoing surgery for colic. J Vet Emerg Crit Care 2009;19:528–35.

61. Hubbell JA, Muir WW. Anesthetic-associated complications. In: Muir WW, Hubbell JA, editors. Equine anesthesia: monitoring and emergency therapy. 2nd edition. St Louis (MO): Saunders Elsevier; 2009. p. 397–417.

62. Hardy J. Monitoring anesthesia. In: Muir WW, Hubbell JA, editors. Equine anesthesia: monitoring and emergency therapy. 2nd edition. St Louis (MO): Saunders Elsevier; 2009. p. 149–70.
63. Aharonso-Raz K, Singh B. Pulmonary intravascular macrophages and endotoxin-induced pulmonary pathophysiology in horses. Can J Vet Res 2010;74:45–9.
64. Blaze CA, Robinson NE. Apneic oxygenation in anesthetized ponies and horses. Vet Res Commun 1987;11:281–91.
65. Robertson SA, Bailey JE. Aerosolized salbutamol (albuterol) improves PaO_2 in hypoxaemic anaesthetized horses—a prospective clinical trial in 81 horses. Vet Anaesth Analg 2002;29:212–8.
66. Gleed RD, Dobson A. Improvement in arterial oxygen tension with change in posture in anaesthetized horses. Res Vet Sci 1988;44:255–9.
67. Hopster K, Kastner SBR, Rohn K, et al. Intermittent positive pressure ventilation with constant positive end-expiratory pressure and alveolar recruitment maneuver during inhalation anaesthesia in horses undergoing for colic, and its influence on the early recovery period. Vet Anaesth Analg 2011;38:169–77.
68. Wilson DV, Soma LR. Cardiopulmonary effects of positive end-expiratory pressure in anesthetized, mechanically ventilated ponies.
69. Wendt-Hornickle EL, Snyder LB, Tang R, et al. The effects of lactated Ringer's solution (LRS) or LRS and 6% Hetastarch on the colloid osmotic pressure, total protein and osmolality in healthy horses under general anesthesia. Vet Anaesth Analg 2011;38:336–43.
70. Boscan P, Steffey EP. Plasma colloid osmotic pressure and total protein in horses during colic surgery. Vet Anaesth Analg 2007;34:408–15.
71. Boscan P, Steffey EP. Plasma colloid osmotic pressure and total protein trends in horses during anesthesia. Vet Anaesth Analg 2007;34:275–83.
72. Jones PA, Tomasic M, Gentry PA. Oncotic, hemodilutional, and hemostatic effects of isotonic saline and hydroxyethyl starch solutions in clinically normal ponies. Am J Vet Res 1997;58:541–8.
73. Jones PA, Bain FT, Byars TD, et al. Effects of hydroxyethyl starch infusion on colloid oncotic pressure in hypoproteinemic horses. J Am Vet Med Assoc 2001;218:1130–5.
74. Hollis AR, Boston RC, Corley KT. Blood glucose in horses with acute abdominal disease. J Vet Intern Med 2007;21:1099–103.
75. Thompson BT. Glucose control in sepsis. Clin Chest Med 2008;29:713–20.
76. Koenig A. Hypoglycemia. In: Silverstein DC, Hopper K, editors. Small animal critical care medicine. St Louis (MO): Saunders Elsevier; 2009. p. 295–9.
77. Suh SW, Hamby AM, Swanson RA. Hypoglycemia, brain energetics, and hypoglycemic neuronal death. Glia 2007;55:1280–6.
78. Hollis AR, Furr MO, Magdesian KG, et al. Blood glucose concentrations in critically ill neonatal foals. J Vet Intern Med 2008;22:1223–7.
79. Sellon DC, Roberts MC, Blikslager AT, et al. Effects of continuous rate intravenous infusion of butorphanol on physiologic and outcome variables in horses after celiotomy. J Vet Intern Med 2004;18:555–63.

Anesthesia for Dystocia and Anesthesia of the Equine Neonate

Lori A. Bidwell, DVM

KEYWORDS

- Anesthesia • Equine • Neonate • Dystocia • Horse • Pregnancy • Parturition

KEY POINTS

- Anesthetic techniques for dystocia should allow fast induction of the mare with minimal cardiovascular and respiratory depressant effects on the mare and neonate.
- The combination of xylazine as premedication followed by ketamine with diazepam for induction results in fast and safe induction for dystocia.
- An infusion of 100–300 mL 5% guaifenesin or the combination of 50 g guaifenesin, 1 g ketamine, and 500 mg xylazine improves relaxation in the mare immediately after induction for dystocia.
- Anesthesia of the neonate is complicated by an immature metabolic function and increased sensitivity to the cardiovascular depressant effects of sedatives and anesthetics.

ANESTHESIA FOR DYSTOCIA

Retrospective studies looking at dystocia correction techniques and survival rates have come to the same conclusion: early referral and short duration of dystocia significantly improve outcome.[1,2] Studies found that in the best-case scenario, survival rates of mares to discharge were between 86% and 91% and for foals between 10% and 43%. In one of the studies, the highest survival rate was found in the high-risk mares that were residents of the hospital near term. Speed of presentation is rarely under the control of the anesthetist, but we do have the ability to anesthetize the mare quickly to increase the potential for a positive outcome. Sedation or anesthetic protocols should be easy to administer and produce relaxation and comfort quickly to efficiently manipulate the fetus.

It is helpful to know if the foal is alive or dead when selecting an anesthetic protocol and delivery technique in a dystocia situation, but there have been occasions when a foal was assumed to be dead but was alive at birth. Selecting a protocol that is of short duration or reversible is advantageous because most drugs administered to

There are no financial or material interests to disclose.

Large Animal Clinical Sciences, College of Veterinary Medicine, Michigan State University, 736 Wilson road, East Lansing, MI 48824, USA

E-mail addresses: loribidwell@hotmail.com; bidwelll@cvm.msu.edu the mare will circulate through the fetus. The entire process of dystocia management should be based on a team approach with a team dedicated to the care of the mare and a team dedicated to support of the neonate after the birth.

Anesthesia of the pregnant mare during parturition is difficult for several reasons. These complicating factors include elevated circulating oxytocin producing vasodilation, the gravid uterus placing pressure on the diaphragm, decreased functional residual capacity, and relaxed esophageal sphincter tone. The results are low blood pressure, difficulty with ventilation and oxygenation, and increased potential for aspiration of gastric content. To make matters worse, the ideal position for manipulating the fetus is to have the mare in the Trendelenburg position. This position involves hoisting the hind legs with shackles while the front end is on the floor (preferably on a padded mattress) in a semilateral position, thus, placing gastric contents and the uterus on top of the diaphragm. Having a hoist attached to the ceiling makes this procedure easier, but a stationary support option has also been suggested.[3]

Although it is helpful to have clinical pathology results (eg, complete blood count, serum chemistry, blood gas, and electrolytes) before anesthesia, this can be acquired after induction. A quick physical examination including auscultation of the heart and chest should be followed by sedation with an α-2 agonist alone or combined with butorphanol (typically 400–500 mg xylazine for a 500 kg mare). Dosing depends on the excitement or depression of the mare. Once the mare's mouth is rinsed and her tail wrapped, she can be walked into an induction stall and anesthesia induced. A fast induction can be performed using the combination of intravenous (IV) ketamine (2.2–2.5 mg/kg) combined with diazepam or midazolam (0.08 mg/kg) IV. Controversy exists over the use of diazepam for induction of a dystocia because of the potential for respiratory depression of the foal at birth. A study was performed in Kentucky comparing the levels of diazepam and its metabolites between the mare and neonate after diazepam administration to the mare for induction for dystocia manipulation. It was determined that there are detectable levels of diazepam and its metabolites in the neonate. Although circulating levels of diazepam were detected, the study concluded that the diazepam levels did not appear to produce consistent respiratory depression in the neonate.[4]

Often, the mare will not relax after induction; therefore, an infusion of between 100 and 300 mL 5% guaifenesin/0.1% ketamine/0.05% xylazine will aid in producing relaxation. **Table 1** has recommended drug dosages for sedation, induction, and infusion. After recumbency is achieved, the mare is intubated and attached to the breathing circuit. Ventilation should be controlled or assisted at 6–8 breaths per minute with a tidal volume of 10 mL/kg. It is likely that the airway pressure will exceed 30 cm H_2O to achieve an adequate tidal volume. Although the high measured airway pressure is concerning to see, it can be disregarded. The pressure is necessary to inflate the lungs with the gastric contents and gravid uterus sitting on the diaphragm. Once the foal is removed, the tidal volume on the ventilator should be adjusted to compensate for the decrease in pressure against the diaphragm. Electrocardiography and direct arterial blood pressure can be used to monitor the mare under anesthesia. Blood pressure readings will record higher-than-true peripheral measurements because of positioning of the mare if a facial artery is used for catheterization.

Once the foal has been removed, the mare can be weaned from the ventilator at 4 breaths per minute until the placenta has been evaluated and the floor has been cleaned or she can be moved into a recovery stall. Sedation in the recovery stall should be avoided, because most mares after foaling do not benefit from any additional cardiovascular depression that can be seen from α-2 agonist or acepromazine administration. Rope-assisted recovery is recommended for these cases, as the

Table 1
Suggested sedative and induction drugs for the pregnant mare

Drug	Dose	Route	Duration
Xylazine	0.2–1.0 mg/kg	IV, IM	20–30 min
Detomidine	0.002–0.040 mg/kg	IV, IM, sublingual	30–60 min
Detomidine infusion	Initial bolus: 0.0075 mg/kg Start infusion at: 0.0006 mg/kg/min	IV, infusion rate is halved every 10–15 min	Sedation lasts approx. 15–30 min after the infusion is stopped
Dexmedetomidine	0.0025–0.005 mg/kg	IV, IM	20–40 min
Acepromazine	0.01–0.04 mg/kg	IV, IM, sublingual	60–240 min
Butorphanol	0.01–0.08 mg/kg	IV, IM	30–50 min
Ketamine	2.2–2.5 mg/kg	IV	15–20 min
Diazepam	0.08–0.1 mg/kg	IV or combined with ketamine IV	15–20 min
Guaifenesin	50–100 mg/kg	IV infusion	20–30 min dose-dependent duration
Guaifenesin, ketamine, xylazine	Guaifenesin: 50 g Ketamine: 1–2 g Xylazine: 500 mg	IV infusion in 1L dextrose or saline	Give to effect, sedation/relaxation duration are dose dependent

postparturient mare is at an increased risk of fracture in recovery because of decreased bone density and weakness.[5,6] Caution should be used when introducing the foal to the mare because she was sleeping during the birth process and may not recognize it as her own.

If manipulation of the live fetus exceeds 20 minutes or manipulation is unsuccessful, cesarean section is recommended. The abdomen of the mare should be clipped and a rough surgical preparation applied during dystocia manipulation to minimize time for surgical preparation. The mare should be moved to the surgical table and ventilation continued. Airway pressure must be monitored during positional changes and when the fetus is removed to avoid excessive or improper ventilation. In addition, arterial blood pressure will drop once the horse is moved into dorsal recumbency and when the fetus is removed. Inhalant anesthetic should be minimized to avoid additional vasodilation and bolus isotonic fluids in an attempt to minimize hypotension during transitions. The positive inotrope dobutamine can be administered as an infusion to effect, or the addition of a vasopressor may be warranted depending on response. Once the fetus is removed, analgesics and anesthetics can be administered as needed for the mare during closure of the uterus and abdomen.

ANESTHESIA OF THE EQUINE NEONATE

Anesthetizing the neonate, particularly the sick neonate, will have inherent increased risk. Electrolyte abnormalities, altered fluid dynamics, hypoglycemia, hypothermia, and anesthetist inexperience are all valid concerns when dealing with foals. Even a seasoned anesthetist can fall under the category of inexperienced when dealing with foals because of the seasonal nature of the patient. Understanding the basics and reviewing them before foaling season are important means to decreasing the risk of anesthetic accidents. Hypoventilation leading to hypoxemia and subsequent cardiac arrest can occur quickly in neonates if the anesthetist is not adequately monitoring the patient. Therefore, anesthesia of the neonate should not be considered simple. Appropriate anesthetic training and monitoring are necessary to minimize risk.

Many procedures can be performed in neonates using sedation and restraint (eg, entropion repair, bandage or splint placement, and catheter placement), but there are others that are more appropriately performed under general anesthesia: rib fracture immobilization, ruptured bladder repair, abdominal exploration, wound and fracture repair, or periosteal elevation. In many cases, injectable general anesthetic techniques can be used, but longer duration procedures benefit from oxygen supplementation and ventilatory support.

A neonate has an immature metabolic ability and sympathetic nervous system, lower mean arterial blood pressure, an increased permeability of the blood–brain barrier, increased vulnerability to hypothermia, and increased sensitivity to anesthetics compared with a 1-month-old foal.[7] From birth through the first 2 weeks of life, a foal should be treated as if incapable of complete hepatic metabolism.[8,9] Drugs that are dependent on hepatic metabolism like opioids, ketamine, benzodiazepines, lidocaine, and α-2 agonists should be used with discretion in neonates.[10]

Complications that can occur in any patient associated with sedatives and inhalant anesthetics are often amplified in neonates. Vasodilation, hypotension, bradycardia, hypothermia, hypoxemia, and hypercapnia can result. Therefore, appropriate blood pressure maintenance and oxygenation become more difficult. In addition, neonates have lower albumin concentrations, increasing the risk of elevated free portions of protein-bound drugs like phenylbutazone and barbiturates. Evidence has shown that diazepam clearance is significantly less in foals 4 days of age versus 21 days and older; therefore, caution should be used in redosing diazepam in neonates because this drug can accumulate.[10] Opioid and α-2 adrenergic receptor location and binding are different in the brain of horses compared with dogs and rats.[11,12] A neonate will become profoundly sedate from an injection of butorphanol compared with an adult horse becoming excited from the same drug. It is unclear if this difference is caused by receptor binding, concentration, or functional differences. An additional physiologic difference between neonates and adults is the minimum alveolar concentration of isoflurane; 0.84% for neonates versus 1.3%–1.6% for adult horses.[13]

Drugs like α-2 agonists and opioids can be used in neonates, but dosing and selection should be appropriate for body size and health status. A neonate will have a more intense and prolonged response to any drug administered. Alpha-2 adrenergic agonists, xylazine and detomidine, have been associated with mild complications, although the high-quality sedation and analgesia often outweigh any negative effects. Xylazine has been reported to produce cardiovascular and respiratory depression, although no significant changes were noted in pH or blood gas tensions.[14,15] Cardiac output depends on heart rate and stroke volume, and foals have a reduced ability to make necessary changes in stroke volume to compensate for decreases in heart rate secondary to drug administration. Therefore, sedatives selected for neonates should have minimal cardiovascular depressant effects. Used alone or in combination by intramuscular (IM) or IV routes, benzodiazepines (diazepam or midazolam), ketamine, propofol, and the opioid agonist-antagonist, butorphanol, are useful choices for sedation or short-term general anesthesia in foals. Butorphanol has been studied in 3- and 12-day-old pony foals at a dose of 0.05 mg/kg IV and IM. The result was sedation rather than increased locomotor activity as is often seen in adults. There were minimal effects on the cardiovascular system and increased time spent nursing.[16] Administration of phenothiazines (eg, acepromazine) is not recommended in pediatric patients because of the potential for significant vasodilation.

Procedures such as bandage change, radiographs, catheter placement, ultrasonographic examination, or procedures to correct entropion can be accomplished in neonates with sedation. In a 30- to 100-kg neonate, a dose of 2–5 mg of butorphanol with 2.5–5 mg of midazolam or diazepam administered IV will result in recumbency that lasts 15–30 minutes. The addition of 100–150 mg ketamine IV or 50–80 mg propofol allows for a more invasive procedure to be performed like a joint flush or urinary catheter placement. Mild to severe hypoxia can occur during sedation or general anesthesia without oxygen supplementation. Oxygen delivered at a rate of at least 3–5 L/min through a nasal canula is recommended.

General anesthesia in neonates presents a unique complication because they respond to pre-anesthetics and inhalant anesthetics with vasodilation and decreased cardiac contractility.[17] Pre-anesthetic examination should include palpation of the pulse, temperature, auscultation of the heart and lungs, and a minimum database that includes packed cell volume, total protein, white blood cell count, and fibrinogen. When presented with a sick neonate, it is important to evaluate glucose and electrolyte concentrations before anesthesia; particularly sodium, potassium, and calcium.[18–20] Glucose levels should be checked before, during, and after anesthesia in the healthy or sick neonate. Although α-2 adrenergic agonist drugs decrease insulin release in adult horses, resulting in elevated glucose levels, the same is not true for neonates. If a neonate requires anesthesia immediately after birth (rib fractures proximal to the heart), a form of hyperimmune plasma can be administered IV under anesthesia to compensate for the lack of colostrum received. Pre-anesthetic fasting is not recommended, although caution should be used if induction occurs soon after the neonate nurses. Intubation with adequate cuff inflation should occur to avoid aspiration.

There are various IV induction techniques that have been used successfully: the combination of ketamine and diazepam or midazolam, ketamine alone, or propofol.[21] A study comparing induction and maintenance techniques in foals 7–15 days old found that the combination of diazepam, ketamine, and isoflurane produced less cardiopulmonary depression than xylazine, ketamine, and isoflurane during abdominal surgery.[15] Although inhalant anesthetic induction through nasotracheal intubation can be used for a depressed foal, the administration of a small amount of ketamine with resulting sympathomimetic effects might be more appropriate for induction. The higher concentrations of inhalant anesthetic required for nasotracheal induction produce more profound vasodilation. Recommended drug doses are listed in **Table 2**.

Table 2
Recommended sedation and induction doses for foals[a]

Drug	Dose
Xylazine	0.5–0.1 mg/kg IV 1–2 mg/kg IM
Detomidine	0.005–0.01 mg/kg IV 0.01–0.03 mg/kg IM
Romifidine	0.04–0.06 mg/kg IV
Butorphanol	0.02–0.04 mg/kg IV, IM, subcutaneously
Propofol	2 mg/kg IV (induction) 0.05–0.5 mg/kg IV (maintenance bolus)
Ketamine	1–2 mg/kg IV
Diazepam or midazolam	0.04–0.08 mg/kg IV

[a] Most doses are extrapolated from adult equine doses.

Additionally, the mare should remain with the foal during sedation and until complete induction. Removal of the mare during sedation or induction will produce excitement in both the foal and mare. The mare can be sedated with a combination of 15 mg acepromazine and 150 mg xylazine or an equivalent amount of romifidine or detomidine. Sterile ophthalmic lubrication is essential to prevent corneal abrasions in the anesthetized neonate.

Monitoring basics include respiration, mucous membrane color, and pulse quality. The addition of an electrocardiogram, capnograph, pulse oximeter, and invasive or noninvasive arterial blood pressure is recommended. For emergency procedures, arterial blood gases are useful for monitoring oxygenation, acid–base balance, and quality of ventilation. It is not uncommon for a neonate to have $Paco_2$ levels of 60 mm Hg or higher with spontaneous ventilation during elective procedures. This can be corrected by assisting ventilation at 1–2 breaths per minute or controlled ventilation at 8–12 breaths per minute. Isotonic fluids should be administered at a rate of 10–15 mL/kg/h for elective procedures and up to 60–80 mL/kg/h in emergency or shock situations. Renal function is immature; therefore, fluid response should be monitored. Central venous pressure and urine output are ideal for measuring fluid response but impractical in many situations. Instead, the neonate should be monitored for signs of oxygenation or ventilatory changes and edema of the nasal cavities or supraorbital space as indicators of fluid overload. Calculating the required hourly fluid volume before anesthesia and using 1-L fluid bags rather than 3- or 5-L bags can minimize excessive fluid administration.

General anesthesia can be maintained using inhalant anesthetics, intravenous bolus, or constant rate infusion of drugs. Isoflurane and sevoflurane are vapor anesthetics currently used commonly in the United States. Halothane is available in some locations outside of the United States but is not recommended in neonates because of the higher hepatic metabolic requirement (20% vs less than 3% in sevoflurane and isoflurane). Injectable anesthetics include ketamine, diazepam, propofol, and the combination called *triple drip* that includes guaifenesin, ketamine, and xylazine.

Inhalant anesthetics should be minimized to lessen vasodilation. Vaporizer settings are typically started at 2% isoflurane or 3% sevoflurane and then reduced to 1.5% and 2.5%, respectively, within 5 minutes of initiation. Functional residual capacity of the lung is smaller in neonates and, therefore, induction of anesthesia is faster. Eye position, blink reflex, and strap muscle tone in the neck are not predictable in neonates. Menace response is a learned behavior; therefore, the neonate will not necessarily respond. Blood pressure is helpful in determining depth of anesthesia in foals, but vasodilation can occur rapidly despite that a surgical plane of anesthesia has not been achieved. Balancing inhalant anesthesia with injectable agents (ketamine or propofol) is the easiest way to minimize vasodilation. When attempting to place an arterial catheter in a sick or healthy neonate, it is important to place the catheter as quickly as possible because the development of vasodilation makes placement progressively more difficult. Administering a positive inotrope or vasopressor might aid in the placement of the arterial catheter by improving cardiac output or vascular tone. From the author's experience, decreasing the concentration of inhaled anesthetic is often the most effective way to increase blood pressure.

Recovery should occur on a padded mat or on straw in a stall. Attempts should be made to dry and warm the foal. Wet hair combined with vasodilation from anesthetics increase the likelihood of hypothermia and should be avoided if possible.[22] Prewarmed towels are useful for drying the foal and achieving or maintaining normothermia during recovery. Forced air warmers or circulating hot water pads are useful for warming a recovering foal as well. Maintaining the foal in recumbency is easily done by sitting behind the foal with pressure on the back of the neck to prevent early arousal. Tongue tone is a good indicator of depth of anesthesia or sedation. When the foal responds to sounds and can pull its tongue back into its mouth easily, assistance to stand should occur by grabbing the base of the tail and giving the back end support. An ataxic foal is difficult to control from the front end and usually needs assistance in the weaker back end of the body. Caution should always be used because some foals will be stimulated by the assistance and they can buck or kick suddenly. The mare can be reintroduced once the foal is stable, although a handler should restrain the mare during reintroduction to protect the foal from a confused mare.

REFERENCES

1. Byron CR, Embertson RM, Bernard WV, et al. Dystocia in a referral hospital setting: approach and results. Equine Vet J 2003;35:82–5.
2. Norton JL, Dallap BL, Johnston JK, et al. Retrospective study of dystocia in mares at a referral hospital. Equine Vet J 2007;39:37–41.
3. Cruz JF. How to use a thoracic support apparatus for horses placed in the Trendelenburg position. In: Proceedings: the 56th Annual Convention of the American Association of Equine Practitioners. Baltimore (MD): 2010. p. 192–4.
4. Bidwell LB, Embertson RM, Bone NL, et al. Diazepam levels in foals after dystocia birth. In: Proceedings: the 54th Annual Convention of the American Association of Equine Practitioners. San Diego (CA): 2008. p. 286–7.
5. Glade MJ. Effects of gestation, lactation and maternal calcium intake on mechanical strength of equine bone. J Am Coll Nutr 1993;12:372–7.
6. Bidwell LA, Bramlage LR, Rood WA. Equine perioperative fatalities associated with general anaesthesia at a private practice – a retrospective case series. Vet Anaesth Analg 2007;34:23–30.
7. Dunlop CL. Anesthesia and sedation in foals. Perinatology. Vet Clin North Am Equine Pract 1994;10:67–85. WB Saunders.
8. Vaala WE. Aspects of pharmacology in the neonatal foal. Vet Clin North Am Equine Pract 1985;1:51–75.
9. Gossett KA, French DD. Effect of age on liver enzyme activity in serum of healthy quarter horses. Am J Vet Res 1984;45:354–6.
10. Norman WM, Court MH, Greenblatt DJ. Age-related changes in the pharmacokinetic disposition of diazepam in foals. Am J Vet Res 1997;58:878–80.
11. Hellyer PW, Bai L, Supon J, et al. Comparison of opioid and alpha-2 adrenergic receptor binding in horse and dog brain using radioligand autoradiography. Vet Anaesth Analg 2003;30(3):172–82.
12. Thomasy SM, Moeller BC, Stanley SD. Comparison of opioid receptor binding in horse, guinea pig, and rat cerebral cortex and cerebellum. Vet Anaesth Analg 2007;34(5):351–8.
13. Dunlop CS, Hodgson DS, Grandy JL, et al. The MAC of isoflurane in foals. Vet Surg 1989;18:247–54.
14. Robertson SA, Carter SW, Donovan M, et al. Effects of intravenous xylazine hydrochloride on blood glucose, plasma insulin and rectal temperature in neonatal foals. Equine Vet J 1990;22:43–7.
15. Kerr CL, Bouri LP, Pearce SG, et al. Cardiopulmonary effects of diazepam-ketamine-isoflurane or xylazine-ketamine-isoflurane during abdominal surgery in foals. Am J Vet Res 2009;70:574–80.

16. Arguedas MG, Hine MT, Papich MG, et al. Pharmacokinetics of butorphanol and evaluation of physiologic and behavioral effects after intravenous and intramuscular administration to neonatal foals. J Vet Intern Med 2008;22:1417–26.
17. Valverde A, Giguere S, Sanchez LC, et al. Effects of dobutamine, norepinephrine and vasopressin on cardiovascular function in anesthetized neonatal foals with induced hypotension. Am J Vet Res 2006;67:1730–7.
18. Perkins G, Valberg SJ, Madigan JM, et al. Electrolyte disturbances in foals with severe rhabdomyolysis. J Vet Intern Med 1998;12:173–7.
19. Lakritz J, Madigan J, Carlson GP. Hypovolemic hyponatremia and signs of neurologic disease associated with diarrhea in a foal. J Am Med Assoc 1992;200: 1114–6.
20. Behr MJ, Hackett RP, Bentinck-Smith J, et al. Metabolic abnormalities associated with rupture of the urinary bladder in neonatal foals. J Am Vet Med Assoc 1981; 178:263–6.
21. Donaldson LL, Dunlop GS, Cooper WL. A comparison of propofol with ketamine after xylazine and butorphanol as field anesthesia for young foals. In: Proceedings Ann Mtg Am Coll Vet Anes. 1998. p. 11.
22. Insler SR, Sessler DI. Perioperative thermoregulation and temperature monitoring. Anesthesiol Clin 2006;24(4):823–37.

Recovery of Horses from Anesthesia

Stuart C. Clark-Price, DVM, MS

KEYWORDS

- Equine • Anesthesia • Recovery • Assisted recovery

KEY POINTS

- Recovery from anesthesia in one of the most dangerous and unpredictable elements of providing anesthesia to horses.
- Medications that can be administered to horses to improve the quality of anesthesia include acepromazine, α_2-agonists, opioids, ketamine, and propofol.
- Assisted recovery techniques that can be used during recovery from anesthesia for horses vary and include hand recovery and use of head and/or tail ropes, slings, and water pools.
- Horses should be closely monitored throughout the recovery period for the purpose of early detection and intervention to reduce complications.

INTRODUCTION

Recovery from anesthesia can be one of the most problematic and unpredictable phases of an anesthetic plan for equine patients. Equine mortality in healthy patients due to complications during recovery can be as high as 32.6%[1] and is probably higher in systemically ill patients. Known complications include delayed recovery, equine postanesthetic myopathy, reinjury of orthopedic repair, fracture or other injury, hypoxemia, and cardiopulmonary arrest.[2] Developing strategies to improve recoveries based on an individual horse's condition should be considered in the same way that an overall anesthetic plan should be tailored to an individual patient's needs. For example, the recovery of a horse after a castration in a field situation may require only the administration of a sedative and an analgesic and then allowing the horse to recover unassisted whereas a horse recovering from a 4-hour carpal bone fracture repair may be expected to have muscular weakness and incoordination that prolongs the recovery period and requires extensive manpower to assist the horse's move to a standing position.

The recovery period begins when the anesthetic, whether it is intravenous (IV) or inhalant, is discontinued and concludes when a horse is standing and considered

Department of Veterinary Clinical Medicine, College of Veterinary Medicine, University of Illinois, 1008 West Hazelwood Drive, MC-004, Urbana, IL 61802, USA
E-mail address: sccp@illinois.edu

Vet Clin Equine 29 (2013) 223–242
http://dx.doi.org/10.1016/j.cveq.2012.11.001
0749-0739/13/$ – see front matter © 2013 Elsevier Inc. All rights reserved.

stable enough to be led back to its stall, paddock, or pasture. The recovery period can be broken down into 6 phases: transition from anesthesia to recovery, first movement, movement to sternal recumbency, first attempt to stand, initially standing, and stable standing.

Continual assessment and monitoring of horses during recovery are essential to achieve the best possible outcome and minimize complications. Practitioners should have a general knowledge of the recovery process and therapeutic options to improve recovery quality in horses in various situations.

- Recovery can be one of the most problematic and dangerous parts of equine recovery from anesthesia.
- A recovery plan should be developed based on an individual horse's condition to minimize complications.
- The recovery period begins when the anesthetic is discontinued and concludes when a horse is standing and considered stable.

PHASES OF RECOVERY

Recovery of horses generally follows the same order of events and, therefore, the sequence of those events can be somewhat predictable. The first phase is the transition from anesthesia to recovery. During this phase, the anesthetic is discontinued and the horse is prepared for recovery and may be moved to a separate area (padded recovery stall, recovery pool, and so forth). Moving large horses may require the use of a hoist system (**Fig. 1**). Smaller horses and foals can be simply carried by hospital personnel to the site of recovery. Horses that were in lateral recumbency

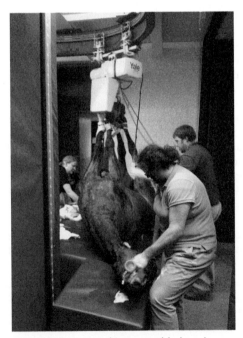

Fig. 1. An anesthetized horse being moved into a padded equine recovery stall with a hoist system. The hoist is connected to a rail system so that the hoist can be removed from the recovery stall after a horse is placed inside for recovery.

during anesthesia should be placed in the same lateral recumbency in a recovery stall. Horses in dorsal recumbency during anesthesia can be placed in either lateral recumbency, although it may be preferential to have the side with a catheter on the upside for easier access. Horses can be placed on towels or other absorbent material to capture sweat and other fluids to prevent puddle formation in the recovery stall. During this time, sedatives, analgesics, or other medications can be administered to smooth recovery or to treat specific conditions. Endotracheal tubes can be left in place for administration of oxygen via insufflation, or ventilation can be assisted with a demand valve until the horse is ventilation sufficiently on its own. Some anesthetists prefer to leave an endotracheal tube in place during recovery to guard against airway obstruction. If the endotracheal tube is removed for recovery, however, phenylephrine (0.25% solution) can be administered into each nostril to reduce upper airway mucous membrane congestion and obstruction.[3] The lower portion of a horse's legs can be wrapped with cotton sheets or purpose-made leg wraps to prevent self-inflicted injury during recovery (**Fig. 2**). The feet of horses can be wrapped with adhesive elastic bandage or the horses can have temporary rubberized shoes placed on their feet to improve traction during attempts to stand, particularly if the flooring surface is wet or slick. The second phase during recovery is defined by a horse's first movement. This lets the anesthetist know that the horse is at or near consciousness. This can be seen as movement of the head and neck, movement of any of the limbs, or even the return of spontaneous swallowing. The onset of this phase is important for the safety of personnel working with and around a recovering horse. In field situations, first movement can be used as a warning for people to move away from a recovering horse to prevent injury, or, in a hospital environment, it can be used as a signal to have personnel leave the recovery stall and/or to close the recovery stall doors. Some anesthetists may use first movement (ie, swallowing) as an indicator to remove an endotracheal tube and administer sedative medications. The third phase of recovery starts when a horse makes attempts to move into sternal recumbency. On occasion, however, some horses may bypass this phase and move directly from lateral recumbency and attempt to stand. In an ideal recovery, the horse moves into and remains in sternal recumbency for a period of time. Horses, in particular those recovering from inhalant anesthesia, may display evidence of disorientation and muscle weakness by flailing with their head and neck and/or limbs while making several attempts to

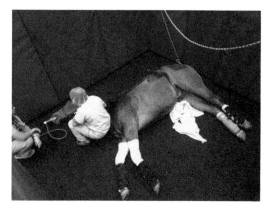

Fig. 2. A horse in a recovery stall after general anesthesia. Protective leg wraps have been applied, a demand valve is used to support ventilation and prevent hypoxemia, and a tail rope is in place to assist the horse to a standing position.

move to sternal recumbency. These horses may benefit from sedation before movement to allow a longer period of time for elimination of anesthetic. The fourth phase begins when a horse makes its first attempt to stand. Most horses attempt to rise with their front limbs first and then rise on their hind limbs once the front limbs are almost fully extended. Some horses adopt a dog-sitting position while attempting to stand. Some horses with certain muscular or neurologic diseases, such as equine postanesthetic myopathy[4] and postanesthetic myelomalacia,[5] assume a dog-sitting position and the anesthetist should evaluate these horses carefully, especially if a horse assumes this position repeatedly with an inability to move or rise on the hind limbs. Fewer horses attempt to stand by rising on the hind limbs first, similar to bovine species. This may indicate, however, that a horse has not yet regained enough coordination or muscular strength to stand. Horses that rise on the hind limbs first my crash around uncontrollably and summersault forward. The fifth phase of recovery begins when the recovering horse initially stands. Horses with good muscle strength and coordination ideally stand quietly while continuing to recover from effects of the anesthetic drugs administered. Some horses, however, stumble around the recovery stall, knuckle over at the pasterns, and have muscle fasciculation, presumably from the anesthetic drugs, and can pose a risk to anyone in the recovery stall. The final phase of recovery occurs when the horse is deemed to have completed recovery and is considered stable enough to be returned to its pen or stall. All of the phases of recovery can have varying presentations depending on the temperament of the horse, the anesthetics used, the length of anesthesia, and the procedure performed.

- There are 6 phases of recovery from anesthesia for horses:
  ○ Transition from anesthesia to recovery
  ○ First movement
  ○ Movement to sternal recumbency
  ○ First attempt to stand
  ○ Initial standing
  ○ Completed recovery

DURATION OF RECOVERY

Duration of recovery can be defined as the period of time from discontinuing anesthetic drug administration to when the horse is considered standing and stable. There are several factors that influence duration of recovery, including duration of anesthesia, hypothermia, hypotension, type of anesthetics used, administration of sedative and analgesic medications after discontinuing anesthetic drug administration, recovery stall environment and design, whether or not a horse's recovery was assisted, breed, individual horse temperament, and age.[6-13] In one study that examined the anesthesia records of 381 horses that underwent general anesthesia with isoflurane, the time to standing ranged from 26 minutes to 92 minutes with an average of 59 minutes.[7] The investigators noted that colic cases and after-hours emergency cases had longer recovery times, and warm-blooded horses and horses that received ketamine intraoperatively had shorter recovery times. Horses receiving only injectable anesthesia may have shorter recovery times than horses receiving inhalant anesthesia, although this is highly dependent on the IV agents used and the duration of inhalant anesthesia. In horses receiving ketamine as an anesthetic agent, recovery can be expected in 30 minutes to 45 minutes, with horses generally standing with only 1 attempt.[14] In most cases, in the author's opinion, horses should show signs of awakening from inhalant anesthesia by

30 minutes to 45 minutes, should show spontaneous movements by 45 minutes to 60 minutes, and make attempts to stand by 60 minutes to 90 minutes. A physical examination, stimulation of the horse, and advanced diagnostics, such as blood gas and electrolyte analysis, should be considered in horses exceeding those times.

- Duration of recovery is the period of time from discontinuing anesthesia to when a horse is standing and stable.
- Recovery time depends on many factors, including type of anesthetic drugs, procedure length, and health status of patient.
- Horses receiving injectable anesthesia can generally be expected to recover in 30 minutes to 45 minutes.
- Horses receiving inhalation anesthesia can generally be expected to recover in 60 minutes to 90 minutes.

RECOVERY FOR FIELD PROCEDURES

Anesthesia for equine patients is probably most commonly performed in field situations due to the ambulatory nature of equine practice. Therefore, total IV anesthesia for quick procedures, such as castrations or simple laceration repair, is used frequently. The majority of horses undergoing field anesthesia are healthy and thus need minimal equipment or assistance during the recovery process. The most important aspect of recovery after field anesthesia is an open area free of obstacles. A large open grass field or pen is suitable for most field recoveries. Natural turf provides some padding for recumbent horses and excellent footing for horses as they stand. Caution should be taken to protect the downside eye of a horse from corneal abrasions from material on the ground by placing a towel under a horse's head. The upside eye should be covered as well in areas of bright sunlight to protect the eye and cornea while the horse is recovering. Additionally, lateral recumbent recovering horses should have halters removed to prevent facial nerve apraxia or use a buckleless rope halter if a halter is necessary to control a horse as it stands.[15]

Solid wall stalls may be used as a recovery area provided the walls are of sufficient height to prevent horses from being able to go over the top. Deeply bedded shaving or straw can be used on the floor of stalls to provide padding during recovery. Placing a large towel under a horse's head is suggested to minimize inhalation of small shavings or straw particles and to prevent corneal abrasions.

Small pens or corals that use pipe panels or wire should be avoided because recovering horses can severely injure their limbs, head, or neck if they slide under or between pipes or receive lacerations if caught in fence wire.[16]

- The most important aspect of recovery after field anesthesia is an open area free of obstacles.
- Natural turf provides some padding and excellent footing for recovering horses.
- Solid wall stalls may be used as a recovery area provided the walls are of sufficient height.
- Horses should not be recovered in small pens or corals that use pipe panels or wire.

RECOVERY FOR IN-HOSPITAL PROCEDURES

Hospitals and clinics that provide advanced surgical services for horses under general or inhalant anesthesia require specific facilities for recovering horses. Recovery stalls with thick padding of the floors and walls should be made available.

RECOVERY STALL DESIGN

There is no consensus in size, shape, or makeup of in-hospital recovery stalls. When building a facility, the location and design of a postsurgical recovery stall should be considered from the start. Recovery stall size should be designed to limit the number of steps a horse can take while recovering to prevent a horse from accelerating and increasing its momentum, such that a potential impact with a stall wall could result in a serious traumatic blunt-force injury. In most cases, stalls of approximately 12 ft by 12 ft (3.6 m by 3.6 m) are sufficient. Hospitals that service a large number of draft-type horses may require a larger stall. Stall shape is easiest to design as square or rectangular. Octagonal or even round stalls may be of benefit, however, because they reduce or eliminate a horse from becoming stuck in a corner while disoriented or uncoordinated during recovery (**Fig. 3**). Reducing the severity of corner angles in a recovery stall may be beneficial and of minimal expense or difficulty during construction or renovation (**Fig. 4**). Recovery stall height depends on factors, such as the size and type of horse seen and the height of the surgical table. A formula has been described for determining the vertical dimension of horses suspended from a hoist and can be used for determining appropriate height of a recovery stall and hoist placement.[17] One of the most important aspects of a postanesthesia recovery stall is adequate floor padding and good footing. A compressible, padded surface for recumbent horses is essential. Thick padding that contours to a horse's body distributes body weight more evenly and possibly reduces the occurrence of complications, such as muscle or nerve injury. A rapidly inflating and deflating air pillow system has been described that may promote higher-quality recoveries (**Fig. 5**).[10] Recovery stall walls should also be thickly padded and of sufficient height (≥8 ft) to prevent any part of a horse from going over the top. Padding of several inches of thickness should cover the walls to provide cushioning in the case of a horse having an impact on a wall. Wall padding that is removable can be desirable to allow thorough cleaning and disinfecting of recovery stalls at regular intervals. Padding should be secured to the wall firmly to prevent dislodging by recovering horses and moving in-between the padding and walls. Removable floor padding can be used also; however, as with wall padding, care must be taken to prevent the padding from moving and allowing a horse from coming in contact with a bare surface. Padding sealed to the floor with a rubber covering is useful and prevents the padding from moving and provides a water

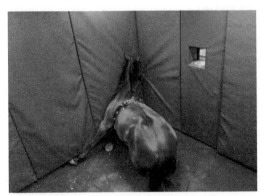

Fig. 3. A horse recovering from general anesthesia stuck in a 90° angle corner of a recovery stall. Recovery stalls that reduce or eliminate severe angles, such as octagons or round stalls, can reduce or eliminate this position and the potential for injury.

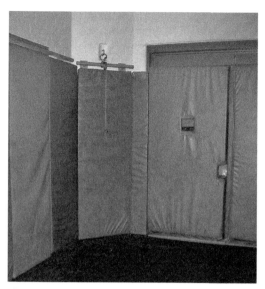

Fig. 4. A padded equine recovery stall. Note that the corners are set so that there are no 90° angles, to reduce the incidence of horses getting stuck in corners. (*Courtesy of* Dr Manuel Martin-Florez, Cornell University, Ithaca, New York.)

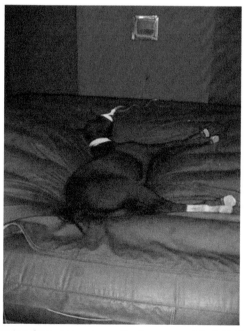

Fig. 5. A horse recovering from general anesthesia on a rapidly inflating and deflating air pillow system. (*Courtesy of* Dr David Hodgson, Kansas State University, Manhattan, Kansas.)

resistant seal. Metal rings or bars should be securely fastened to the walls at various places around the recovery stall at a height of approximately 8 ft to facilitate head and tail ropes for assisted recoveries (**Fig. 6**). Recovery stall doors should be wide enough to allow horses to pass through easily while hoisted or walked through but of sturdy construction. External door bars can be placed to reinforce door stability and allow a place for personnel to stand and view recovering horses (**Fig. 7**). Recovery stalls should have good lighting to allow for proper visibility for viewing recoveries. Some practitioners recommend a light dimming option for recovery stalls; however, darkening a recovery stall does not seem to have an impact on recovery time or quality.[18] An electric hoist on a rail system can be used to facilitate movement of horses from a surgical suite to a recovery stall. Clinician and staff safety should always be a concern around recovering horses and opportunities that enhance safety should be considered when building or remodeling a recovery stall. Windows, platforms, or video cameras for remote viewing should be available for continual observing of horses recovering unassisted. Quickly accessible stall exits should be available for personnel working directly with recovering horses while preventing horses from escaping. Small door exits for going through or footholds or rope ladders for going over stall doors can be installed. A uniquely designed all-in-one room can be constructed that can be used as an induction, surgery, and recovery room (**Fig. 8**).

- Recovery stall should be approximately 12 ft by 12 ft.
- Increasing corner angles in recovery stalls may be beneficial and limit horses becoming stuck.
- Proper floor padding and good footing may be the most important factors in a recovery stall.
- Recovery stall walls should have padding and rings for head and tail ropes.
- Personnel safety is important and remote viewing options and quick stall exits should be available.

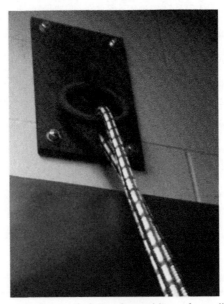

Fig. 6. A metal ring securely fastened above the padding of a wall in an equine recovery stall to facilitate the use of ropes. The ring is set at a height of 8 ft.

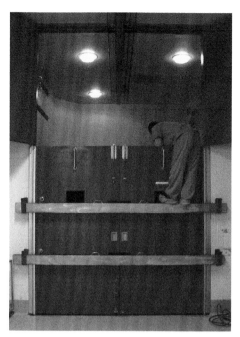

Fig. 7. Reinforced doors to an equine recovery stall with aluminum bars. The bars a wide enough and have a nonslip surface to allow someone to observe a horse while it recovers from anesthesia. (*Courtesy of* Dr Manuel Martin-Flores, Cornell University, Ithaca, New York.)

IMPACT OF ADMINISTERED MEDICATIONS ON RECOVERY QUALITY

One of the more heavily investigated areas of equine recovery is determination of medications that can be administered to smooth out or improve the quality of recovery. Horses may become awakened and aware of their surroundings while still under the influence of inhalant anesthetic during recovery (see article on Inhalant Anesthetics by Brosnan). The idea is that a medication can be administered to calm or sedate a horse during which time the horse can continue to eliminate inhalant anesthetics so that when the horse attempts to stand, any lingering effects from the anesthesia (muscle weakness, incoordination, shivering, and excitement) can be minimized and the overall experience of the horse improved.[11] Additionally, the anesthetic agents used during the intraoperative period can have beneficial or adverse effects on recovery quality.

Inhalant anesthetic agents are the cornerstone for providing general anesthesia in horses. Unfortunately, they are also one of the causes of complications regarding recovery. In general, inhalant anesthetic use results in greater incoordination and muscle weakness than use of total IV anesthetic techniques.[19] Early on and in some parts of the world, halothane was the main inhalant anesthetic used in horses. Since the clinical introduction of isoflurane, however, studies have demonstrated shorter times to sternal recumbency, shorter times to standing, and higher-quality recoveries compared with halothane.[20–22] One report demonstrated that horses anesthetized with isofluane has quicker times to sternal recumbency and standing but that those horses recovery were less composed than horses that were anesthetized with halothane.[12] The inhalant anesthetic sevoflurane is a newer agent that has less tissue

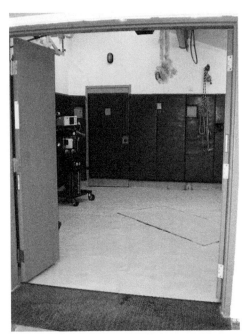

Fig. 8. A unique all-in-one room that serves as an induction room with a swing gate (not visible in photo), a surgical suite with hydraulic table that rises from the floor, and a padded recovery stall with hoist. (*Courtesy of* Dr Joseph Coli, Comstock Equine Hospital, Reno, Nevada.)

solubility than isoflurane and is, therefore, eliminated quicker and can result in faster recoveries.[23] Unfortunately, this has not translated into clinically improved recoveries. Differences in recovery times or quality have not been demonstrated in adult horses anesthetized with sevoflurane compared with isoflurane.[24] Additionally, foals of 1 month to 3 months of age showed no difference in induction or recovery characteristics using sevoflurane versus isoflurane.[25] The use of adjunctive sedatives and analgesic medications probably negates any difference that the use of isoflurane or sevofluane may demonstrate clinically and, therefore, the use of one over another cannot be recommended.

Acepromazine has a long history of use and is currently the only phenothiazine tranquilizer commonly used in equine patients. Administration of acepromazine can reduce anxiety, reduce avoidance behavior, and sedate horses.[26] Additionally, although not analgesic in itself, acepromazine can alter the perception of pain and enhance the analgesic and sedative effects of opioids and α_2-agonists.[26,27] These effects make acepromazine useful during the recovery period, particularly when combined with other sedatives or analgesic medications to facilitate recovery.[19,28,29] Acepromazine typically has a longer onset of action (10–15 minutes) when administered IV than α_2-agonists and even longer when administered intramuscularly (20–40 minutes).[26] Doses of 0.01 mg/kg IV to 0.04 mg/kg IV can be administered shortly before or when entering the recovery stall to allow sufficient time of onset. Acepromazine can cause hypotension through peripheral α blockade and should be used with caution in hypotensive or systemically compromised patients.[29]

The number of available α_2-agonist drugs has grown over the past several years and, because of their rapid onset and reliable action, have become a popular medication to administer during the recovery period of horses.[26] Xylazine is probably the most commonly used sedative during the recovery period and has been recommended to sedate horses that try to rise to quickly and improve recovery.[14,19] Xylazine administration increases time to sternal recumbency and time to standing while decreasing the number of attempts to sternal recumbency and standing.[11,13] Recovery quality was higher in horses that received xylazine compared with horses that received no postanesthetic sedation.[11,13] Detomidine has a greater potency and longer duration of action than xylazine[30] and has been used as a constant rate infusion both for standing sedation[31] and as a supplement for general anesthesia.[32] Detomidine infusion during anesthesia at 5 μg/kg/h does not affect the duration or quality of recovery.[32] When administered at recovery, however, detomidine improves recovery quality and increases time to standing while reducing the number of attempts to stand.[11] Romifidine is similar to detomidine in levels and duration of sedation but with less ataxia than that seen with xylazine or detomidine.[30] The reduction in ataxia may make romifidine a favorable choice over xylazine as a postanesthetic sedative to improve recovery quality in horses,[33] although in another report,[34] xylazine and romifidine did not differ in recovery quality or duration in horses but did improve recovery quality, increase recovery time, and reduce the number of attempts to stand compared with horses did not receive any sedative medications at recovery.[11] Dexmedetomidine and, previously, medetomidine have been traditionally used for small animal patient sedation and preanesthetic administration, but it has been use in horses as a constant rate infusion during anesthesia and it improves recovery.[35,36] When using dexmedetomidine, however, care must be taken to dose it appropriately because equipotent doses to xylazine can cause marked ataxia that may complicate recovery.[37]

The use of opioids in horses continues to be somewhat controversial and there are few reports of their use to improve recovery quality. Opioid administration in horses has the potential to have serious adverse effects, such as excitement and increased locomotor activity, and is probably best administered in conjunction with acepromazine or an α_2-agonist.[26] Butorphanol and morphine are the opioids with the most evidence to support their use during recovery. Morphine dosed at 0.1 mg/kg showed no difference in recovery scores or increase in incidence of postanesthesia complications compared with horses that did not receive morphine,[37] and horses that received morphine as a premedication and an intraoperative infusion needed fewer attempts to attain sternal recumbency and standing and had a shorter time to standing after first movement than horses that did not receive morphine.[38] It is difficult to recommend the use of opioids for the purpose of improvement in recovery quality; however, the author routinely uses opioids in horses in conjunction with sedatives for analgesic purposes.

Lidocaine infusions have become more commonplace for horses during and after anesthesia, particularly in horses recovering from abdominal exploratory for gastrointestinal accidents. Lidocaine infusions have been shown to reduce clinical signs and cytokines associated with endotoxemia[39] and reduce inhalant anesthetic requirements during general anesthesia.[40] Lidocaine infusion has been shown to have an effect on the quality of recovery in horses, resulting in higher levels of ataxia during recovery, and it has, therefore, been recommended that intraoperative infusions be discontinued 30 minutes prior to the end of the surgical period to minimize recovery effects.[41]

Ketamine is probably the most commonly used injectable anesthetic in horses. Ketamine has been used as an infusion alone or in combination with other drugs to reduce the minimum alveolar concentration of inhalant anesthetics or to maintain short-term IV anesthesia.[42] Recovery from IV anesthesia is generally shorter in duration and higher in quality than recovery from inhalant anesthetics for horses,[42] although this may be secondary to total duration of anesthesia. Although there are scant reports in the literature, anecdotal reports support administration of ketamine during the recovery period to reanesthetize a horse and allow it more time to eliminate inhalant anesthetic. One report showed improved quality of recovery when xylazine and ketamine were infused for 30 minutes after discontinuation of sevoflurane.[43] More investigation is warranted before ketamine administration during recovery can be recommended on a routine basis.

The use of propofol to improve equine recovery quality has been well reported and is gaining traction in academic and specialty practice.[43–47] The use of propofol as an induction agent in adult horses is problematic and potentially dangerous because excitement can occur[47]; however, it can be useful as an adjunctive anesthetic agent and result in calm and smooth recoveries. Propofol, in combination with xylazine, has been shown to produce quality recoveries and can be useful in cases where a high-quality recovery is particularly important.[43] Propofol is a powerful respiratory depressant and, therefore, oxygenation and ventilation must be carefully monitored in horses when used.[43,45,46] In horses where an atraumatic and smooth recovery is paramount, such as long bone fracture repair, a propofol and xylazine combination in conjunction with the use of a sling has been described.[45]

- Sedative, analgesic, and anesthetic medications can be administered to horses during the recovery period to allow more time to eliminate inhalant anesthetic and result in a higher quality recovery (**Table 1**).
- Acepromazine can be administered as a sole agent or in combination with other medications (α_2-agonists) to reduce anxiety and calm horses during recovery but can produce hypotension particularly at higher doses.
- α_2-Agonists (xylazine, detomidine, romifidine, and dexmedetomidine) are frequently administered to horses during recovery from anestheisa. Xylazine is most commonly used although the use of romifidine shows promise. Dexmedetomidine may cause excessive ataxia and should be used with caution.
- Opioid medications can be used to improve analgesia. Lower doses are recommended to avoid excitement and may work best when combined with other sedative/analgesic medications, such as acepromazine or α_2-agonists.
- Lidocaine infusions during anesthesia provide benefits to anesthetized horses but may cause ataxia during recovery and should be discontinued 30 minutes before moving to a recovery stall.
- Reanesthetizing horses with ketamine after general anesthesia during recovery may allow for increased elimination of inhalant anesthesia and higher-quality recoveries.
- Propofol can be administered to horses to smooth out the recovery period and can be used in combination with α_2-agonists and assisted recovery methods when a high recovery quality is paramount. Oxygenation and ventilation should be monitored closely when using propofol.

ASSISTED RECOVERY

The decision of whether or not to perform assisted recovery depends on many factors, and no clear consensus exists on when to perform assisted recovery and which method is best. For the majority of healthy horses with uncomplicated anesthesia and procedures, an unassisted recovery is probably acceptable, although it is standard practice in some hospitals to assist every recovery with a minimum of a head and tail ropes. Horses with severe systemic disease or compromise, significant

Table 1
Postanesthetic drugs administered during recovery that have been used to improve the quality of recovery of horses after general anesthesia

Drug	Dosage	Notes	References
Acepromazine	0.01–0.2 mg/kg IV	Duration of onset may be as long as 15 min, reduces excitement, large doses may cause hypotension	Driessen et al,[28] 2011; Hubbell and Muir,[19] 2009; Driessen,[48] 2006
Xylazine	0.1–0.4 mg/kg IV	Prolongs recovery time, analgesic	Hubbell and Muir,[19] 2009; Driessen,[48] 2006; Santos et al,[11] 2003
Detomidine	0.002–0.01 mg/kg IV	Same as xylazine	Hubbell and Muir,[19] 2009; Santos et al,[11] 2003
Romifidine	0.008–0.01 mg/kg IV	Same as xylazine	Bauquier and Kona-Boun,[34] 2011; Santos et al,[11] 2003
Butorphanol	0.01–0.02 mg/kg IV	Analgesic, can cause excitement, can be combined with a sedative	Driessen,[48] 2006
Morphine	0.05–0.15 mg/kg IV	Analgesic, can cause excitement, can be combined with a sedative	Hubbell and Muir,[19] 2009; Clark,[53] 2008
Ketamine	0.3 mg/kg IV bolus followed by 0.06 mg/min infusion for 30 min	Administered in conjunction with a xylazine bolus and infusion	Wagner et al,[43] 2012
Propofol	0.75 mg/kg bolus followed by 0.125 mg/kg/min infusion	Administered in conjunction with a xylazine bolus and infusion, respiratory depression may occur	Wagner et al,[43] 2012

orthopedic disease, or an injury where weight loading of a limb can compromise a repair; elderly or exhausted horses; horses with prolonged anesthesia times; postpartum mares; and draft horses should receive some degree of assisted recovery. The method chosen to use to assist a horse is dictated by clinician preference, staff experience, facility capabilities, and available equipment and resources. Some veterinarians advocate physically holding a horse to the ground until the horse has eliminated enough anesthetic that is can safely stand in a coordinated manner. This method cannot be recommended, however, because of the unnecessary risk of personal injury.

ASSISTED RECOVERY METHODS

The simplest method of assisted recovery for horses is a hand recovery. This consists of 1 or more persons assisting a horse to stand and could be done by holding onto a halter placed on a horse or lifting the horse by the base of the tail as it stands.

This method works well for foals, ponies, and small horses (<200 lb or 90 kg) but is not recommended for larger horses because there is a great deal of risk of injury to those assisting a horse.

The use of a tail rope run through a wall ring or over a stall door is a simple and effective method to provide support to horses that need some assistance to rise up on their pelvic limbs (**Fig. 9**).

The use of head and tail ropes is similar to the use of a tail rope alone but a second rope is used and tied to a halter to control the horse's head during recovery (**Fig. 10**).

Sling recovery has been described and is advocated for traumatic recovery of horses from general anesthesia.[19,45,48,49] Advantages of sling and lift devices include controlled movement of a horse from a recumbent position to standing, reduced, or balanced weight bearing, particularly on limbs with orthopedic injury. Disadvantages include intolerance of the sling by a horse, expense of equipment and facilities that can accommodate a sling, equipment failure, injury to surgical site, and increased and trained personnel. There are several lift and sling devices, including the large animal vertical lift system, the sling-shell system, the Liftex large animal sling, and the Anderson sling. These devices are described in detail by Driessen.[48]

The use of a purpose-built tilt table for returning recovering horses to a standing position has been described.[8] Overall, most horses recovered with minimal incidence of serious complications; however, a small percentage of horses failed to adapt to the system and required transfer to a recovery stall. Disadvantages of this system include cost of the table, the number of personnel required, and longer recovery times. The use of a tilt table could be considered for facilities that have such a system, particularly for horses that have a higher potential for catastrophic injury after orthopedic procedures.

A hydropool system can be used for recovery of horses where difficult recoveries can be anticipated (**Fig. 11**).[50] The pool described is 12 ft long, 4 ft wide, and 8.5 ft

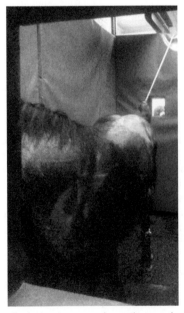

Fig. 9. A horse standing with the assistance of a tail rope during recovery from general anesthesia.

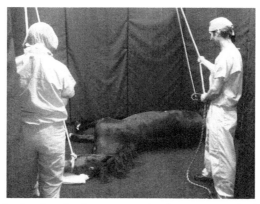

Fig. 10. The use of a head and tail rope to assist the recovery of a horse after general anesthesia.

deep with a hydraulic floor and a water heater and jet system to provide water up to 100°F flowing around the horse at various speeds for a therapeutic effect. The pool is used by lowering an anesthetized horse into the pool and then raising the floor to the level of the horse's feet when it is determined to be strong enough to stand and then continuing to raise the floor until the horse is at the level of the surrounding floor at which time the horse is walked out. Disadvantages of this system included the cost of a specialized pool, personnel requirements, and reported complications that included pulmonary edema and incisional infections.

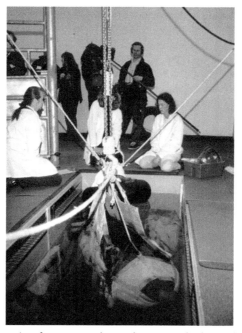

Fig. 11. A horse recovering from general anesthesia in a hydropool system. (*Courtesy of* Dr Stephen Greene, Washington State University, Pullman, Washington.)

Another water-based recovery system for postanesthesia horses has been described.[51] The pool-raft system uses a pool 22 ft wide and 11 ft deep and a custom modification of a US Navy life raft to accommodate 4 horse limbs. The raft use is limited to horses with a distance between the fore and hind limbs of up to 4.6 ft. Anesthetized horses are sling lifted into the raft, which is then lowered into the pool, and the raft secured to the pool deck. The horse's head is placed on a smaller raft to prevent aspiration of water. Horses judged to be awake are lifted out of the pool and moved to a padded recovery stall in a sling. This system is considered for decreasing complications associated with recovery in high-risk horses. Disadvantages of this system include the cost of the pool and raft system as well as large personnel requirements.

- The decision to assist the recovery of a horse after anesthesia depends on several factors, including clinician experience and preference, personnel available, facilities, surgical procedure performed, patient health status and temperament, and economics.
- Several options exist for assisted recovery, although an unassisted recovery may be acceptable in certain cases.
- Methods for assisted recovery range from a simple hand recovery and use of head and tail ropes to advanced options requiring specific facilities.
- Personnel safety should always be taken into account when choosing a method for assisted recovery and should never be performed alone.

COMPLICATIONS DURING RECOVERY

Similar to other phases of anesthesia for horses, complications can arise at any time during recovery. Complications during recovery can be particularly troublesome because monitoring is usually minimized in a potentially moving animal and thus recognition of problems may not be recognized. Complications that can occur during the recovery period include hypotension, hypoxemia, respiratory obstruction, pulmonary edema, orthopedic and other traumatic injury, muscle and nerve injury, and myelomalacia.[1,2,4,5,14,19,26] Constant and vigilant observation of horses during recovery by experienced personnel is essential. In certain circumstances, adverse events during recovery require intervention, such as administration of medications or obtaining blood samples for diagnostic tests. A system for unobtrusive drug administration and blood sampling has been described.[52]

Detailed description and treatment options of all possible complications that can occur during recovery from anesthesia in horses are beyond the scope of this article and have been reviewed previously.[15,19] Traumatic injury and failure of orthopedic repair are among the most concerning complications and are a major focus of this article and a main reason for interventions that improve recovery quality. Other complications that manifest during recovery have their origins in the anesthetic period and are resultant of blood pressure and tissue perfusion management and proper position and include myopathy, neuropathy, and possibly myelomalacia. Delayed awakening and prolonged recovery are unusual in healthy adult horses but may be seen in horses that are anesthetized for long durations (>3 hours), anesthetized for emergencies (colic), or are exhausted or fatigued. Hypoxemia, hypotension, acid-base disturbances, airway obstruction, and pulmonary edema can delay recovery and can be identified by clinical signs, physical examination, physiologic parameter measurement, and blood sample analysis. Hypothermia and hypoglycemia should also be considered, particularly in foals. Targeting treatment to identified problems should be performed in an effort to improve the recovery of individual horses with the goal of getting a horse to a standing position.

- Continual observation and monitoring of horses during recovery are necessary to quickly identify current and impending adverse events to allow for intervention.
- Complications that can occur during the recovery include traumatic injury, failure of a surgical repair, delayed recovery, and physiologic disturbances.

REFERENCES

1. Johnston GM, Eastment JK, Wood JL, et al. The confidential enquiry into perioperative equine fatalities (CEPEF): mortality results of phases 1 and 2. Vet Anaesth Analg 2002;29(4):159–70.
2. Bidwell LA, Hubbell JA, Muir WW. Anesthetic risk and euthanasia. In: Muir WW, Hubbell JA, editors. Equine anesthesia monitoring and emergency therapy. 2nd edition. St Louis (MO): Saunders Elsevier; 2009. p. 439–46.
3. Lukasic VM, Gleed RD, Scarlett JM, et al. Intranasal phenylephrine reduces post anesthetic upper airway obstruction in horses. Equine Vet J 1997;29(3):236–8.
4. Clark-Price SC, Gutierrez-Nibeyro SD, Santos MP. Anesthesia case of the month. EPAM. J Am Vet Med Assoc 2012;240(1):40–4.
5. Jouber KE, Duncan N, Murray SE. Post-anesthetic myelomalacia in a horse. J S Afr Vet Assoc 2005;76(1):36–9.
6. Valverde A, Rickey E, Sinclair M, et al. Comparison of cardiovascular function and quality of recovery in isoflurane-anaesthetised horses administered a constant rate infusion of lidocaine or lidocaine and medetomidine during elective surgery. Equine Vet J 2010;42(3):192–9.
7. Voulgaris DA, Hofmeister EH. Multivariate analysis of factors associated with post-anesthetic times to standing in isoflurane-anesthetized horses: 381 cases. Vet Anaesth Analg 2009;36:414–20.
8. Elmas CR, Cruz AM, Kerr CL. Tilt table recovery of horses after orthopedic surgery: fifty-four cases (1994-2005). Vet Surg 2007;36:252–8.
9. Ringer SK, Kalchofner K, Boller J, et al. A clinical comparison of two anaesthetic protocols using lidocaine or medetomidine in horses. Vet Anaesth Analg 2007;34:257–68.
10. Ray-Miller W, Hodgson DS, McMurphy RM, et al. Comparison of recoveries from anesthesia of horses placed on a rapidly inflating-deflating air pillow or the floor of a padded stall. J Am Vet Med Assoc 2006;229(5):711–6.
11. Santos M, Fuente M, Garcia-Iturralde R, et al. Effects of alpha-2 adrenoceptor agonists during recovery from isoflurane anaesthesia in horses. Equine Vet J 2003;35(2):170–5.
12. Donaldson LL, Dunlop GS, Holland MS, et al. The recovery of horses from inhalant anesthesia: a comparison of halothane and isoflurane. Vet Surg 2000;29(1):92–101.
13. Matthews NS, Hartsfield SM, Mercer D, et al. Recovery from sevoflurane anesthesia in horses: comparison to isoflurane and effect of postmedicaton with xylazine. Vet Surg 1998;27(5):480–5.
14. Hubbell JA. Horses. In: Tranquilli WJ, Thurmon JC, Grimm KA, editors. Lumb & Jones' veterinary anesthesia and analgesia. 4th edition. Ames (IO): Blackwell Publishing; 2007. p. 717–29.
15. Muir WW, Hubbell JA. Anesthetic-associated complications. In: Muir WW, Hubbell JA, editors. Equine anesthesia monitoring and emergency therapy. 2nd edition. St Louis (MO): Saunders Elsevier; 2009. p. 397–417.
16. Barber SM. Management of neck and head injuries. Vet Clin North Am Equine Pract 2005;21(1):191–215.

17. Clutton RE, Chase-Topping M, Squires R, et al. Vertical dimensions of suspended horses. Equine Vet J 2010;42(8):758–61.
18. Clark-Price SC, Posner LP, Gleed RD. Recovery of horses from general anesthesia in a darkened or illuminated recovery stall. Vet Anaesth Analg 2008; 35(6):473–9.
19. Hubbell JA, Muir WW. Considerations for induction, maintenance, and recovery. In: Muir WW, Hubbell JA, editors. Equine anesthesia monitoring and emergency therapy. 2nd edition. St Louis (MO): Saunders Elsevier; 2009. p. 381–96.
20. Durongphongtorn S, McDonnell WN, Kerr CL, et al. Comparison of hemodynamic, clinicopathologic, and gastrointestinal motility effects and recovery characteristics of anesthesia with isoflurane and halothane in horses undergoing arthroscopic surgery. Am J Vet Res 2006;67(1):32–42.
21. Matthews NS, Miller SM, Hartsfield SM, et al. Comparison of recoveries from halothane vs isoflurane anesthesia in horses. J Am Vet Med Assoc 1992; 201(4):559–63.
22. Auer JA, Garner HE, Amend JF, et al. Recovery from anaesthesia in ponies: a comparative study of the effects of isoflurane, enflurane, methoxyflurane and halothane. Equine Vet J 1978;10(1):18–23.
23. Steffey EP, Mama KR. Inhalation anesthetics. In: Tranquilli WJ, Thurmon JC, Grimm KA, editors. Lumb & Jones' veterinary anesthesia and analgesia. 4th edition. Ames (IO): Blackwell Publishing; 2007. p. 355–93.
24. Leece EA, Corletto F, Brearley JC. A comparison of recovery times and characteristics with sevoflurane and isoflurane anaesthesia in horses undergoing magnetic resonance imaging. Vet Anaesth Analg 2008;35:383–91.
25. Read MR, Read EK, Duke T, et al. Cardiopulmonary effects and induction and recovery characteristics of isoflurane and sevoflurane in foals. J Am Vet Med Assoc 2002;221(3):393–8.
26. Muir WW. Anxiolytic, nonopioid sedative-analgesics, and opioid analgesics. In: Muir WW, Hubbell JA, editors. Equine anesthesia monitoring and emergency therapy. 2nd edition. St Louis (MO): Saunders Elsevier; 2009. p. 185–209.
27. Doherty TJ, Geiser DR, Rohrback BW. Effect of acepromazine and butorphanol on halothane minimum alveolar concentration in ponies. Equine Vet J 1997;29: 374–6.
28. Driessen B, Zarucco L, Kalir B, et al. Contemporary use of acepromazine in the anaesthetic management of male horses and ponies: a retrospective study and opinion poll. Equine Vet J 2011;43(1):88–98.
29. Clark-Price S, Divers TJ. Anesthesia for field emergencies and euthanasia. In: Orsini JA, Divers TJ, editors. Equine emergencies. 3rd edition. St Louis (MO): Saunders-Elsevier; 2008. p. 661–70.
30. Lemke KA. Anticholinergics and sedatives. In: Tranquilli WJ, Thurmon JC, Grimm KA, editors. Lumb & Jones' veterinary anesthesia and analgesia. 4th edition. Ames (IO): Blackwell Publishing; 2007. p. 203–39.
31. Goodrich LR, Clark-Price SC, Ludders J. How to attain effective and consistent sedation for standing procedure in the horse using constant rate infusion. Proceedings of the 50th Annual Convention of the American Association of Equine Practitioners 2004. p. 229–32.
32. Schauvliege S, Marcilla MG, Verryken K, et al. Effects of a constant rate infusion of detomidine on cardiovascular function, isoflurane requirements and recovery quality in horses. Vet Anaesth Analg 2011;38(6):544–54.
33. Robinson KJ, Brosnan RJ, Nguyen K, et al. Comparison of the effects of alpha-2-agonists romifidine and xylazine on quality of recovery from general

anesthesia in horses. In: Proceedings of the 15th Internation Veterinary Emergency and Critical Care Symposium. Chicago: 2009. p. 716.

34. Bauquier SH, Kona-Boun JJ. Comparison of the effects of xylazine and romifidine administered perioperatively on the recovery of anesthetized horses. Can Vet J 2011;52(9):987–93.

35. Marcill MG, Schauvliege S, Segaert S, et al. Influence of a constant rate infusion of dexmedetomidine on cardiopulmaonary function and recovery quality in isoflurane anaesthetized horses. Vet Anaesth Analg 2012;39(1):49–58.

36. Bryant CE, England GC, Clarke KW. Comparison of the sedative effect of medetomidine and xylazine in horses. Vet Rec 1991;129(19):421–3.

37. Mircica E, Clutton RE, Kyles KW, et al. Problems associated with perioperative morphine in horses: a retrospective case analysis. Vet Anaesth Analg 2003; 30(3):147–55.

38. Clark L, Clutton RE, Blissitt KJ, et al. The effects of morphine on the recovery of horses from halothane anaesthesia. Vet Anaesth Analg 2008;35(1):22–9.

39. Peiro JR, Barnabe PA, Cadioli FA, et al. Effects of lidocaine infusion during experimental endotoxemia in horses. J Vet Intern Med 2010;24(4):940–8.

40. Rezende ML, Wagner AE, Mama KR, et al. Effects of intravenous administration of lidocaine on the minimum alveolar concentration of sevoflurane in horses. Am J Vet Res 2011;72(4):446–51.

41. Valverde A, Gunkelt C, Doherty TJ, et al. Effect of a constant rate infusion of lidocaine on the quality of recovery from sevoflurane or isoflurane general anaesthesia in horses. Equine Vet J 2005;37(6):559–64.

42. Doherty T, Valverde A. Management of sedation and anestheisa. In: Doherty T, Valverde A, editors. Manual of equine anestheisa & analgesia. Ames (IO): Blackwell Publishing; 2006. p. 206–59.

43. Wagner AE, Mama KR, Steffey EP, et al. Evaluation of infusions of xylazine with ketamine or propofol to modulate recovery following sevoflurane anesthesia in horses. Am J Vet Res 2012;73(3):346–52.

44. Rezende ML, Boscan P, Stanley SD, et al. Evaluation of cardiovascular, respiratory and biochemical effects, and anesthetic induction and recovery behavior in horses anesthetized with a 5% micellar microemulsion propofol formulation. Vet Anaesth Analg 2010;37:440–50.

45. Steffey EP, Brosnan RJ, Galuppo LD, et al. Use of propofol-xylazine and the Anderson sling suspension system for recovery of horses from desflurane anesthesia. Vet Surg 2009;38:927–33.

46. Steffey EP, Mamma KR, Brosnan RJ, et al. Effect of administration of propofol and xylazine hydrochloride on recovery of horses after four hours of anesthesia with desflurane. Am J Vet Res 2009;70(8):956–63.

47. Oku K, Yamanaka T, Ashihara N, et al. Clinical observations during induction and recovery of xylazine-midazolam-propofol anesthesia in horses. J Vet Med Sci 2003;65(7):805–8.

48. Driessen B. Assisted recovery. In: Doherty T, Valverde A, editors. Manual of equine anestheisa & analgesia. Ames (IO): Blackwell Publishing; 2006. p. 338–51.

49. Taylor EL, Galuppo LD, Steffey EP, et al. Use of the Anderson Sling Suspension System for recovery of horses from general anesthesia. Vet Surg 2005;34: 559–64.

50. Tidwell SA, Schneider RK, Ragle CA, et al. Use of a hydro-pool system to recover horses after general anesthesia: 60 cases. Vet Surg 2002;31(5): 455–61.

51. Sullivan EK, Klein LV, Richardson DW, et al. Use of a pool-raft system for recovery of horses from general anesthesia: 393 horses (1984-2000). J Am Vet Med Assoc 2002;221(7):1014–8.
52. Clutton RE. Device for unobtrusive drug administration and blood sampling in horses recovering from anaesthesia. Vet Rec 2008;163:303–4.
53. Clark L, Clutton RE, Blissitt KJ, et al. The effects of morphine on the recovery of horses from halothane anaesthesia. Vet Anaesth Analg 2008;35(1):22–9.

Index

Note: Page numbers of article titles are in **boldface** type.

A

Vet Clin Equine 29 (2013) 243–255
http://dx.doi.org/10.1016/S0749-0739(13)00010-2
0749-0739/13/$ – see front matter © 2013 Elsevier Inc. All rights reserved.

vetequine.theclinics.com

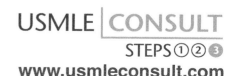

Our issues help you manage *yours*

Every year brings you new clinical challenges.

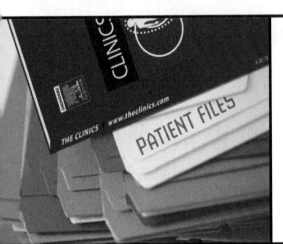

Every **Clinics** issue brings you **today's best thinking** on the challenges you face.

Whether you purchase these issues individually, or order an annual subscription (which includes searchable access to past issues online), the **Clinics** offer you an efficient way to update your know how...one issue at a time.

DISCOVER THE CLINICS IN YOUR SPECIALTY!

Veterinary Clinics of North America: Equine Practice.
Publishes three times a year.
ISSN 0749-0739.

Veterinary Clinics of North America: Exotic Animal Practice.
Publishes three times a year.
ISSN 1094-9194.

Veterinary Clinics of North America: Food Animal Practice.
Publishes three times a year.
ISSN 0749-0720.

Veterinary Clinics of North America: Small Animal Practice.
Publishes bimonthly.
ISSN 0195-5616.

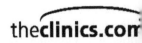

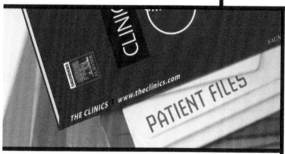

Moving?

Make sure your subscription moves with you!

To notify us of your new address, find your **Clinics Account Number** (located on your mailing label above your name), and contact customer service at:

Email: journalscustomerservice-usa@elsevier.com

800-654-2452 (subscribers in the U.S. & Canada)
314-447-8871 (subscribers outside of the U.S. & Canada)

Fax number: 314-447-8029

Elsevier Health Sciences Division
Subscription Customer Service
3251 Riverport Lane
Maryland Heights, MO 63043

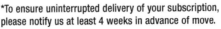

Printed and bound by CPI Group (UK) Ltd, Croydon, CR0 4YY

03/10/2024

01040439-0011